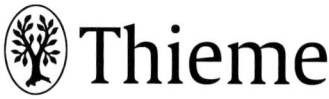

Therapeutic Energy Application in Urology

Standards and Recent Developments

Edited by

Ch. Chaussy
G. Haupt
D. Jocham
K. U. Köhrmann
D. Wilbert

Georg Thieme Verlag
Stuttgart · New York

*Bibliographic Information published by
Die Deutsche Bibliothek*

Die Deutsche Bibliothek lists this publication in the Deutsche Nationalbibliografie; detailed bibliographic data is available on the internet at http://dnb.ddb.de.

© 2005 Georg Thieme Verlag KG
Rüdigerstraße 14
70469 Stuttgart, Germany
http://www.thieme.de
Thieme New York, 333 Seventh Avenue
New York, NY 10001, USA
http://www.thieme.com

Printed in Germany

Cover design by Thieme Verlagsgruppe
Typesetting by Druckerei Sommer, Feuchtwangen
Printing and Bookbinding by Grafisches Centrum Cuno
   GmbH & Co. KG, Calbe

ISBN 3-13-134171-8 (GTV)
ISBN 1-58890-428-8 (TNY)   1 2 3 4 5 6

Important note: Medicine is an ever-changing science undergoing continual development. Research and clinical experience are continually expanding our knowledge, in particular our knowledge of proper treatment and drug therapy. Insofar as this book mentions any dosage or application, readers may rest assured that the authors, editors, and publishers have made every effort to ensure that such references are in accordance with **the state of knowledge at the time of production of the book.**

Nevertheless, this does not involve, imply, or express any guarantee or responsibility on the part of the publishers in respect to any dosage instructions and forms of applications stated in the book. **Every user is requested to examine carefully** the manufacturers' leaflets accompanying each drug and to check, if necessary in consultation with a physician or specialist, whether the dosage schedules mentioned therein or the contraindications stated by the manufacturers differ from the statements made in the present book. Such examination is particularly important with drugs that are either rarely used or have been newly released on the market. Every dosage schedule or every form of application used is entirely at the user's own risk and responsibility. The authors and publishers request every user to report to the publishers any discrepancies or inaccuracies noticed. If errors in this work are found after publication, errata will be posted at www.thieme.com on the product description page.

Some of the product names, patents, and registered designs referred to in this book are in fact registered trademarks or proprietary names even though specific reference to this fact is not always made in the text. Therefore, the appearance of a name without designation as proprietary is not to be construed as a representation by the publisher that it is in the public domain.

This book, including all parts thereof, is legally protected by copyright. Any use, exploitation, or commercialization outside the narrow limits set by copyright legislation, without the publisher's consent, is illegal and liable to prosecution. This applies in particular to photostat reproduction, copying, mimeographing, preparation of microfilms, and electronic data processing and storage.

Editorial

There is increasing evidence that the introduction of ESWL was one of the key points for the ongoing development in the field of therapeutic energy application in Urology. The editors of this book are excited that it was possible to call together almost to the day 25 years after the first clinical application of ESWL another consensus meeting which covers recent developments and strategies in the treatment of stone disease and the actual status of the technologies. The different energies like focused Ultrasound, Cryotherapy, Radiofrequency, Laser and Brachytherapy were extensively discussed in the working group "Alternative Energies".

The organisational structure of the meeting paralleled that of previous meetings in 1993, 1995 and 1997 with an initial plenary session to phrase the topics and questions for the committees to work out the answers which at last were discussed in a final plenary session.

Main topics of the invited five groups have been new developments in shockwave technology and alternative energy sources, the definition of standards and future prospects. Besides the nowadays inevitable discussion about economic impact of new technologies the beneficial effect and direct impact on the patients fate was supposed to be one of the leading subjects of discussions and concerns.

Purpose of this meeting was to evaluate the status quo and assess the progress in the selected topics verifying the consent, realising the dissent and defining further research targets by dissemination of data and ideas given in the contributions of the individual authors and study groups.

The editors wish to express their gratitude to all authors who contributed their work and time before, during and after the meeting. Only with this support it was possible to publish the results of this consensus meeting timely.

Special thanks are also due to the Georg Thieme Publishers who made particular effort for rapid editing and printing to have this book out in time for the World Congress of Endourology 2005.

This book has been produced for timely information of all physicians interested and involved in the innovative application of energy in medicine and for engineers who contribute new ideas for continuous development and improvement in the field of minimal invasive therapy for a variety of diseases.

Munich, April 2005

Christian G. Chaussy

Contents

Editorial V

Shockwave Lithotripsy: Basics, Facts and Prospects

Progress in Lithotripter Technology 1
J. J. Rassweiler (Chairman), T. Bergsdorf, S. Ginter, B. Granz, A. Häcker, A. Lutz, O. Wess, D. Wilbert

Two *Ex Vivo* Models for the Evaluation of SW-Induced Renal Injury 16
A. Häcker, T. Bergsdorf, P. Alken, Ch. Chaussy

The Light Spot Hydrophone – LSHD: A New Level of Precise Ultrasonic Shock Wave Measurement 20
B. Granz, R. Nanke

Shock Wave Lithotripsy (SWL) and Focal Size 26
O. Wess

Treatment of Urinary Stones

Consensus 36
K. U. Köhrmann (Chairman), R. Hofmann, T. Knoll, D. Neisius, C. Türk, G. Haupt

Lower Pole Stones 39
D. Neisius

Proximal Ureteral Stones 44
P. Olbert, R. Hofmann

Distal Ureteral Stones 49
C. Türk

Endourological Techniques – Clinical Pathways 55
T. Knoll, P. Honeck

Statement of the "German Society for Shock Wave Lithotripsy" about "Outpatient versus Inpatient" ESWL 64
K. U. Köhrmann, C. Chaussy

Diagnosis and Metaphylaxis in Urolithiasis

Diagnostic Approach 65
W. L. Strohmaier

Metabolic Evaluation and Metaphylaxis of Stone Disease 72
M. Straub, A. Hesse

Pediatric Aspects of Nephrolithiasis and Nephrocalcinosis 86
B. Beck, B. Hoppe

Energy Application for Non-Surgical Urological Therapies

Consensus 92
S. Thüroff (Chairman), A. Blana, M. Braun, B. Brehmer, A. Häcker, R. Muschter, S. Neubauer, U. Witzsch, Ch. Chaussy

Technical Principles of High Intensity Focused Ultrasound (HIFU) 95
A. Blana, A. Häcker

Status of High Intensity Focused Ultrasound (HIFU) in Urology in 2005 98
S. Thüroff, Ch. Chaussy

Cryotherapy of the Prostate 103
U. K. F Witzsch, M. Braun

Prostate Brachytherapy 106
S. Neubauer, P. Derakhshani, G. Spira

TUMT for Benign Prostatic Hyperplasia 117
R. Berges

Radiofrequency (RF) Therapy of the
Kidney: Indications, Technique, and
Results 122
B. Brehmer, G. Jakse

Cryotherapy of Renal Cell Carcinomas 126
U. K. F. Witzsch

Extracorporeal Application of High
Intensity Focused Ultrasound (HIFU) for
Renal Tumor Thermoablation: Technical
Principles and Clinical Application 128
A. Häcker, M. S. Michel, K. U. Köhrmann

**Extracorporeal Shock Wave Therapy
(ESWT) in Urology**

Consensus 131
S. Lahme (Chairman),
G. Hatzichristodoulou, E. W. Hauck

Etiology and Clinical Implications
of Peyronie's Disease 132
G. Hatzichristodoulou, E. W. Hauck,
S. Lahme

ESWT in Peyronie's Disease 137
E. W. Hauck, G. Hatzichristodoulou,
S. Lahme

ESWT in Orthopedics

Physical-Technical Principles of ESWT 144
M. Maier, T. Tischer, L. Gerdesmeyer

Basic Research in Orthopedic
Extracorporeal Shock Wave Application —
An Update 154
T. Tischer, L. Gerdesmeyer, M. Maier

**Manufacturers' Update
on Lithotripter Concepts**

Dornier MedTech: Products
and New Developments —
An Overview 164
H. Hermeking

Siemens Medical Solutions: LITHOSKOP:
A New Era in Stone Therapy and Overall
Urology 167
M. Lanski

Storz Medical: Shock Waves for Stone
Treatment and Tissue Engineering 172
O. Wess

Wolf: Innovative Piezoelectric Shock
Wave Systems — PIEZOLITH 3000 and
PIEZOSON 100 *plus* 175
S. Ginter, W. Krauß

Participants 178

Index 181

Shockwave Lithotripsy: Basics, Facts and Prospects

Progress in Lithotripter Technology

J. J. Rassweiler, T. Bergsdorf, S. Ginter, B. Granz, A. Häcker, A. Lutz, O. Wess, D. Wilbert

Actual Lithotripter Concepts

Today, mainly two types of lithotripters are provided by the manufacturers [1–8].

"ESWL-tables" with an optimized design used for the previously underestimated mid-range to low-end machines. Such devices (e. g., Siemens Modularis, Dornier Compact Delta and Sigma, Storz Modulith SLK, Wolf Piezolith 3000, Direx Nova Ultima, Medstone STS-T, HMT LithoDiamond) consist of a treatment table, a shock wave source with either lateral or coaxial ultrasound, and an isocentric C-arm as main localization system (Tables **1** and **2**). Such systems might be attractive for low volume departments.

"Uro-lithotripters" with a single fluoroscopic localization system especially designed for urological purposes (e. g., Phillips LithoDiagnost, Siemens Lithostar Multiline, Storz Modulith SLX, Modulith SLX-F2, Dornier Lithotripter S, Dornier Lithotripter SII). However, these machines only possess a limited capacity for diagnostic examinations (e. g., plain X-ray: KUB, IVP). The manufacturers offer the use of ultrasound scanners, but in reality this is very optional. Some of the uro-lithotripters provide dual imaging with a combination of both fluoroscopic and ultrasonic localization in addition (Siemens Lithoskop, Dornier Lithotripter S, Dornier Lithotripter SII, Storz Modulith SLX, Modulith SLX-F2). Such machines are mainly intended for high volume stone centers, although they can be considered as a very economic workstation even in medium-sized departments with a sufficient endourological workload.

Mechanism and Theories of Stone Disintegration

Increasing perfection through three lithotripter generations has led to systems of high fragmentation efficiency and minimal side effects. Despite this success, there was only limited agreement on the relevant fragmentation mechanisms. However, recent studies mainly promoted by manufacturers (e. g., Storz-Medical, Siemens, Dornier) led to distinct agreement about the physical parameters responsible for either stone fragmentation or renal trauma. Based on the current physical literature, four different mechanisms of stone fragmentation are discussed (Fig. **1**).

Tensile and shear stresses

The fragmentation of stones needs tensile stress or strain. SW pulses are pressure waves consisting of a positive and a negative pressure part. Both parts can act in different ways. The positive part can only result in significant tensile stress if it is narrower in spatial extension in the stone than the dimension of the stone itself; thus creating pressure gradients, shear stress, and finally, tensile stress and strain. This is especially the case if the focus diameter is small compared to the stone diameter, resulting in a crater-like fragmentation or erosion, as observed with most sharply focusing sources. In addition, compression can also induce tensile stress at the tips of pre-existing flaws, leading to tensile cracks [9–11]. Waves of duration shorter than the travelling time in the stone are transmitted into the stone and reflected at the low impedance stone-water rear interface with pressure inversion; thus, splitting off stone material by the tensile stress in the reflected wave, known as the Hopkinson effect.

Cavitation

In addition to the direct strain action on the stone, the negative pressure wave causes cavitation in the water surrounding the stone and, also, within the water in the microcracks and cleavage interfaces of the calculus. Cavitation erosion is especially observed at the anterior and posterior sides of artificial stones *in vitro* [11–14]. Cavitation may lead to the fragmentation of materials that are resistant to tear and shear waves (e. g., cystine, cholesterol). Suppression of cavitation, e. g., by use of highly viscous media (such as bile) or hyperpressure, significantly re-

Table 1 Characteristics of recently introduced lithotripters

Machine	SW generation	Aperture [mm]	Localization X-ray	Ultrasound	Clinical application
Dornier Compact Sigma	electromagnetic (flat coil, EMSE 140f)	140	parallel isocentric X-ray C-arm and isocentric C-arm of shock wave source	lateral ultrasound	2003
Compact Delta	electromagnetic (flat coil, EMSE 140f)	140	parallel isocentric X-ray C-arm and isocentric C-arm of shock wave source	lateral ultrasound	1997
Lithotripter S	electromagnetic (flat coil, EMSE 220f EMSE 220f-XXP)	220	isocentric X-ray C-arm	lateral ultrasound	1997
Lithotripter S II	electromagnetic (flat coil, EMSE 220f EMSE 220f-XXP)	220	isocentric X-ray C-arm	lateral ultrasound	2003
Siemens Multiline	electromagnetic (flat coil, System M)	145	in-line fluoroscopy	in-line ultrasound (optional)	1994
Modularis	Electromagnetic (flat coil, System C/Cplus)	130	Isocentric C-arm	lateral ultrasound	1998
Lithoskop	electromagnetic (flat coil, System Pulso)	168	parallel isocentric in-line fluoroscopy C-arm (double C)	in-line ultrasound	2005
Storz Modulith SLX	electromagnetic (cylinder)	300	in-line fluoroscopy	in-line ultrasound	1995
Modulith SLK	electromagnetic	178	off-line fluoroscopy (Lithotrack-navigation)	in-line ultrasound	1998
Modulith SLX-F2	electromagnetic (dual focus)	300	in-line fluoroscopy	in-line ultrasound	2004
Xinin Compact CS	electromagnetic (self-focusing)	120	–	lateral ultrasound	2001
Wolf Piezolith 3000	piezoelectric (double layer)	360	isocentric C-arm	coaxial ultrasound	2000
Edap-Technomed LT02-X	Piezoelectric	500	in-line C-arm	coaxial ultrasound	1997
Vision	electrohydraulic (Diatron III)	220	isocentric C-arm	lateral ultrasound	2001
Medstone STS-T	Electrohydraulic	150	isocentric C-arm	lateral ultrasound (very optional)	1999
Direx Nova Ultima	electrohydraulic (Trigen-technology, turnable)	150	isocentric-C-arm	lateral ultrasound (very optional)	2000
Duet	two electrohydraulic sources (!)	150	isocentric C-arm	lateral ultrasound	2001
Integra	Electromagnetic (trapezoid, hollow)	220	in-line fluoroscopy	lateral ultrasound	2004
HMT Healthtronics LithoDiamond	10,000 SW/electrode	200	isocentric C-arm	–	2002

Table 2 Localization principles of the actual lithotripter concepts

Concept	Lithotriptor features
Uro-lithotripter	multifunctional table with integrated C-arm (Siemens Lithostar Multiline) or X-ray system (Storz Modulith SLX), but restricted functions for diagnostic purposes (e. g., IVP, retrograde pyelogram); unrestricted use (Siemens Lithoskop, Storz Modulith SLX-F2, Dornier Lithotripter S, Dornier Lithotripter S II)
Third generation lithotripter	multifunctional table with dual localization systems and all options for urological X-ray diagnostics and therapy (e. g., Storz Modulith SL 20, Siemens Lithostar Plus 2, Dornier Lithotripter U 50, Phillips LithoDiagnost M)
ESWL tables	Treatment table for endourology plus shock wave source with adjustable isocentric C-arm (e. g., Siemens Modularis, Wolf Piezolith 3000, Dornier Compact Delta and Compact Sigma, Medstone STS)

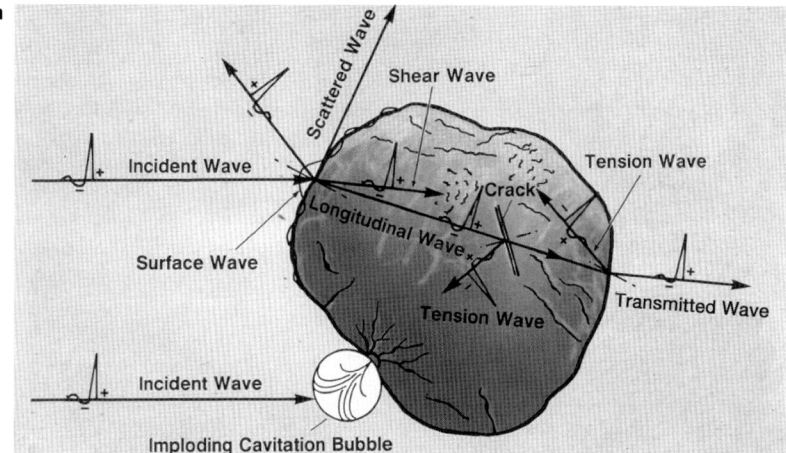

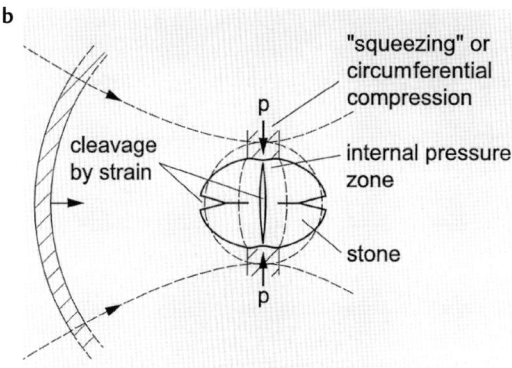

Fig. 1 Theories of stone disintegration. a Tear and shear forces and cavitation. b Quasi-static squeezing (adapted from Eisenmenger 2001).

duces the disintegrative efficacy of shock waves. This indicates a substantial contribution of fragmentation by cavitation in the disintegration process after the initial spalling effect. In recent *in vitro* experiments, it has been shown, that the stone fragmentation is significantly enhanced by a second shock wave applied during the collapse of the cavitation bubbles generated by the first lithotripter shock wave [15]. However, until now, manufacturers could not reproduce these results in different settings (e. g., use of double layer piezo-electric crystals; modified acoustic lens of electromagnetic shock wave source).

Cavitation seems to be an important factor of shock wave-induced tissue injury [16], e. g., vascular lesions or by release of free radicals.

4 Progress in Lithotripter Technology

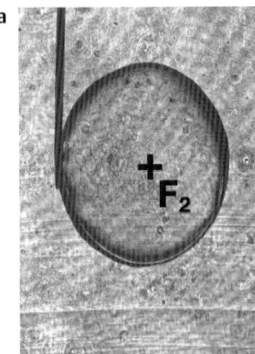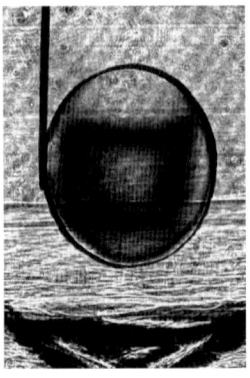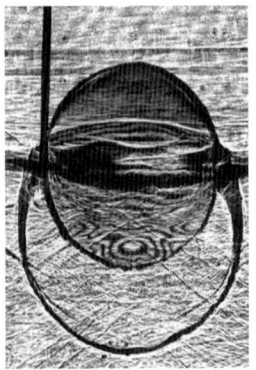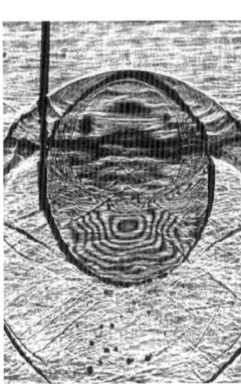

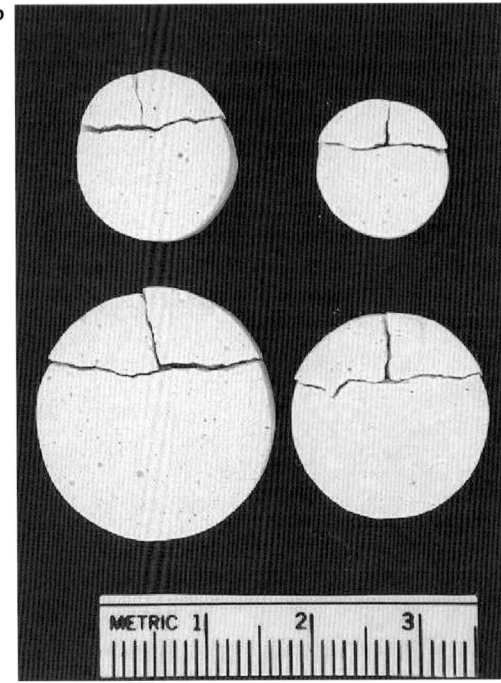

Fig. 2 Observation of shock wave front passing a test stone (adapted from Zhong 2001). **a** High-speed photography, translucent stone-model. **b** Initial fracture line in calcified test stone, perpendicular or parallel to shock wave front.

Quasistatic squeezing

Experiments with test stones revealed that the disintegration does not depend on the maximal shock wave pressure or the rise time, which both have significant impact on the tear and shear forces, but much more on the shock wave energy. Earlier observations of first cleavage planes, either parallel or perpendicular to the wave propagation lead to a third theory called "squeezing" — a theory of fragmentation described by Eisenmenger [11].

The positive part of the pressure wave acts on the stone by quasistatic squeezing (Fig. **1b**). This induces a binary fragmentation with first cleavage surfaces that are either parallel or perpendicular to the wave propagation. This mechanism of squeezing suggests, for high stone fragmentation efficiency in ESWL, focal diameters of up to 20 mm (to be larger than the stone) with pulse durations up to 2 microseconds, but not necessarily a steep shock front. The focal positive pressure should be reduced to the lower pressure range of 10 MPa to 30 MPa, because this is completely sufficient to overcome the breaking threshold of maximal 2 MPa for human and artificial calculi.

This theory stimulated the discussion about the importance of a large focal size and a lower focal pressure (e. g., in the HM3) compared to the small focal size with high pressure due to the large aperture in the newly designed systems. Experimental studies with translucent test stones and high-speed photography were able to demonstrate that the passage of the shock wave front results in a high orthogonal pressure zone in the second third of the stone (Fig. **2**). However, Zhong [8] explained this spalling by reflection of the positive wave at the backfront of the stone (i. e. the Hopkinson effect).

Moreover, studies with piezolelectric and electromagnetic shock wave sources also could not reproduce the theory of quasistatic squeezing: If the stone is positioned before or behind the focal zone (–6 dB), the disintegration efficacy is reduced despite a still existing peak pressure of more than 30 MPa in this area. This phenomenon is more pronounced when harder test stones are used. Finally, if two stones are placed along the blast path of a shock wave front directly in the focal zone, only the proximal one is fragmented, whereas the second one, which should be "squeezed" by the surrounding shock wave, remains untouched. All these experiments support that the tear and shear forces including the wave reflection at the distal border of the stone (spalling effect) are the most important mechanisms for stone disintegration.

Dynamic fatigue

Dynamic fatigue has been proposed as a general theory for stone comminution and tissue injury in SWL (17). The theory is based on the observation that stone fragmentation inflicted by the lithotripter shock waves accumulates during the course of the treatment, leading to eventual destruction of the stone configuration. The stone fracture process is therefore characterized as an evolutionary process consisting of three phases:
- initiation (e. g., based on spalling effect),
- propagation (associated to cavitation), and
- coalescence or collapse (due to the increasing fragility).

Finally, microcracks are produced by the mechanical stresses associated with the lithotripter shock waves that may result in a sudden break-off of the calculus once the molecular structure of the stone is completely destroyed. The theory relates physical properties of the stone, e. g., fracture toughness, acoustic speed, density and void dimensions, to shock wave parameters, e. g., peak pressure, pulse width, pulse profile and number of shocks for fragmentation.

In summary, none of these theories is able to explain exclusively the entire phenomenon of shock wave-induced stone fragmentation, but they play an important role in the understanding of this complex process.

Relevance of Different Physical Parameters for Stone Disintegration

The International Electrotechnical Commission (IEC) recently presented a draft for the standardized measurement of shock waves. Herein, all relevant parameters describing a shock wave physically are listed and defined (Table 3).

Measurement of shock wave pressure

In addition to this, physicists from Siemens and the University of Erlangen have developed a new light spot hydrophone (Fig. **3b**) using the shock-wave-induced changes of reflection of a 35 mW laser light source focused on the front side of a glass block [18]. This system proved to be as precise as the laser-fiber hydrophones (Fig. **3a**) proposed by Staudenraus [19], but were significantly easier in handling. It has to be mentioned that, in the year 2005, pressure measurements with other probes (e. g., PVDF) are no longer considered as relevant by the leading manufacturers. Only laser-based hydrophones are the standard for precise measurements of time profiles of shock waves.

The impact of the theory of quasistatic squeezing

Concerning the relevance of these physical parameters for stone disintegration, various groups tried to reproduce the theory of quasistatic squeezing, because this would be in favor of a larger focal zone. However, the theory could not be confirmed because:
- different focal zones had no impact on stone disintegration,
- primary fragmentation occurred orthogonal to the shock wave front, but not in the middle of the stone, and
- if two stones are focused with a total diameter less than the focal zone, only the first stone breaks.

All these observations are consistent with the experimental work of Zhong [10], who presented the theory of the spalling effect resulting in primary stone fragmentation due to reflec-

Table **3** Shock wave parameters

Parameter	Unit
Peak pressure (p+)	MPa
Negative pressure (p−)	MPa
Rise time (t_r)	ns
Pulse width (T_{p+} or T_{p-})	µs
Intensity/Energy density (PII)	mJ/mm^2
Focal energy (E_f)	J

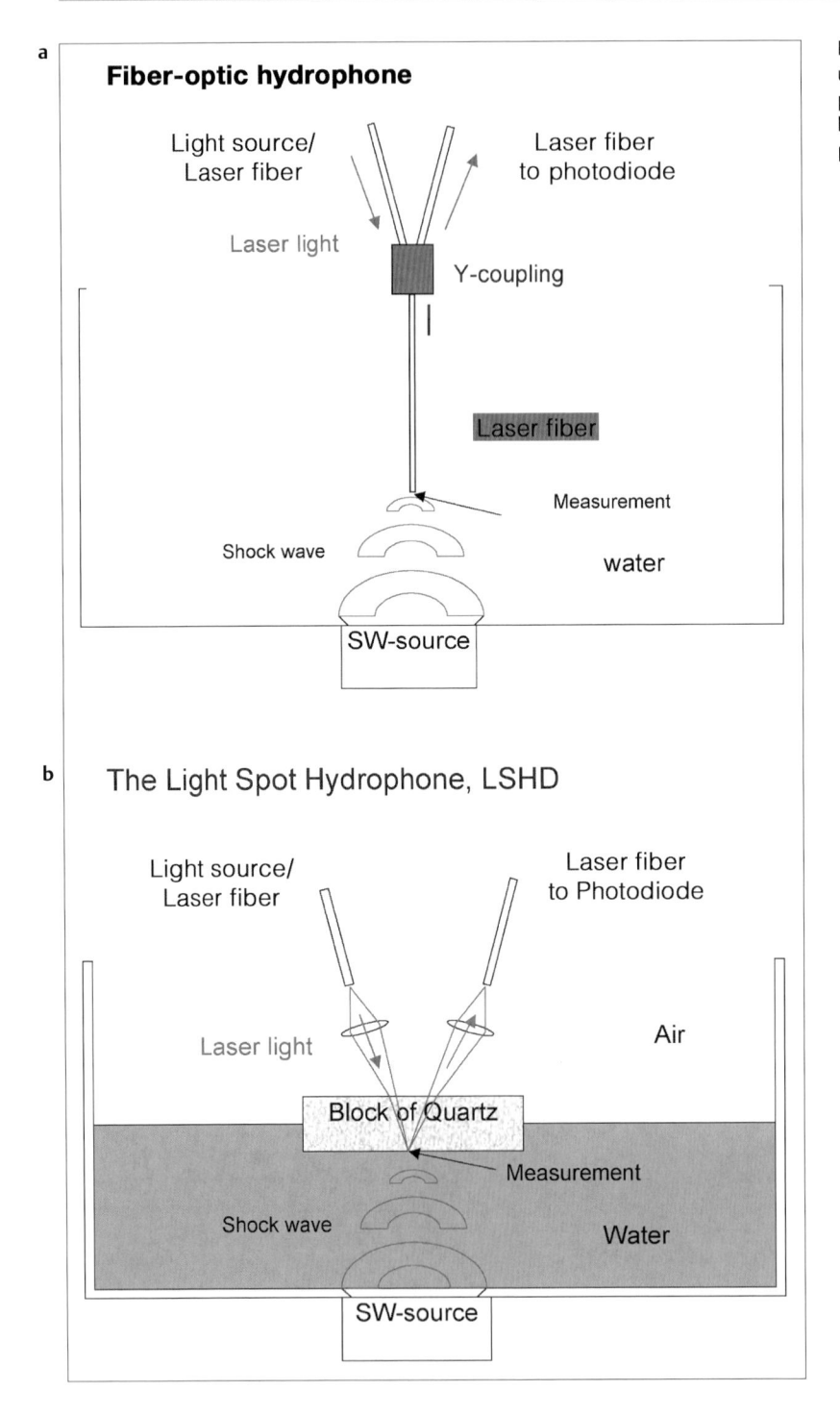

Fig. 3 Hydrophones in use. **a** Fiberoptic hydrophone (Staudenraus). **b** Light-spot hydrophone (Granz).

tion of the shock wave front at the backside of the stone (Fig. **2**). Interestingly, in accordance to the theory of quasistatic squeezing, the shock wave front surrounds the ellipsoid-shaped stone, but fragmentation is induced due to high energy density zones at the distal third, and not in the middle of the stone (Fig. **1b**) as the squeezing theory would impose, Only, if round-shaped stone models are used, due to geometrical reasons first fracture lines occur in the middle of the stone.

The importance of shock wave energy

On the other hand, in accordance with Eisenmenger [11], the peak pressure may play only a minor role for stone disintegration as long as the threshold of 10 to 30 MPa is exceeded. Thus, the peak pressure has been overestimated in the recent years. Further experiments confirmed the early findings of Granz (20) that the focal shock wave energy represents the most important physical parameter for stone fragmentation (Fig. **4**). This would be also in accordance with the *in vitro* study of Teichmann [21] where only lithotripter with high energy output (e. g. Modulith) or larger focal size (e. g. Siemens Lithostar with System C) were able to meet the efficacy of the unmodified HM3-80nF-generator. Furthermore, a comparison of three different Dornier EMSEs of the same geometry — EMSE 220F, EMSE 220F-XP and EMSE 220F-XPP — showed that disintegration does not correlate with maximum pressure, but rather with energy [33].

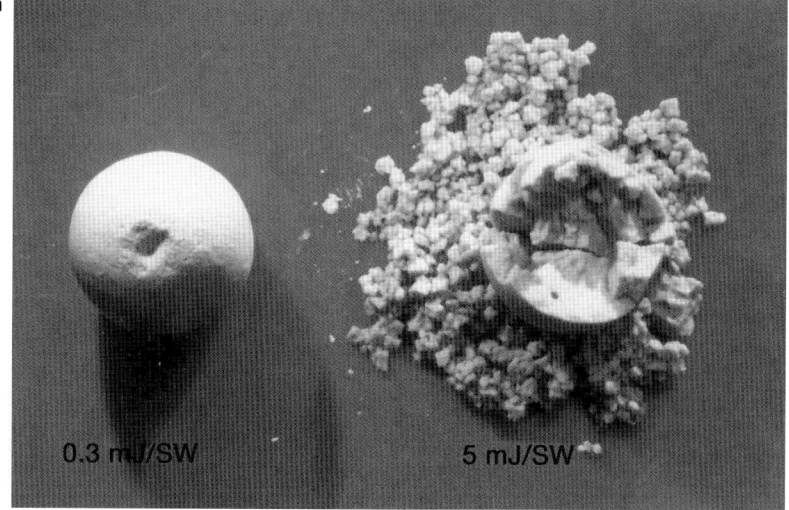

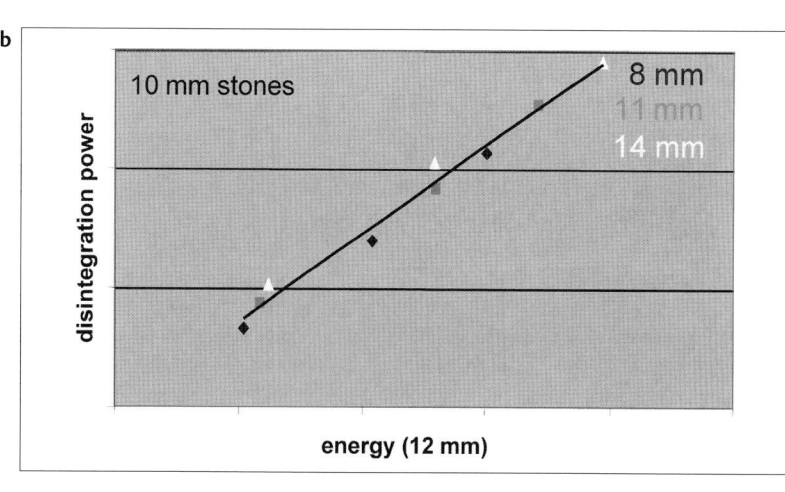

Fig. **4** Demonstration of the impact of different physical shock wave parameters for stone disintegration (with permission from Dr. Ralf Nanke, Dr. Bernd Granz, Jens Fehre, Siemens. Erlangen).
a Stone model demonstrating the importance of shock wave energy for stone disintegration (same peak pressure: p+ = 20 mPa; 1000 impulses with 0.3 vs. 5 mJ/SW). Graph demonstrating that stone disintegration depends on energy and not on focal size (three different electromagnetic sources)

Interestingly, this correlates well with recent results of an animal study concerning the sequence of shock wave energy for optimal fragmentation by Preminger's group [22]. Using the same overall number of impulses, increasing levels of generator voltage (18 to 22 kV) proved to more efficacious and less traumatic than a decreasing sequence (22 to 18 kV). This means that high peak pressure alone is not the decisive parameter characterizing fragmentation efficiency. If the threshold for stone disintegration is overcome, lower pressure levels may be sufficient for initial fragmentation. Higher peak pressures (i.e., leading to more cavitation due to associated higher negative pressure) may play a role only in the final process of stone disintegration.

On the other hand, we see that energy density is connected with side effects, like tissue trauma. This results in the requirement for a focus with moderately high energy levels, but with low maximum energy density or equivalently, a focus with a high ratio of energy versus energy density.

Technical realization of larger focal zones

Whereas in the last century, there was a trend to increase the peak pressure of the shock wave source, novel research programs of the different lithotripter manufacturers aimed at an increase of the focal zone. There exists a consensus that the focal zone of a shock wave source has not to be larger than the stone. Therefore, a small focal zone is still favorable if the stone is small and not moving. However, in the clinical situation with considerable respiratory movement of kidney and stone, with a larger focal zone, the chance of a successful hit increases as well as the delivered amount of shock wave energy on the calculus. According to this, several manufacturers modified their shock wave sources to enlarge the focal size (Fig. 5):

- double-layer of piezoelectric elements,
- switchable pulse width of the electromagnetic cylinder,
- change of coil modification, and
- modulation of shock wave front by variation of acoustic lens.

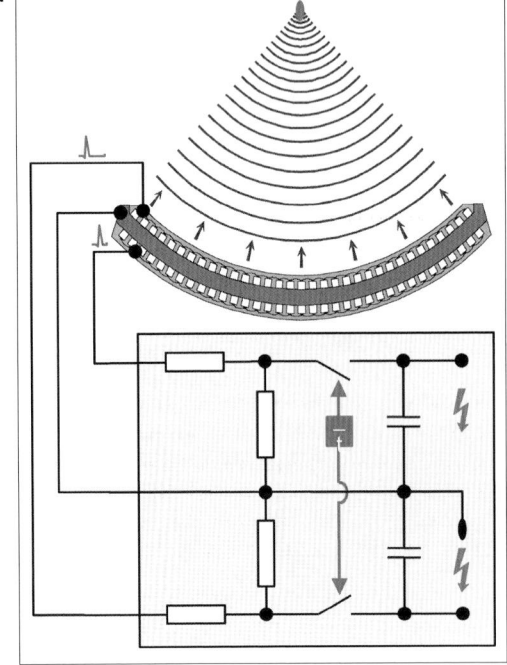

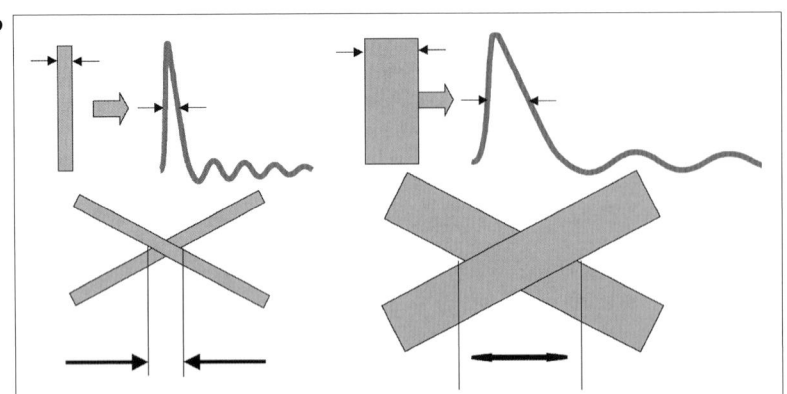

Fig. 5 Technical principles of enlargement of the focal size. a Double-layer arrangement of piezoelectric elements (Richard Wolf). b Extension of pulse width of electromagnetic cylinder (Storz-Medical).

Physicists at Richard Wolf developed a *double-layer arrangement of the piezoelectric elements* enabling a reduction of the aperture from 50 to 30 cm associated with a significant increase of the focal zone (Piezolith 3000). This system (Fig. **5a**) is very sophisticated, because the synchronization of the travelling of two shock waves realized by special thyristors coordinating the two electrical circuits is not trivial. Additionally, the double-layer technology enables further modifications, such as the variation of delay, pulse forming, which may become important in the future. To date, however, a better fragmentation could not be realized.

Recently Storz-Medical introduced a lithotripter enabling the use of two different focal sizes (Modulith SLX-2F). Technically, this can be realized by *two different pulse durations of the shock wave* using the same generator and a paraboloid reflector (Fig. **5b**). Actually, the manufacturer recommends the larger focal zone (50 × 9 mm) for renal calculi and the smaller focal zone (28 × 6 mm) for ureteral stones or stones which may require highest energies. This device offers both treatment strategies to be selectable by the operator.

Dornier MedTech Systems also modified their EMSE 220 to the EMSE 220 XXP by enlargement of the pulse width to achieve a similar *in vitro* disintegrative efficacy as the HM3 (Fig. **6**). Due to the longer pulse the acoustic focal energy of the EMSE was increased, whereas the maximum p+ was not increased. As a consequence the −6 dB focus which is related to the maximum pressure value became broader. In another experiment the focal zone of an EMSE 220 was increased by a different shock wave lens but the applied electric power remained constant. This resulted in a decreased fragmentation *in vitro*. A beneficial contribution of the squeezing effect could not be observed in this test [33].

The research department of Siemens has developed a new electromagnetic shock wave source for their upcoming device (Siemens Lithoskop). The application of increased amounts of shock wave energy was mainly realized by the *optimization of the coil configuration* used in the electromagnetic element [23, 24].

An electromagnetic self-focusing shock wave source with a large focal diameter (up to 20 mm), a longer pulse duration (up to 2 µs), and a relatively low peak pressure (10 MPa to 30 MPa) has been under clinical evaluation. First clinical results of this device were promising (25). However, these results represent only a single center study in China and are restricted to ultrasound localization with limited access to ureteral stones. Further studies are necessary to reconfirm these data. Like the piezoelectric double layer system, the self-focusing system theoretically enables pulse forming (e.g., by use of different coils), but such systems have not yet been realized.

Finally, Direx presented another electromagnetic lithotripter with trapezoid cone-shaped cylinder and a paraboloid reflector (Integra), offering a variable focal area selectable from 6 to 18 mm. However, there are no clinical data available yet.

Since recent investigations did not prove any impact of the focal size on stone disintegration,

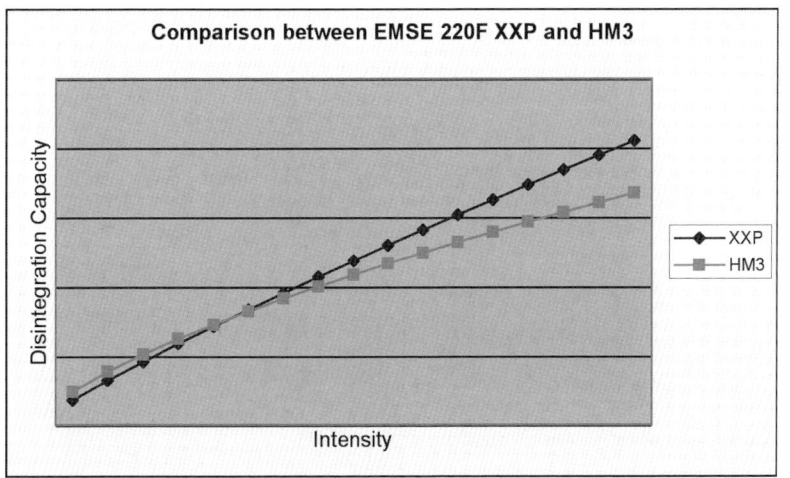

Fig. **6** Comparison of disintegrative efficacy of modified electromagnetic shock wave source (EMSE 220 F-XXP) to Dornier HM3.

clinical results must be awaited to finally determine the relevance of different focal sizes [26].

Combination of SW sources

Several strategies have been proposed to improve the efficiency of shock wave lithotripsy. The first one is based on the idea that forced collapse of cavitation bubbles by a shock wave can significantly enhance the damage to a nearby solid surface, and thus stone fragmentation. Recent studies using a piezoelectric annular array shock wave generator that can be retrofitted on an HM-3 lithotripter have demonstrated that stone fragmentation *in vitro* can be significantly improved when optimal shock wave-bubble interaction is produced [27]. Further studies are underway to evaluate the effectiveness of this method *in vivo*, and to assess the impact of this modification on tissue injury.

With respect to this idea, the recently presented Direx Duet lithotripter might be interesting, because in this device *two electrohydraulic shock wave sources* are integrated. Theoretically, in a synchronized mode, this could result in a reinforced wave (i.e., doubling the aperture for given energy) or, in an asynchronized mode, at least reduce the shock wave-induced trauma. However, recent theoretical studies showed no improvement of disintegrative efficacy when shock waves were delivered under an angle of 90° setting. Theoretically, only if completely synchronized and less than 45°, best at 180° there might be a positive effect [23]. Technically, there exists the problem that exact synchronization of impulses with the electrohydraulic system (spark gap) is very difficult due to the variation of pulses (jitter effect). In accordance to this, preliminary clinical data with this device could not demonstrate an improvement of shock wave efficacy, mainly because dual application was not feasible due to an inappropriate shock wave window for the second source.

Improved Application

Despite all the technical modifications, the following few basic principles to be observed during clinical application of ESWL are of utmost importance for successful results. Vice versa, application mistakes may have more impact on the outcome than any technical improvements. With the Dornier HM3, application is very simple:

- patients were in a complete water bath as optimal coupling medium,
- stone localization was accomplished with two X-ray converters,
- the focal zone was very large compensating for respiratory movements, and
- treatment was carried out under epidural or general anesthesia

In contrast to this, new lithotripters use a water cushion with ultrasonic gel, a single fluoroscopic localization system (e.g., coaxial C-arm; Table **1**) and the focal zones are smaller. Evidently, such systems require a more careful application.

Optimal coupling

Coupling with water cushion may result in a 5% attenuation of shock wave energy. However, this can increase by more than 10-fold if the coupling media and area are not handled carefully:
- the skin should be shaved at the entrance area,
- the coupling medium (gel, oil or water) should be put on the entire area, and
- only coupling oils or gels recommended by the manufacturer should be used (i.e., no Vaseline because of its high viscosity)

Devices using real-time coaxial ultrasound provide the ability of real-time control of the coupling in the central part of the source. They can exclude peripheral coupling errors only when the transducer is retracted in a remote position.

Optimal localization and monitoring

The stone has to be placed in the center of the focal zone; however, respiratory movement may dislodge the calculus considerably. Sophisticated systems with respiratory belts and triggering of SW impulses (e.g., Siemens Lithostar) have been abandoned mainly due to the increased treatment time and irregular shock wave delivery. Immobilization of the stone by high-frequency ventilatory respiration anesthesia turned out to be too invasive. Conclusively, a larger focal zone has the advantage to reduce the rate of incorrectly hitting impulses. If lithotripters with smaller focal zones are used, real-time coaxial ultrasound localization may be the optimal alternative to guarantee adequate coupling and localization of the stone.

Definition of focal zone

In this context, the definition of the focal zone may become important. There is consensus that the classical focal zone definition (–6 dB) has only a minor relevance to describe the energy output or, respectively, the disintegrative efficacy of a shock wave source. The main reason for this is the fact that this focal zone definition depends only on the peak pressure – focal zone minus 6 dB – whereas the disintegrative efficacy depends on the applied energy including a minimal pressure of about 30 MPa. Therefore, the manufacturers have defined further parameters such as the distribution of shock wave energy around the focal zone with specific threshold values (e. g., 5 MPa and 10 MPa).

Minimizing shock wave induced renal trauma

Animal experiments as golden standard [28] are very expensive and only available in limited number. Therefore, several *in vitro* models have been introduced consisting mainly of artificially perfused kidneys [29]. Basically, the following morphological findings can be summarized. Shock wave-induced damage of renal parenchyma primarily occurs at vessels and tubular cells. Depending mainly on the energy density, first venules are damaged in the medulla (grade I lesion), followed by rupture of arterioles in the cortex (grade II/III lesion). The main physical reasons for this are cavitation (e. g., for ecchymosis) and tear and shear forces, depending on the following factors:
- sudden changes (jumps) of impedance in the tissue penetrated by the shock wave;
- nuclei of cavitation in the parenchyma, blood, urine or bile; and
- elasticity and resistance of the tissue exposed to shock waves

Recently, in cooperation with Siemens Medical Solutions an *in vitro* test system was established aiming at a quantitative judgment of the renal vascular damage [309]. The isolated porcine kidney was perfused with a ferroxide solution (Berlin blue) during shock wave application, enabling morphological and histopathological investigation of the renal vascular damage. Based on the introduction of a lesion score, it could be shown that the energy density (ED+) represented the only parameter with proven statistical correlation in regard to tissue damage (Fig. 7). Another, similar model using barium sulfate perfusion at the end of shock wave application may also be used accordingly [31].

There is no doubt that, in the last decade, peak pressure has been overestimated as the main factor for stone fragmentation. Future developments are focused on the optimization of the focal size to deliver adequate amounts of energy to disintegrate the stone avoiding at the same time high levels of energy density representing the main physical parameter for the induction of tissue trauma. However, the exact impact of the focal zone on the outcome of ESWL has yet to be determined in future clinical studies.

Overall, it is most likely that further optimization of the pressure waveform, distribution, and sequence of the lithotripter shock waves is needed in order to maximize stone comminution while minimizing tissue injury in SWL.

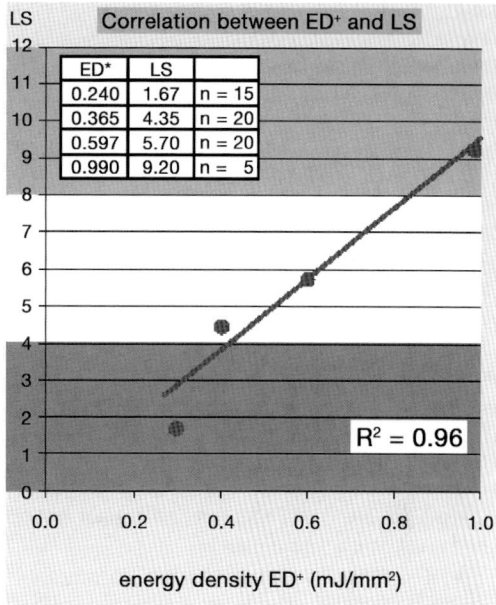

Fig. 7 Correlation of energy density (mJ/mm^2) to renal lesion in a perfused porcine model (LS = lesion score).

Localization Systems

Treatment strategies in ESWL are to a great extent influenced by the imaging system available in a lithotripter.

Fluoroscopy

Fluoroscopic localization is the preferred modality. It allows visualization of all radio-opaque calculi with almost no limitations with respect to localization (i.e., ureter). There have been significant technical innovations introduced by the lithotripter companies:

Isocentric C-arm: Most manufacturers have modified the stone localization systems to the use of an isocentric C-arm. Such systems can be easily connected to any type of shock wave source.

AP and CC projection versus AP and lateral projection: For X-ray localization at least two projections are required with an angle between the two axes of projection of about 30° to allow proper positioning of the shock wave source. In existing lithotripters either AP and cranial caudal (CC) projections are realized (e.g., Dornier Compact Delta, Dornier Compact Sigma, Dornier Lithotripter S, Dornier Lithotripter S II) or AP and lateral projections (e.g., Storz Modulith SLX-F2; Siemens Lithoskop). In case of CC projection generally two angles of projection are possible (+/– 30°). In case of lateral projection only one axis is realized in general.

Fluoroscopy passing by versus passing through the shock wave source: The X-ray projections have to be chosen in a way that the shock wave source is out of the path of the X-rays as much as possible. Today different manufacturers offer different solutions sometimes with a variation of solutions in their own product family.

Fluoroscopy passing by the shock wave source: In this case the axes are chosen so that the X-rays by-pass the shock wave source leading ideally to unrestricted fluoroscopy (e.g., Dornier Compact Delta, Dornier Compact Sigma, Wolf Piezolith 3000).

Fluoroscopy passing through the shock wave source (in-line fluoroscopy): In this case the shock wave source has openings to allow the X-rays to pass through them leading to X-ray imaging which is limited by the openings in the shock wave source. In the case of AP projection this leads to a projection axis for X-ray imaging which is in-line with the axis of shock wave propagation, therefore it is also called in-line fluoroscopy. The naming may lead to the perception that in-line fluoroscopy is associated with the same advantages as in-line ultrasound. However, it is associated with a considerable reduction of the field of view limited by the opening inside the shock wave source through which the X-rays have to pass.

Only lithotripters with a single fluoroscopic localization system (e.g., Siemens Lithostar Multiline, Siemens Lithoskop, Storz Modulith SLX, Modulith SLX-F2) present in-line fluoroscopy as another alternative. In the recent Siemens Lithoskop both modalities are technically combined. The shock wave source is aligned on a C-arm parallel to the fluoroscopic C-arm, which enables in-line fluoroscopy via the centrally perforated electromagnetic source.

Digital imaging: Nowadays, the price and applicability of the lithotripter are mainly defined by the quality of the localization system. All manufacturers now provide excellent digital upgradeable systems, e.g., for uro-lithotripters the fluoroscopic system consists of a high-quality digitized X-ray imaging system mounted on a rotatable C-arm with preferably isocentrically integrated shock wave source.

Lateral projection for stone localization: On the x- and y-axes, p.a. projection (with the X-ray source posterior to the patient) is performed to reduce radiation exposure to the patient (e.g., as introduced in the Dornier MFL 5000). For the z-axis *lateral projection* has several advantages over cranio-caudal projections (e.g., as previously used in the Siemens Lithostar). This concerns:
– minimizing the localization error due to respiratory movement of the kidney and ureter,
– providing better image quality (especially if air bags are used) due to the shorter distance to the object, and
– reducing the X-ray exposure to the patient.

Such concepts are realized in two most recent lithotripters (Storz Modulith SLX-F2; Siemens Lithoskop).

Use of air bags: Interestingly, the use of air bags in the X-ray beam, a concept known from the Dornier HM3 and Wolf Piezolith 2300, has been reincorporated in some devices (e.g., Storz Modulith SLX-F2). Evidently, the quality of imaging is improved and the fluoroscopic time may be shortened.

A similar improvement of the image can be achieved by displacing the inner tubing in the lens towards the patient during fluoroscopy (e.g., Siemens Multiline, Siemens Lithoskop).

3D-navigation: Recently, Storz-Medical presented a new computer-aided system to reduce the radiation exposure of the patient: the Litho-

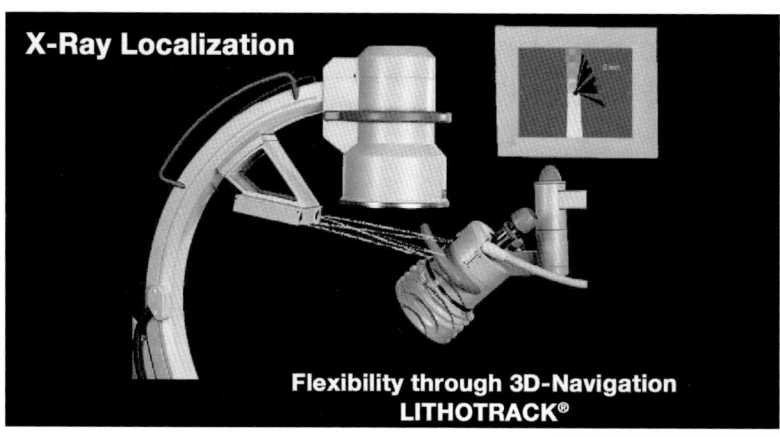

Fig. 8 Lithotrack for 3D X-ray navigation (Storz Modulith SLK).

track in the Modulith SLK (Fig. 8). The system works similar to 3D-navigation devices in other clinical settings. The position of the SW head is controlled by a stereocamera. The correct position of the SW source can be controlled by virtual reality without the need of continuous fluoroscopy.

In summary, the quality of fluoroscopic imaging has been improved significantly and several technical innovations enable a marked reduction of radiation exposure.

Ultrasound

Advantages: Sonographic localization represents the cheapest localization modality with no side-effects. There is no doubt that sonographic localization of most renal calculi is possible and treatment success can be adequately assessed due to real-time scanning without X-ray exposure. In an exploratory study by Dornier Medtech in which the efficacy achieved by using a lithotripter with X-ray localization was compared to the same lithotripter with isocentric ultrasound localization, no differences in efficacy were found between both the two localization modalities. Therefore, the localization error due to deviations caused by the variation in acoustical parameters may not be clinically relevant as far as the efficacy of ESWL is concerned. Nevertheless, theoretically a localization error due to deviation and coupling errors should be minimized if a coaxial scanner is used. This might be a beneficial point in the treatment of children and infants. Moreover, this localization modality may be helpful for ESWT (e. g., for Peyronie's disease). In dedicated ESWT devices, ultrasound is used routinely (Dornier Epos Ultra).

Disadvantages: Stone localization is difficult and almost impossible in some areas, i. e., in the middle third of the ureter or with an indwelling ureteral catheter (double J-stent). Determination of the size of each individual stone fragment may be inadequate due to superimposed fragments or artifacts. Ultrasound depends mainly on the proficiency of the operator, which may entail a longer training period. Thus, even for most of the previous promoters (Wolf, Edap) ultrasound localization represents only the second choice.

Technical aspects: In-line ultrasound represents the most accurate localization modality, whereas the deviation of lateral ultrasound may amount to 4 mm (e. g., Siemens Lithoskop). The clinical relevance of this finding, however, has not been demonstrated. The lateral ultrasound offers easier handling of the system avoiding interfering structures like ribs. Simultaneous real-time use of both fluoroscopic and ultrasonic localization are available in all present day lithotripters by Dornier and in the Siemens Lithostar Modularis consisting of an isocentric C-arm and a lateral isocentric ultrasound transducer. For the operator, a movable source is preferred rather than moving the patient to the ultrasound source. Nevertheless, ultrasonic stone localization requires optimal training of the treating urologist.

Perspectives of SWL Technology

Further developments are already focusing on the improvement of the disintegrative efficacy of the lithotripters. There is evidence that the amount of shock wave energy delivered to the stone and not peak pressure represents the main factor for stone disintegration. The impact of a variable focal size will be determined soon. Further technological improvements may concern an optimization of the wave form avoiding high energy density and negative pressure with cavitation-associated tissue trauma. Finally new imaging technology might be applicable for extracorporeal shock wave lithotripsy like 3D-ultrasound for stone targeting or duplex-sonography [34, 35] to determine early stone fragmentation [32].

References

1. Köhrmann KU, Rassweiler JJ, Manning M, Mohr G, Henkel TO, Jünemann KP, Alken P. The clinical introduction of a third generation lithotriptor: Modulith SL 20. J Urol 1995; 153: 1379–1383
2. Flam TA, Chice R, Dancer P et al: Electroinductive lithotripsy increases precision and efficacy at F 2. Experimental data and clinical application with the Sonolith 4000. J Endourol 1993; 7: S178 (abstract No. W.XI-6)
3. Dann T, Schneller J, Knipper A, Jocham D. Litho Diagnost M a new multifunctional urologic workstation. J Endourol 1993; 7: S178 (abstract No. W.XI-4)
4. Tailly G. The Dornier Lithotripter U/15/50: A multifunctional and multidisciplinary workstation. J Endourol 1998; 12: 301
5. Tailly GG. Consecutive experience with four Dornier lithotripters: HM4, MPL9000, Compact and U/50. J Endourol 1999; 13: 329–338
6. Rassweiler JJ, Renner C, Chaussy C, Thüroff, S. Treatment of renal stones by extracorporeal shock wave lithotripsy. Eur Urol 2001; 39: 187–199
7. Rassweiler JJ, Saltzman B, Tailly G, Timoney A, Zhong P. Shock Wave Lithotripsy Technology. In: Segura J, Conort P, Khoury S, Pak C, Preminger GM, Tolley D (eds): Stone Disease. 1st International Consultation on Stone Disease. Health Publications, Pars, 2003, pp 289–356
8. Tailly GG. Two years experience with the EMSE 220F-XXP. A new gold standard? J. Endourol 2004; 18 (Suppl): A26 (abstract MP1/15)
9. Zhong P, Preminger GM. Mechanisms of differing stone fragility in extracorporeal shock wave lithotripsy. J Endourol 1994; 8: 163–168
10. Zhong P, Xi XF, Zhu SL, Cocks FH, Preminger GM. Recent developments in SWL physics research. J Endourol 1999; 13: 611–617
11. Eisenmenger W. The mechanisms of stone fragmentation in ESWL. Ultrasound Med Biol 2001; 27: 683–693
12. Crum LA. Cavitation microjets as a contributory mechanism for renal calculi disintegration in ESWL. J Urol 1988; 140: 1587–1590
13. Sass W, Dreyer HP, Kettermann S, Seifert J. The role of cavitational activity in fragmentation processes by lithotripters. J Stone Disease 1992; 4: 193–198
14. Delius M, Brendel W. A mechanism of gallstone destruction by extracorporeal shock waves. Naturwissenschaften 1988; 75: 200–201
15. Zhou Y, Cocks FH, Preminger GM, Zhong P. Innovations in shock wave technology: updates in experimental studies. J Urol 2004; 172: 1892–1898
16. Fischer N, Müller HM, Gulhan A, Sohn M, Deutz FJ, Rübben H, Lutzeyer W. Cavitation effects: Possible cause of tissue injury during extracorporeal shock wave lithotripsy. J Endourol 1988; 2: 215–220
17. Lokhandwalla M, Sturtevant B. Fracture mechanics model of stone comminution in ESWL and implications for tissue damage. Phys Med Biol 2000; 45: 1923–1940
18. Granz B, Nanke R, Fehre J, Pfister T, Engelbrecht R. Light spot hydrophone, innovation in lithotripsy. Medical Solutions 2004; 1: 86–87
19. Staudenraus J, Eisenmenger W: Fibre-optic probe hydrophone for ultrasonic and shock wave measurements. Ultrasonics 1993; 31: 267–273
20. Granz B, Köhler G. What makes a shock wave efficient in lithotripsy. J. Stone Disease 1992; 4: 123–128
21. Teichmann JMH, Portis AL, Parker PJ, Bub WL, Endicott RC, Denes B, Perale MS, Clayman RV. In vitro shock wave lithotripsy comparison. J Urol 2000; 164: 1259–1264
22. Springhart WP, Sung JC, Sur RL, Murguet CM, Machoney ME, Zhong P, Preminger GM. Treatment strategy improves in vivo stone comminution and tissue injury in shock wave lithotripsy. J Endourol 2004; 18 (Suppl): A12 (abstract BR3/2)
23. Mihradi S, Homma H, Kanto Y. Numerical analysis of kidney stone fragmentation by short pulse impingement. JSME Int J 2004; 47: 581–587
24. Granz B, Lanski M, Nanke R, Mahler M, Rohwedder A, Chaussy C, Thüroff S. Lithostar Modularis – a proven system with new innovative features. Electromedia 2003; 71: 53–57
25. Eisenmenger W, Du XX, Tang C, Zhao S, Wang Y, Rong F, Dai D. The first clinical results of "wide-focus and low pressure" ESWL. Ultrasound Med Biol 2002; 28: 769–774
26. Ng CF, McLornan L, Thompson TJ, Tolley DA: Comparison of piezoelectric lithotriptors using matched pair analysis. J Urol 2004; 172: 1887–1891

27 Xi X, Zhong P. Improvement of stone fragmentation during shock wave lithotripsy using a combined EH/PEAA shock wave generator — in vitro experiments. Ultrasound Med Biol 2000; 26: 457–467
28 Rassweiler J, Köhrmann KU, Back W, Fröhner S, Raab M, Weber A, Kahmann F, Marlinghaus E, Jünemann KP, Alken P. Experimental basis of shock wave-induced renal trauma in the model of the canine kidney. World J Urol 1993; 11: 43–53
29 Koehrmann KU, Back W, Bensemann J, Florian J, Weber W, Kahmann F, Rassweiler J, Alken P. The isolated perfused kidney of the pig: New model to evaluate shock wave-induced lesions. J Endourol 1994; 8: 105–110
30 Chaussy C, Bergsdorf T, Thüroff S, Chmelar C. The isolated perfused pig kidney — a reliable tissue model for the evaluation of renal tissue injury. A comparison of two shock wave systems. J Urol 2004; 171 (Suppl): 391
31 Haecker A, Leistner R, Knoll T, Koehrmann KU, Alken P, Michel MS, Marlinghaus EH. Ex vivo evaluation of renal injury of a new electromagnetic shock wave generator with user selectable dual focus size. BJU Int 2004; 94 (Suppl): 8 (abstract MP-2.02)
32 Rassweiler JJ, Tailly GG, Chaussy C. Progress in lithotriptor technology. EAU Update Series 2005; 3: 17–36
33 Forssmann B, Ueberle F, Bohris C. Towards a new EMSE generation. J. Endourol 2002; 16 (Suppl 2): 18–21
34 Bohris C, Bayer T, Lechner C. Hit/Miss monitoring of ESWL by spectral Doppler ultrasound. Ultrasound in Medicine and Biology 2003; 29: 705–712
35 Bohris C, Bayer T. Doppler Ultrasound for Hit/Miss Monitoring in ESWL. In: Chapelon JY, Lafon C (eds): Conference Proceedings, 3rd International Symposium on Therapeutic Ultrasound, 22–25 June, 2003, INSERM U556, Lyon, France, pp 169–172

Two *Ex Vivo* Models for the Evaluation of SW-Induced Renal Injury

A. Häcker, T. Bergsdorf, P. Alken, Ch. Chaussy

Introduction

For renal and ureteral stone disease, shock wave lithotripsy (SWL) has been proved to be an effective and safe method with a low risk for clinically significant long-term sequelae. Acute side effects of SWL are pain and gross hematuria and renal hemorrhage due to parenchymal and vascular injury. In the pathogenesis of these adverse events, damages to vascular and tubule cells are considered to be the primary event, with a following disturbance of the microcirculation and ischemic changes in the supplied parenchyma. Technical parameters of the shock wave generator that determine the extent of the vascular and parenchymal injury have not yet been completely clarified to date.

The aim of this report is to characterize and compare two different experimental settings of *ex vivo* perfused kidneys for the evaluation of SW-induced renal injury.

Materials and Methods

Kidney preparation

Kidney preparation was performed identically in both models. Kidneys were obtained from freshly slaughtered pigs. Perirenal fat was removed, the renal capsule was kept intact on the renal surface. Renal artery, vein, and ureter were cannulated, then perfused with cold (4 °C) 0.9 % NaCl solution (+ 5,000 IU heparin) under physiological pressure conditions (~ 80 mmHg), in order to flush the kidney free of blood and to achieve a fast cooling of the renal parenchyma. These prepared kidneys were stored in cold (4 °C) physiological saline solution.

Model 1: histopathologic evaluation

The kidneys were warmed up slowly to 25 °C before they were positioned in a water bath with degassed water (25 °C). The exchangeable shock wave source (electromagnetic shock wave system M/C/experimental, Siemens Medical Solutions, Erlangen, Germany) was directly integrated into the water bath, to achieve an energy loss-free coupling of the acoustic energy into the renal tissue (Fig. 1). A laser crosshair in the water bath, representing the focal spot of the SW system, enabled the localization of the renal collecting system (upper/lower pole). All treatments were performed with a fixed SW frequency of 120 SW/min under continuous arterial perfusion with Berlin Blue solution (Berlin Blue pigment dye diluted in isotonic NaCl solution) for six minutes, realized with a peristaltic pump (Ureteromat Perez-Castro, Storz), producing an adjustable flow of perfusion fluid. A real-time pressure transducer was integrated in the arterial arm, to monitor the perfusion pressure (~ 80 mmHg). Each kidney was used for two shock wave experiments (upper/lower pole).

After the shock wave exposure, the two poles of the kidney were separated and the superficial, macroscopic lesions were documented with a digital camera. For the histopathological examination, a tissue block (containing the complete shock wave exposed area) from the shock wave entry and shock wave exit was excised and fixed with formalin. The blocks were cut perpendicular to the renal surface into 2 mm slices and stained with hematoxylin and eosin. These samples were investigated by a pathologist with regard to localization, morphology, and extent of dye extravasation, indicating the renal vascular trauma.

To achieve a semiquantitative judgement of the investigated shock wave trauma, the histopathological report was transferred into a score system, judging the localization (extent) and grade (severity) of shock wave induced vascular lesion (Fig. 2).

The localization was categorized into 4 different groups (**L0–L3**):
- **L0:** no paravasation of pigment dye,
- **L1:** subcapsular lesions,
- **L2:** extravasation in the peripheral part of renal parenchyma, and
- **L3:** distribution of vascular lesions over the whole parenchyma.

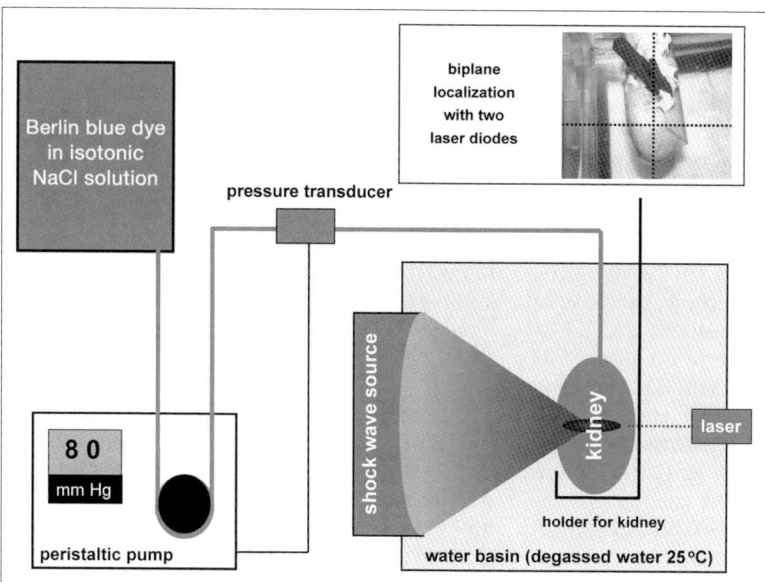

Fig. 1 Experimental setting for the histopathological model.

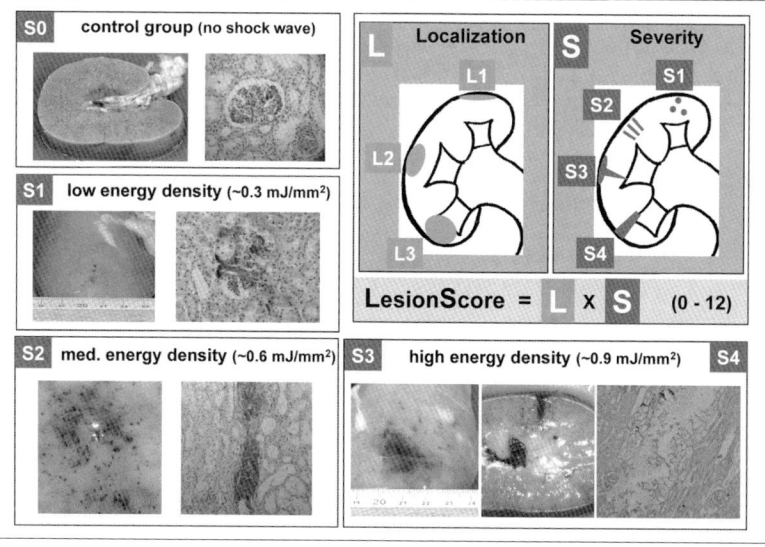

Fig. 2 Results of the histopathological model.

The grade of tissue trauma was classified according to the severity of vessel lesions into 5 different groups (**S0–S4**):
- **S0**: macroscopic and histopathological examination indicates only intravasal deposition of pigment dye; there is no evidence for vessel lesions,
- **S1**: spotted extravasation of dye (petechiae) is visible on the renal surface or in the renal cortex, corresponding to rupture of small vessels,
- **S2**: a string-shaped paravasation of dye along the cortical vessels and tubuli indicates the rupture of bigger vascular structures,
- **S3**: extensive extravasation of dye leads to dehiscence of renal tissue and subcapsular deposition of Berlin Blue, and
- **S4**: disrupture of renal parenchyma and string-shaped loss of parenchyma with massive extravasation of dye as a direct destructive effect of high energy shock waves.

Finally, the localization score (0–3) and severity score (0–4) of every tissue sample were multiplied, to generate the lesion score (0–12), characterizing the total extent of shock wave-induced renal vascular trauma.

Model 2: radiological evaluation

The kidneys were heated to 37 °C in degassed water before the trial started. For coupling the shock waves, the kidneys were immersed into degassed water at a temperature of 25 °C. The kidneys were continuously perfused at 100 mL/min. with isotonic sodium chloride solution through the renal arteries at a pressure between 80–120 cm H_2O by a commercial medical perfusion pump (Fresenius Inc., Germany). Shock waves were applied vertically under ultrasonographic control (B mode, 3.5 MHz transducer) in the center of the cortex of both kidney poles. After application of the SW, a barium sulfate ($BaSO_4$) suspension was perfused through the renal artery. The kidneys were cut into plane-parallel slices of 5 mm thickness by a rotary knife. Vessels and extravasation were documented by X-ray on mammographic film. The maximal diameter (mm) of the extravasation in the cortex, representing the extent of the vascular lesion, was measured.

Discussion

Animal experiments for the evaluation of shock wave-induced kidney trauma present some important disadvantages. The number of experiments is limited because of the large scale and expensive experimental set-up, the limited availability of specimens, and the protracting process, to pass the ethics committee. Furthermore, the interindividual variance of animals and the experimental conditions confine the evidence of the experimental results [1, 2]. A direct comparison of different lithotripters is not possible.

The isolated, perfused *ex vivo* porcine kidney model may neutralize these limitations. These *ex vivo* kidneys are unlimitedly available and large numbers of repetitive trials are possible at very low cost. Our preliminary results have shown that macroscopic and histological examination of shock wave exposed kidneys reveal typical renal vascular and parenchymal injuries, comparable to earlier animal experiments [3, 4]. These correlations are also be found again in the human shock wave application (CT and MRI examination after ESWL treatment) [5, 6].

Using the histopathological model, the renal vascular trauma was characterized by extravasal deposition of Berlin blue dye; the localization

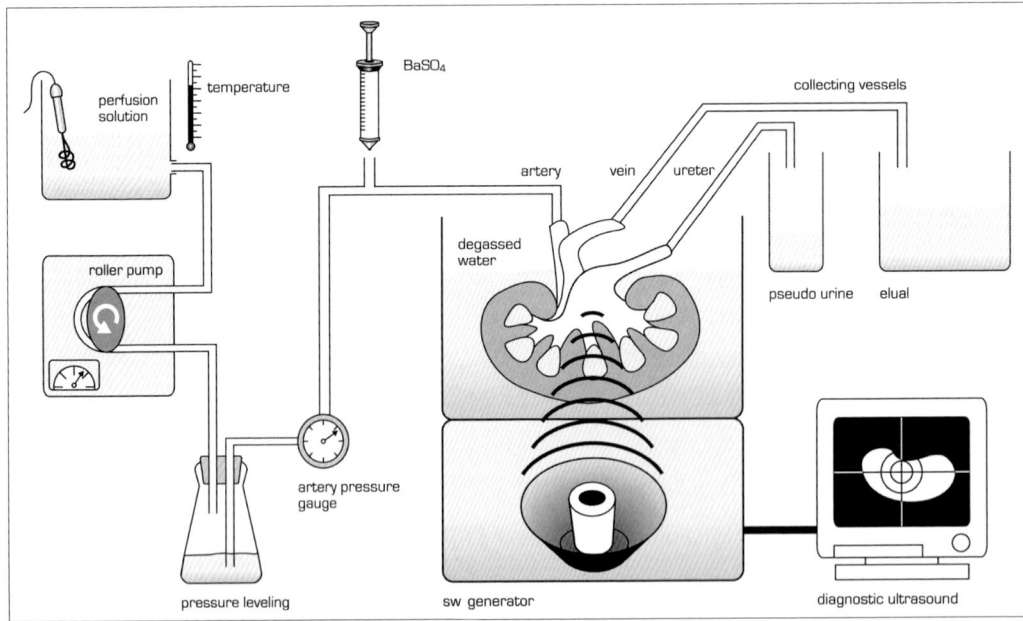

Fig. 3 Experimental setting for the radiological model.

and morphology of dye paravasation was in relation to the applied shock wave parameters. Depending on the strategy of histopathological examination (cross sections through parenchyma), the distribution of paravasation was specified vertically (from capsule to renal calix). The introduction of the "lesion score" enabled a semiquantitative judgement of the renal vascular injury, induced by high energy shock wave; and statistical analysis of correlations between shock wave parameters and resulting tissue trauma became feasible. The perfusion solution (Berlin blue dye in isotonic NaCl solution) has different acoustic characteristics (e.g., absorption of shock wave energy, induction of cavitation) in comparison to blood and therefore will have an effect on the degree of renal tissue damage. This might be a restriction of this experimental set-up, but on the other hand this factor was constant for all experiments. In contrast, the radiological model measures the maximum extent of the barium extravasate in mm, which is an objective measurement procedure. However, a semiquantitative judgement is not possible.

General limitations of both *ex vivo* models have to be mentioned. The findings are not directly transferable to *in vivo* conditions. The isolated perfused kidney is not a reproduction of the conditions in the human body, but a rational experimental set-up, to create a "tissue phantom." The acoustic characteristics of tissue in the shock wave path, which absorbs and reflects shock wave energy are not considered, as well as respiratory movements of the kidney, arterial hypertension, and pre-existing diseases of the kidney. Additionally, the kidneys are isolated and denervated and therefore there is no influence of the vegetative innervation.

Conclusions

Both experimental set-ups are suitable instruments to evaluate high energy shock wave-induced renal vascular trauma by means of radiological or histopathological investigation. Further trials and diversifications of the model, such as interposition of tissue layers in the shock wave path or simulation of respiratory movements, are mandatory to prove the validity of these experimental findings. The ease of use and low running costs might encourage the development of a standardized "tissue phantom" which was previously not available.

References

[1] Blomgren P, Connors B, Lingeman J, Willis L, Evan A. Quantitation of shock wave lithotripsy-induced lesion in small and large pig kidneys. Anat Rec 1997; 249: 341–348

[2] Clayman R. Relationship between kidney size, renal injury, and renal impairment induced by shock wave lithotripsy. J Urol 2000; 164: 1860

[3] Connors B, Evan A, Willis L, Blomgren P, Lingeman J, Fineberg N. The effect of discharge voltage on renal injury and impairment caused by lithotripsy in the pig. J Am Soc Nephrol 2000; 11: 310–318

[4] Delius M, Enders G, Xuan Z, Liebicht H-J, Brendel W. Biological effects of shock waves: kidney damage by shock waves in dogs – dose dependence. Ultrasound in Med & Biol 1988; 117–122

[5] Recker F, Ruebben H, Neuerburg J, Bex A, Deutz F, Hofstaedter F. Magnetic resonance imaging of acute and long-term alterations following extracorporeal shock wave lithotripsy in rats. Urol Int 1990; 45: 28

[6] Rubin J, Arger P, Pollack H, Banner M, Coleman, Mintz M, VanArsdalen K. Kidney changes after extracorporeal shock wave lithotripsy. CT evaluation. Radiology 1987; 162: 21–24

The Light Spot Hydrophone — LSHD: A New Level of Precise Ultrasonic Shock Wave Measurement

B. Granz, R. Nanke

Introduction

Lithotripsy with extracorporeally generated, focused ultrasonic shock waves is the method of choice for the therapeutic treatment of concrements in urology. The therapeutic effect is a result of the high pressure pulse amplitude and the energy content of the focused shock wave hitting the kidney or the ureter stone [1]. Since the beginning of the lithotripter development, engineers have struggled with the precise measurement of these helpful properties: pulse shape and amplitude and focus energy content. The requirements for the hydrophones are impressive: amplitudes from a few MPa up to 150 MPa, linearity in this range, bandwidth from approx. 10 kHz to 15 MHz, small sensitive area, absolute calibration, easy to operate, and stable against cavitation. But unfortunately a shock wave able to destroy kidney stones does the same with hydrophones. On the other hand, the lithotripter development engineer requires a hydrophone that should survive the measurement procedure in the laboratory with some hundred measurement events.

Current Hydrophone Situation

In the beginning, lithotripter shock wave field measurements were performed with PVDF membrane hydrophones developed for diagnostic ultrasound [2], followed by the more stable needle hydrophones [3], and the capacitively coupled membrane hydrophone [4] especially developed for shock wave measurements. PVDF as a piezoelectric material for hydrophones is frequently used because of its high bandwidth properties [5]. And even in the standard IEC 61846 it is stated that the shock wave hydrophone should be equivalent to a 25-µm thick polymer (PVDF) hydrophone [6].

However, PVDF hydrophones suffer from the poor adhesion of the metallic contacts and from the hydrophobic behavior of the polymer surface. This results in a poor lifetime of the membrane PVDF hydrophone in the presence of high amplitude pressure pulses, and in a poor ability to measure the negative part of the pulse.

In other words, shock waves destroy PVDF hydrophones, and the energy measurement is not reliable.

With the fiberoptic hydrophone [7], a system with the potential also to represent the negative part of the shock wave came onto the field. The tip of an optical fiber connected to a laser is used as a hydrophone. The sensor effect is based on the alteration of the laser light reflectivity at the tip with the pressure of the water in which the tip is immersed. The shock wave measurement with the fiberoptic hydrophone obtains good results in pulse and energy presentation, with the drawback that the optical fiber with a diameter of about 100 µm tends to break frequently during the measurement of the shock wave's focal distribution. This results in a tedinous redismantling, recutting, recalibration, and repositioning procedure of the tip of the fiber. All this makes the measurement of the shock wave's focal distribution to a time-consuming task.

The Light Spot Hydrophone

Basic considerations

For the development of a new shock wave hydrophone, we put the properties — stability, broad bandwidth, positive and negative pressure pulse presentation, dynamic range — in our ranking as first place. This resulted in the design of a novel optical hydrophone with improved performance. The optical fiber will be exchanged by a free optical beam and the tip of the fiber by a light spot of this optical beam which is reflected at an extended glass surface immersed in water. The light spot at the glass-water interface will be the sensitive zone of the set-up, giving the hydrophone its new name: light spot hydrophone — LSHD.

Design considerations

The variation of the optical refractive index of water with the travelling ultrasonic pressure pulse is well-known and used, e. g., for Schlieren optical presentations of the ultrasonic field [8]. At a glass-water interface of a glass block, this variation can be measured by the alteration of the reflected light intensity of a light beam coming through the glass block. High sensitivity can be achieved for an incident light beam at an angle close to the angle of total reflection [9]. But this set-up is extremely non-linear. This means, the sensitivity is strongly amplitude-dependent.

For the LSHD, we consider the case where the angle of the incident light beam is close to normal to the glass interface of a glass block. In this case, the angle of the light beam is negligible and the reflected light intensity is a function only of the refractive index of the water. If the pulse impinges the glass-water interface, the light reflectivity $R(p)$ at this location varies synchronously with the pressure-pulse waveform, and the reflected light intensity shows the same temporal dependence as the pressure pulse.

$$R(p) = \left(\frac{n_w(p) - n_g}{n_w(p) + n_g}\right)^2 \qquad (1)$$

where $n_w(p)$ is the pressure dependent refractive index of water, and n_g the refractive index of the glass block. These optical indices can be found in optical tables and publications, e. g., [10], for the index $n_w(p)$. The reflected light intensity is converted by a photodetector (photodiode with amplifier) to a voltage, which is measured with a digital oscilloscope.

Calculation of the sensitivity

In our set-up we use the following notations:
- S = Sensitivity of the hydrophone, the measured voltage for a given pressure propagating in water, as end of cable sensitivity,
- U = the voltage measured at the oscilloscope,
- R = the optical reflectivity at the glass-water interface,
- p = the actual pressure at the glass-water interface, and
- k = a system-dependent constant which contains all system properties relevant for the measured reflected light intensity, like light source intensity, light intensity losses by connectors or lenses, photodetector efficiency.

The sensitivity is

$$S = \frac{U}{p} \quad \text{or} \quad S = \frac{dU}{dp} \qquad (2)$$

We can rewrite this sensitivity by:

$$S = \frac{dU}{dp} = \frac{dU}{dR} \cdot \frac{dR}{dp} \qquad (3)$$

The measured voltage at the oscilloscope is:

$$U = k \cdot R \qquad (4)$$

The voltage depends only on the reflectivity R and on a factor k which contains all other system properties. For zero pressure, this means without incident pressure pulse, the constant k can be calculated from U and the reflectivity R from Equation (1), this voltage is called U(DC). If the reflectivity changes because of an incident pressure of the pulse then the voltage changes as well:

$$dU = k \cdot dR \quad \text{or} \quad \frac{dU}{dR} = k \qquad (5)$$

This is the first term in the sensitivity formula of Equation (3).

The second term $\frac{dR}{dp}$ can be calculated from Equation (1) using optical tables and the published data for $n_w(p)$. We will see $\frac{dR}{dp}$ that is not constant, it changes by 6% for an actual pressure p at the interface of 100 MPa compared to zero.

As a result, the sensitivity S in Equation (2) can be calculated only by using optical tables and a single measurement of a voltage U at zero pressure, which represents all system properties. By monitoring and recording this voltage U during the measurement, this system delivers on-line calibration control and on-line calibration documentation.

The actual pressure p at the interface is the sum of the incident pressure amplitude plus the reflected pressure amplitude of the same phase. With the quartz glass used, the pressure amplitude reflectivity is 0.79, according to the acoustic impedance mismatch between the glass and water.

Bandwidth estimation

If we consider the bandwidth of a piezoelectric hydrophone, e.g., a PVDF membrane hydrophone, the bandwidth is limited by the sensitive thickness of the hydrophone, and the sensitivity decreases if the hydrophone thickness is larger than half the wavelength of the ultrasound pulse. For a 25 µm PVDF membrane this results in a bandwidth of about 40 MHz.

For a light spot reflected at a glass-water interface this sensitive thickness originates from the optical tunnel effect. The depth of the intrusion of the reflected part of the light at the interface into the water is considered here as the sensitive thickness [7]. The depth of the intrusion is in the order of half the optical wavelength λ [11]; in the case of a light beam with λ = 783 nm this results in a sensitive thickness of 0.29 µm in water, which is about two orders of magnitude smaller than the 25 µm requirement in the standard 61846. The equivalent bandwidth of the light spot can be estimated to 2.5 GHz. Consequently the resulting measurement bandwidth for the LSHD is only dependent on the bandwidth of the photodetector which converts the temporal shape of the reflected light intensity into an electrical signal.

Construction of the light spot hydrophone

The light spot hydrophone — LSHD consists mainly of two parts, the optical head and the control unit with all optoelectronics. Both parts are connected by optical fibers guiding the light from a laser diode to the optical head and the reflected light back to the photodetector.

The optical head

The optical head is built on a base plate which can be connected to a 3D positioning set-up for the 3D measurement of the acoustic field. Two lens systems are fixed on the plate; their properties are calculated for optical free beam configuration (Freistrahl-Optik) in air. The first lens system focuses the laser light to a spot at the remote surface of a glass block in front of the lens. The second focuses the reflected light of the spot into the optical fiber connected to the photodetector. The angles of the incident and reflected beam are close to normal to the glass surface, in the current set-up they are ± 7°. The optical properties and the light polarization-dependent effects of the LSHD are presented in detail in [12]. By proper adjustment of the lens systems, a light spot diameter of 100 µm and smaller can be achieved, the result of the diameter is documented. This light spot is fixed with reference to the base plate, by 3D translating, the base plate, the light spot at the glass surface moves to the intended 3D position for the lateral and axial field measurement.

The glass block can be translated in one dimension parallel to the base plate, and parallel to the glass front surface. By translating the glass block, the 3D position of the light spot remains fixed, only the glass surface moves with reference to the light spot, offering the light spot a new area of glass material to proceed with the measurement.

By mounting the optical head in the measurement set-up, only the front side of the glass block and part of it is immersed in the water. The rear side of the glass block with the optical beam and the lenses are kept in air. The measurement set-up is shown in Fig. 1.

The glass block

For the glass block material we choose pure quartz glass because of its distinctive good adhesion to water [13] and its high theoretical tensile strength: more than 1000 MPa [14]. Realistic tensile strengths are in the region of 70 to 100 MPa because of impurities and water imbedded in the quartz crystal. With increasing purity of the material the price rises. A good trade-off is quartz glass "Herasil 3" [15]. The mechanical and optical material properties are well documented. At λ = 783 nm, the refractive index n_g = 1.4538, the speed of sound c = 5700 m/s and the density ρ = 2.2 g/cm^3 result in an acoustic impedance of 12.5 MRayl.

The dimensions of the glass block with 90 × 60 mm^2 (front surface) × 30 mm (thickness) are so large that the diffracted and reflected waves from the edges and the rear side will be delayed for more than 10 µs and thus do not contribute to the measured pulse. This means the actual acoustic pressure pulse is presented one-to-one in a time period of 10 µs, there is no need for the correction of ringing or overshoot.

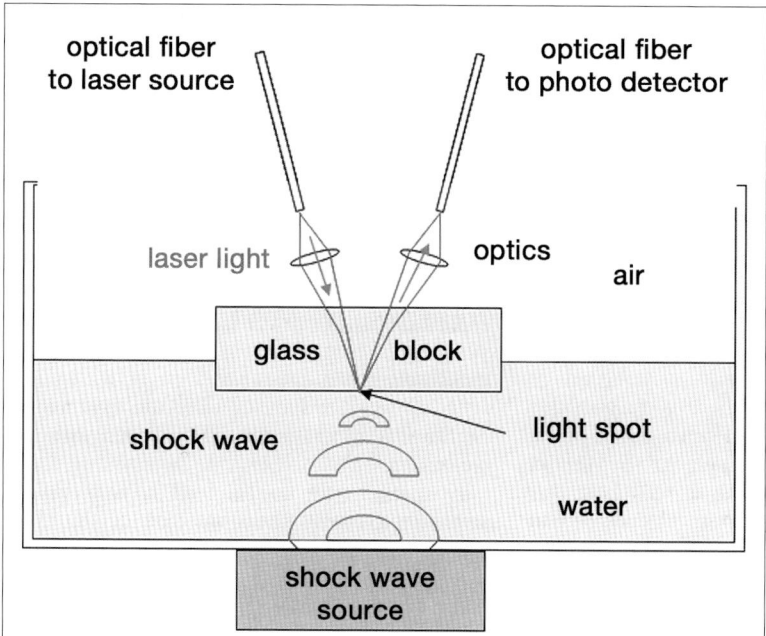

Fig. 1 Measurement set-up of the light spot hydrophone (LSHD).

The optoelectronics with calibration control

The optoelectronics are compiled in a control box which contains all electronic and optical components. These are electric power supply, laser diode with a power of 35 mW at λ = 783 nm, and photodetector consisting of a fast photodiode and a transimpedance amplifier. The transimpedance amplifier has two outputs, the first, AC coupled, for the broadband (40 MHz) amplified pressure pulse signal, the second, less sensitive, for the DC voltage signal U(DC), measured at zero pressure for calibration control (see Calculation of sensitivity, above).

There are two optical ports: one output, from the laser source connected to the first lens system at the optical head with a single mode fiber, and one input to receive the reflected light, connected with the second lens system with a larger multimode fiber (for details see [12]).

There are three electronic ports (BNC connectors). The first, the 50 Ω output of the broadband pulse signal, the second, a high impedance output for the DC level for calibration control, and a third output that monitors the acoustic power of the laser diode.

Results

Sensitivity and calibration

According to the Equations (3) and (5) above, the sensitivity S can be calculated to

$$S = \frac{dU}{dp} = k \cdot \frac{dR}{dp} \qquad (6)$$

For a U(DC) of 0.3 V and a reflectivity at the glass-water interface at zero pressure of R = $2 \cdot 10^{-3}$, k = $1.5 \cdot 10^2$ V. The second term can be calculated close to zero pressure to $4.7 \cdot 10^{-6}$ 1/MPa and to $4.2 \cdot 10^{-6}$ 1/MPa for an incident pressure of 100 MPa (actual pressure = 179 MPa).

Additionally, the term has to be multiplied with the factor 1.79 for the actual pressure at the interface, and with a factor of 8 for the ratio the different amplification factors for the voltages of the DC value and the pressure pulse signal of the transimpedance amplifier. In total:

$$S = 1.5 \cdot 10^2 \cdot 4.7 \cdot 10^{-6} \cdot 1.79 \cdot 8 \; \frac{V}{MPa} =$$

$$10^{-2} \; \frac{V}{MPa} = 10 \; \frac{mV}{MPa}$$

This resulting value of the sensitivity is based on the calibration control U(DC). It had been verified by two procedures. First, with a second liquid instead of water at the glass interface, with a known optical refractive index n(liquid), which is identical to the refractive index of water at a certain pressure. The second procedure had been carried out by the German Physikalisch-Technische Bundesanstalt (PTB) by a precise measurement with the substitution method in the range 0.5 to 15 MHz. This resulted in a PTB calibration certificate, demonstrating that the frequency-dependent sensitivity is in compliance with the requirements of the standard IEC 61846. As also the other requirements of the IEC standard: sensor diameter < 1 mm, and equivalence to a 25 µm PVDF hydrophone are fulfilled, the LSHD is a focus and a field hydrophone in the sense of IEC 61846.

Measurements with the LSHD

Immersing the front side of the glass block in the measurement water tank results in the sensitivity by the measurement of the value U(DC). The translation of the glass block with respect to the light spot proves the quality of the glass material, over a distance of 30 mm with 3 mm translation steps the deviation in U(DC) and thus in reflectivity from the average is below 0.5 %.

With the LSHD, we measured the ultrasonic field parameters of the new shock wave source of the Siemens LITHOSKOP®, the Pulso™, together with the Siemens shock wave sources of the LITHOSTAR Multiline and Modularis to verify the data. The glass block proved to be stable for hundreds of shock waves in the region up to 70 MPa. Tiny surface defects due to cavitation are detected by alteration of U(DC) of more than 10 % by one shot. This effect could be solved by translating the block for about 5 mm. With the measurements up to 120 MPa, sometimes defects in the volume of the glass block occurred, reducing U(DC) to 50 to 100 percent. Again this can be solved by translating the glass block. For large defects, the glass block is exchanged, without moving the optical head and with it the light spot, so the measurement can proceed without readjustment.

The highly reproducible shock wave generated by the electromagnetic shock wave source and the new highly reproducible hydrophone LSHD even enable pulse averaging to increase the signal to noise ratio. An overlay of 5 consecutively measured pulses at 70 MPa revealed almost identical curves for the first p+, the p−, and the second p+ half-wave of the pulses [16].

This demonstrates the striking properties of the new hydrophone: its one-to-one presentation of the shock wave over the full length without the need of correction of ringing or overshoot. This is presented in Fig. 2 for a pulse in the focus. All these properties also apply for the measured pulses off-axis, which contribute more to the focal energy of the shock wave. This enables the precise and fast measurement of all shock wave field data with high reliability.

The single shot pressure equivalent noise proved to be about 0.5 MPa. Electronics and optics are described in detail in [12].

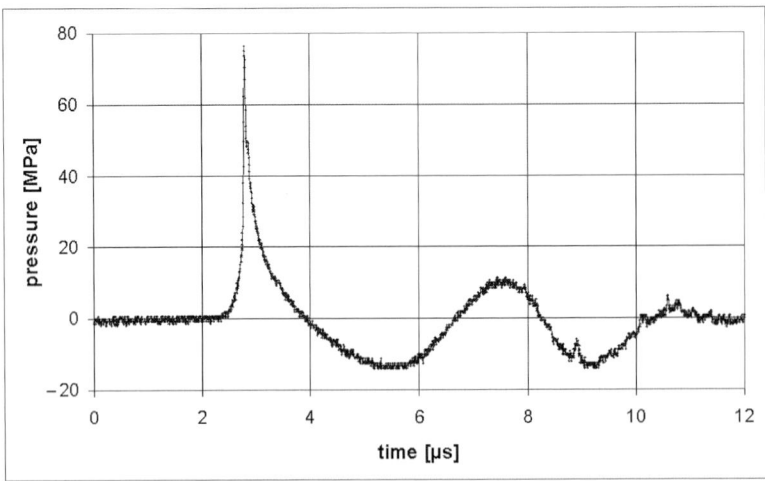

Fig. 2 Example of a measured shock wave pulse in the focus of a lithotripter.

Conclusion

With its bandwidth, sensitive area size and sensitive thickness, the new shock wave hydrophone LSHD complies with the requirements of the standard IEC 61846 for a field and a focus hydrophone. The unique potential of the light spot to move across the glass interface enables to proceed with the measurement even if the glass is partially damaged, thus, the required measurement time is reduced drastically. The calibration control delivers on-line the current absolute amplitude calibration. The data for the calibration control are confirmed by a PTB certificate. The high reproducible one-to-one presentation of the pulses over their full lengths without the need of correction enables precise pulse shape and energy measurements for the reliable classification of lithotripter shock wave sources.

This light spot hydrophone LSHD had been developed in a close cooperation between Siemens Medical Solutions and the Lehrstuhl für Hochfrequenztechnik, University of Erlangen, both in Erlangen, Germany.

References

[1] Granz B, Köhler G. What makes a shock wave efficient in lithotripsy? J Stone Disease 1992; 4: 123–128

[2] Coleman AJ, Saunders JE. A survey of the acoustic output of commercial extracorporeal shockwave lithotripters. Ultrasound in Med & Biol 1989; 3: 213–227

[3] Platte M. A polyvinylidene fluoride needle hydrophone for ultrasonic applications. Ultrasonics 1985; 23: 113–118

[4] Granz B, Holzapfel R, Köhler G. Measurement of shockwaves in the focus of a lithotripter. Proceedings of the 1989 IEEE Ultrasonics Symposium, pp 991–994

[5] DeReggi AS, Roth SC, Kenney JM, Edelmann S, Harris GR. Piezoelectric polymer probe for ultrasonic applications. J Acoust Soc Am 1981; 69: 853–859

[6] "Ultrasonics – Pressure Pulse Lithotripters – Characteristics of Fields," Standard IEC 61846, 1998

[7] Staudenraus J, Eisenmenger W. Fibre-optic probe for ultrasonic and shockwave measurements in water. Ultrasonics 1993; 31: 267–273

[8] Osterhammel K. Optische Untersuchung des Schallfeldes kolbenförmig schwingender Quarze. Akust Z 1941; 6: 73–86

[9] Paltauf G, Schmidt-Kloiber H. Measurement of laser-induced acoustic waves with a calibrated optical transducer. J Appl Phys 1997; 82: 1525–1531

[10] Yadev HS, Murty SN, Sinha KHC, Gupta BB, Dal Chand. Measurement of refractive index of water under high dynamic pressures. J Appl Phys 1973; 44: 2197–2200

[11] Drexhage KH. Monomolecular layers and light. Scientific America 1970; 222: 108–119

[12] Engelbrecht R et al. Robust light spot hydrophone with calibration control for the measurement of medical ultrasound shockwaves. In: Proceedings, 12th Int. Conf. Sensor 2005 (Nuremberg 2005). AMA Service GmbH, Wunstorf, 2005. To be published

[13] Wolf KL. Physik und Chemie der Grenzflächen, Springer, Berlin, 1957

[14] Doremus RH. Glass Science, 2nd ed, John Wiley & Sons, New York, 1994

[15] Heraeus Quarzglas GmbH, Germany, data sheet "Quarzglas für die Optik," June 2003

[16] Granz B et al. Light spot hydrophone, innovation in lithotripsy. MEDICAL SOLUTIONS, June 2004; 86–87

Shock Wave Lithotripsy (SWL) and Focal Size

O. Wess

Introduction

Shock waves in medicine were first introduced by Chaussy and co-workers in 1980 for *in vivo* kidney stone fragmentation [1]. The legendary HM3 spark gap lithotripter was developed by Dornier engineers Forssmann, Hepp, and Hoff utilizing the pioneering electrohydraulic principle of shock wave generation. The method was simple and efficient. Breaking and removing kidney stones without open surgery was fascinating and justified some side effects such as minor skin lesions and, rarely, perirenal and subcapsular hematomas. Synchronizing shock waves with the cardiac cycle (ECG-triggering) was imperative due to the strong interaction of shock waves with the heart rate causing up to 80% dysrhythmias [2]. Heavy pain sensations during shock wave delivery made general anesthesia (GA) or peridural anesthesia (PDA) mandatory.

Since the early 1980s technical developments have made modern lithotripsy devices more comfortable and side effects were significantly reduced. Fragmentation efficiency, however, was only slightly improved [3]. Some still consider the old HM3 as being the "gold standard" in lithotripsy due its "large focal area." Is a large focal size a prerequisite for fragmentation efficiency and is it necessarily accompanied by side effects? We have analyzed the impact of focal size and distribution of shock wave fields on the performance of lithotripters.

Materials and Methods

Physical and technical aspects of shock wave generation and focusing are analyzed with respect to optimal shock wave field parameters for medical use. The field distribution of large aperture systems (cylinder paraboloid configuration) is compared to the original HM3 focal zones.

Shock wave efficacy and side effects

Stone fragmentation is based on acoustic energy delivered by high energy shock waves to the stone. A certain amount of energy is required to achieve sufficient fragmentation results. Technically, the goal is to transmit the appropriate energy without causing significant side effects.

Hematomas have to be considered as being potentially associated with SWL. The risk of perirenal or intrarenal hematoma is estimated to be between 0.1% and 0.6% (detected by the ultrasound technology of the 1980s) [4–6]. Using MRI or CT instead of ultrasound 20 to 25% hematomas [7, 8] are reported. Even though only a few of these require surgical intervention, side effects of shock waves are rare but not negligible.

Whenever shock wave energy surpasses a certain level, the risk of side effects is real. We also have to consider shock wave energy passing laterally and behind the target area. In case of electrohydraulic or spark gap technology, there is an unfocused part of the primary shock wave which is vagabonding through the patient. The focused and unfocused shock wave fields of an electrohydraulic generator are shown in Fig. 1.

Under typical treatment conditions the shock wave field is transmitted into the patient's body and has an impact on several tissue layers and organs as shown in Fig. 2.

Focused shock waves not only interact with the target stone but dispose a significant amount of energy to a wide area of tissue including the superficial skin area in the coupling region (Fig. 2). Depending on the targeted treatment area and the direction of shock wave transmission also the heart muscle may be exposed to focal shock wave energy causing extrasystoles.

Even under precisely controlled targeting conditions the interaction of the unfocused field with the heart and other organs is almost inevitable.

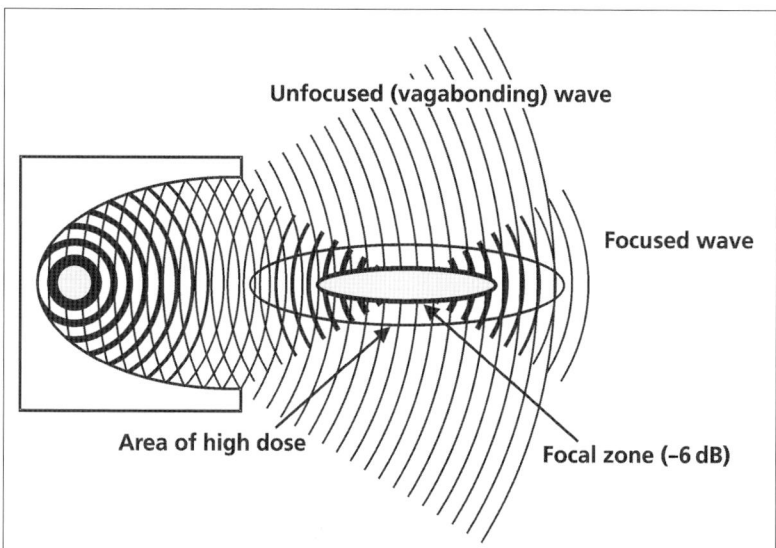

Fig. 1 Unfocused and focused shock wave field of an electrohydraulic generator.

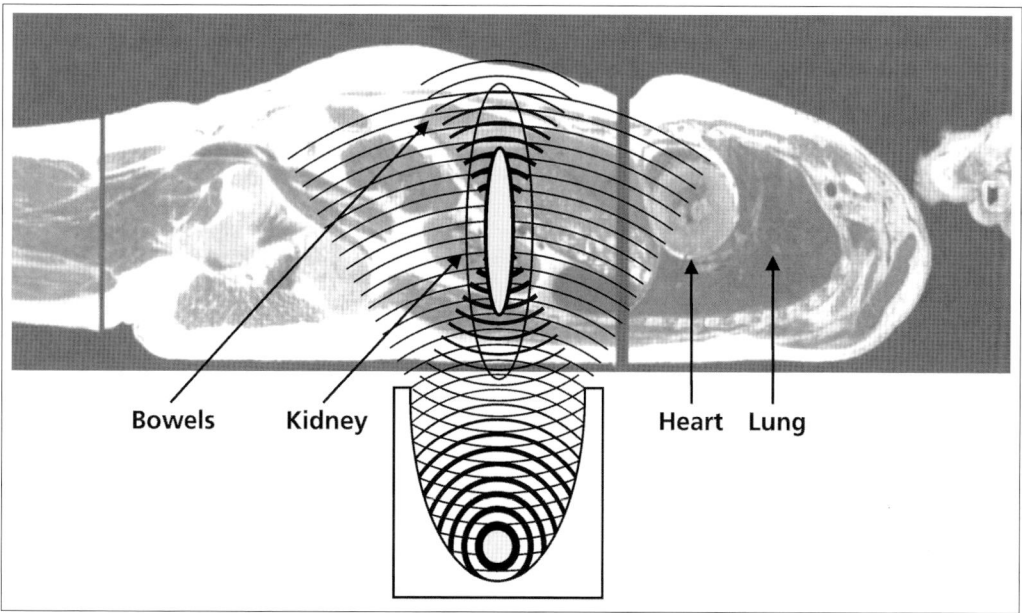

Fig. 2 Tissue and organs affected by shock waves of an electrohydraulic spark gap generator.

Focal zone and treatment zone

The shock wave field is the decisive factor characterizing the performance of a lithotripsy device.

There are several parameters such as peak pressure, pulse length, and energy content required to describe shock wave fields in detail. The "focal zone" is one of the key parameters which deserve a closer look since focal zone and treatment zone are often mixed up although they clearly have to be differentiated.

Fig. 3 shows a focused shock wave field. The spatial energy distribution can be measured by

28 Shock Wave Lithotripsy (SWL) and Focal Size

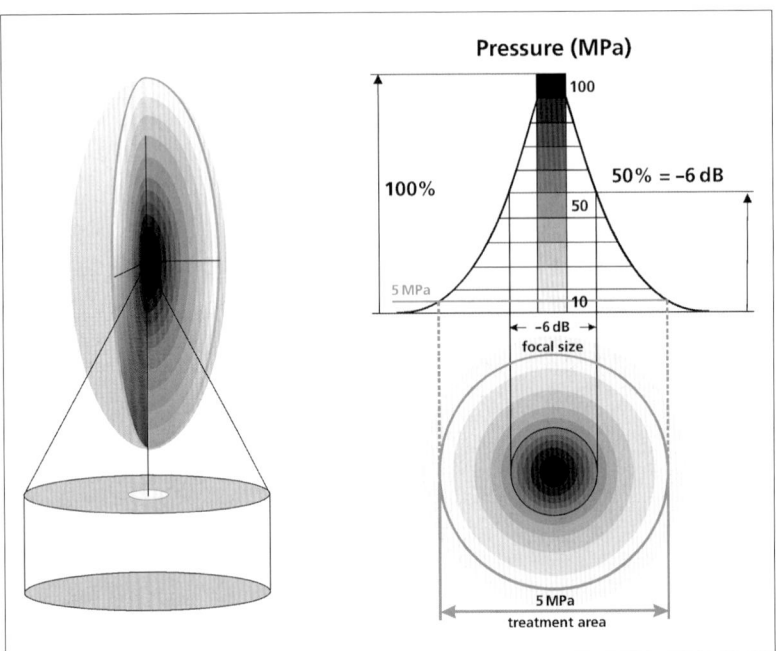

Fig. 3   –6 dB-focus and 5 MPa treatment zone.

pressure probes which are scanned through the field. The energy is concentrated around a center (focus) and dissipates with decreasing amplitudes to distant areas.

The peak pressure can be adjusted to various levels.

–6 dB-focal area

The –6 dB-focal area is defined by pressures being equal or higher than 50% of the actual peak pressure. In case of a peak pressure of 100 MPa (as displayed in Fig. **3**) the line of 50% is defined by the 50 MPa isobar. Since 50% is equivalent to –6 dB, this focus is called the –6 dB-focus. Selecting another peak pressure of, e. g., 40 MPa, the –6 dB isobar (50% value) would equal 20 MPa. This example shows no relationship between the dimensions of the focal zone and energy content. The –6 dB-focus does not reflect the shock wave energy contained in the focal area. It, therefore, does not stand for fragmentation efficiency. The –6 dB-focal size simply defines the "quality" of focusing and is, taken as a single measure, but not as useful parameter to quantify the fragmentation performance of a lithotriptor.

Treatment area

An additional parameter is required to characterize an area of efficient shock wave interaction. This parameter must be closely linked to the energy content of the shock wave field. By definition of the Working Group Technical Developments — *Consensus Report of the German Society of Shock Wave Lithotripsy* [9], the pressure value of 5 MPa (50 bar) is considered as a limit above which shock waves are assumed to generate some medical effects. Pressure values below 5 MPa are deemed to have no or only minor effects in medical treatment. In case of shock waves for stone fragmentation a limit of 10 MPa is accepted as the fragmentation threshold.

We call this area the "treatment zone" of a shock wave generator. Even if a threshold of medical efficiency of shock waves is not precisely known, there is no doubt that higher shock wave energies create higher effects and/or side effects.

Treatment zones may be significantly larger or smaller than the focal (–6 dB) zone depending on the energy level selected. The discrepancy between the two zones is due the fact that the treatment zone is related to a defined pressure value (5 MPa or 10 MPa, respectively) whereas the definition of the –6 dB-focal zone relates to any variable peak pressure and therefore does not reflect energy and, hence, efficiency.

Focal zone and fragmentation

The spatial dimensions of the treatment zone will significantly change with the selected energy settings as shown in Fig. 4. The area of efficient stone fragmentation is not a fixed quantity but will be larger at high energy settings compared to low settings. In contrast, depending on the particular shock wave generator, the −6 dB-focus may stay almost unchanged or may even become smaller with higher energy settings if the peak pressure is increased.

Fig. 4 shows the varying axial and lateral dimensions of the treatment zone (light grey), compared to −6 dB-focal zones (dark grey).

Ideal, conventional, and optimized focal sizes

Ideally, shock wave energy should only be disposed to the target stone or the region of interest and nowhere else. This would optimize efficacy and reduce side effects to the possible limits. The ideal focus can be defined as a small spherical volume of exactly the target size. (For a typical kidney stone a sphere with a diameter of 12 mm might be an appropriate size.) For anatomical reasons a spherical focus is not achieved due to limited access windows and aperture restrictions of the shock wave source. Conventional shock wave systems, such as the HM3, feature a significantly larger focal zone. As a consequence, pressure amplitudes are either far below optimum values required for fragmentation or, if increased to achieve optimum fragmentation, generate excessive strain to surrounding tissue.

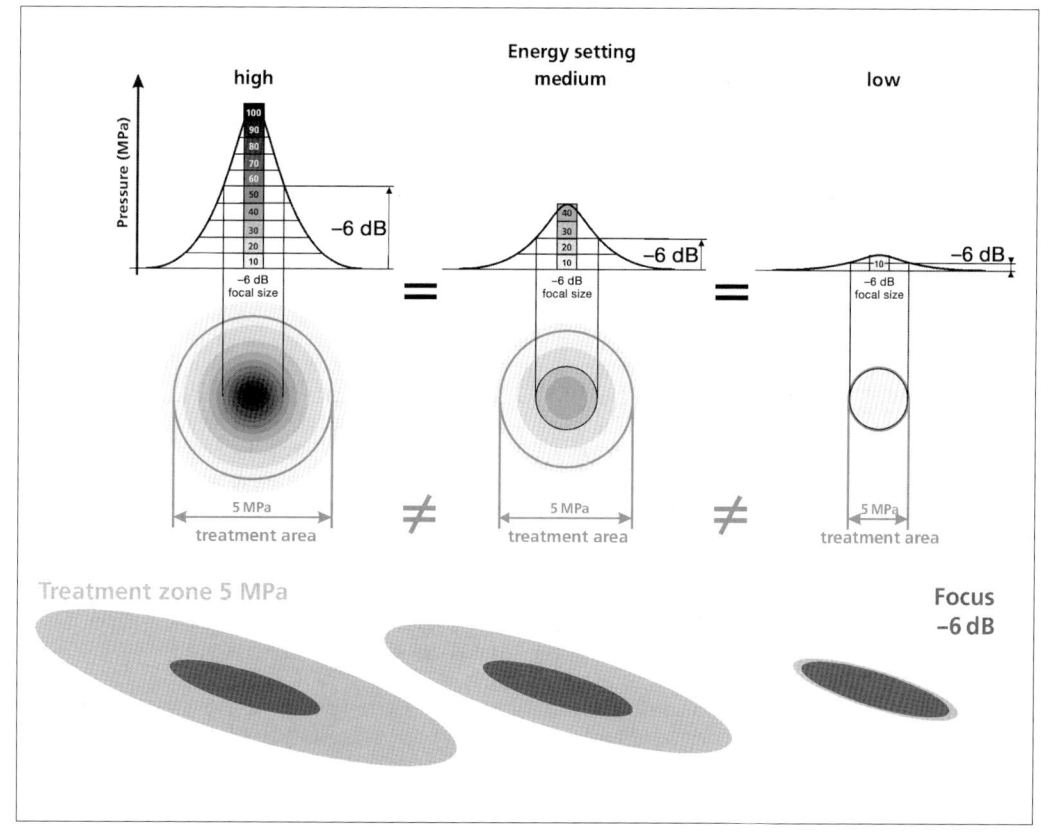

Fig. 4 High, medium, and low energy settings and corresponding decreasing treatment (5 MPa) areas. Note that the −6 dB-focus may remain unchanged although the disposed shock wave energy is significantly reduced.

Bony structures and gas-filled organs such as lung tissue provide only limited access windows to reach the target area. For human anatomy, an aperture angle of approximately 90° is a natural limit for focusing shock waves to a precise target area of a few millimeters. Smaller aperture angles of 50–60° limit the focusing qualities of a shock wave generator to lower energy densities and thus limit fragmentation reserves for hard and impacted stones.

An increased aperture angle (90° vs. 62° at HM3) significantly modifies the shock wave field and focal energy distribution. Not only shock wave transmission from skin to target zones within the body is performed with essentially less tissue lesions but energy concentration and consequently fragmentation efficiency can be strongly enhanced simultaneously. The advantage of larger apertures is based on the physics and characteristics of waves in general.

Gentle transmission and simultaneous concentration of shock wave power for optimum energy density in the treatment area is achieved by enlarging aperture angles to the limits given by human anatomy. Based on the strategy of optimal field parameters, utmost protection against side effects is guaranteed by restricting to the minimal values required for fragmentation. Optimal field distributions also provide energy reserves for fragmentation of extraordinary hard stones. The field needs to be precisely controlled by a wide range of energy levels in order to provide exactly the individually required dose on the target. Full benefit of efficiency and low side effects are simultaneously guaranteed only if energy settings are selected to reach just the required level.

Based on the principle of electromagnetic shock wave generation Storz Medical developed a specific generator configuration (Fig. **5**). The source is characterized by a cylindrical coil (instead of a flat coil such as in usual electromagnetic sources) and a parabolic reflector (instead of an acoustic lens) for focusing. This technique allows for the design of extremely large apertures (300 mm), extraordinary focal depths (165 mm), and aperture angles of 84°. This type of shock wave source matches ideally with all the above stated criteria of an optimum source.

The cylinder source not only provides favorable shock wave field distributions but also the widest energy range from very low to very high peak pressures (up to 100 MPa and more, if required). Shock wave delivery is stable and reproducible compared to conventional spark gap technology.

The techniques of large aperture systems allow the development of different treatment strategies. If very gentle treatment with minimal side effects is required, the peak pressure is adjusted just to the sufficient fragmentation level, not higher (Fig. **6**).

In cases of very hard or impacted stones within the ureter, e. g., higher shock wave energies and peak pressures may be required. Due to the excellent focusing qualities of large aperture systems the available shock wave energy can be concentrated to a small area around the focus center.

This new option of individually matched treatment strategies needs to be carefully selected in order to avoid tissue lesions when applied incorrectly. However, it offers additional treatment options not available with conventional techniques.

Due to the possibility of boosted energy application, an efficient localization system is required to provide precise control over the treatment position during shock wave exposure.

Tissue areas affected by this type of shock wave source are shown schematically in Fig. **7**. Compared to electrohydraulic systems, energy distribution is concentrated around the focus avoiding the unfocused vagabonding wave associated with spark gap technology.

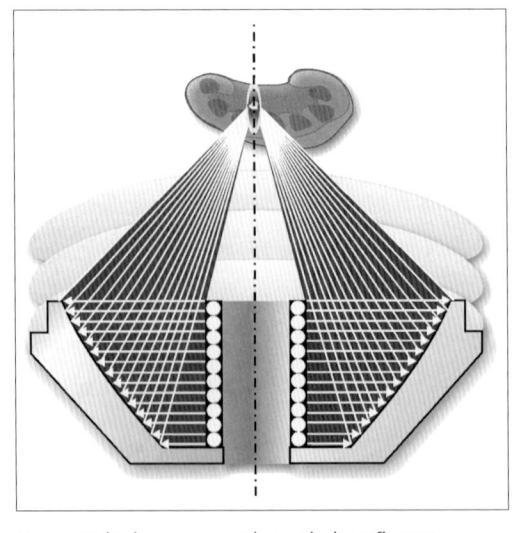

Fig. **5** Cylinder source with parabolic reflector.

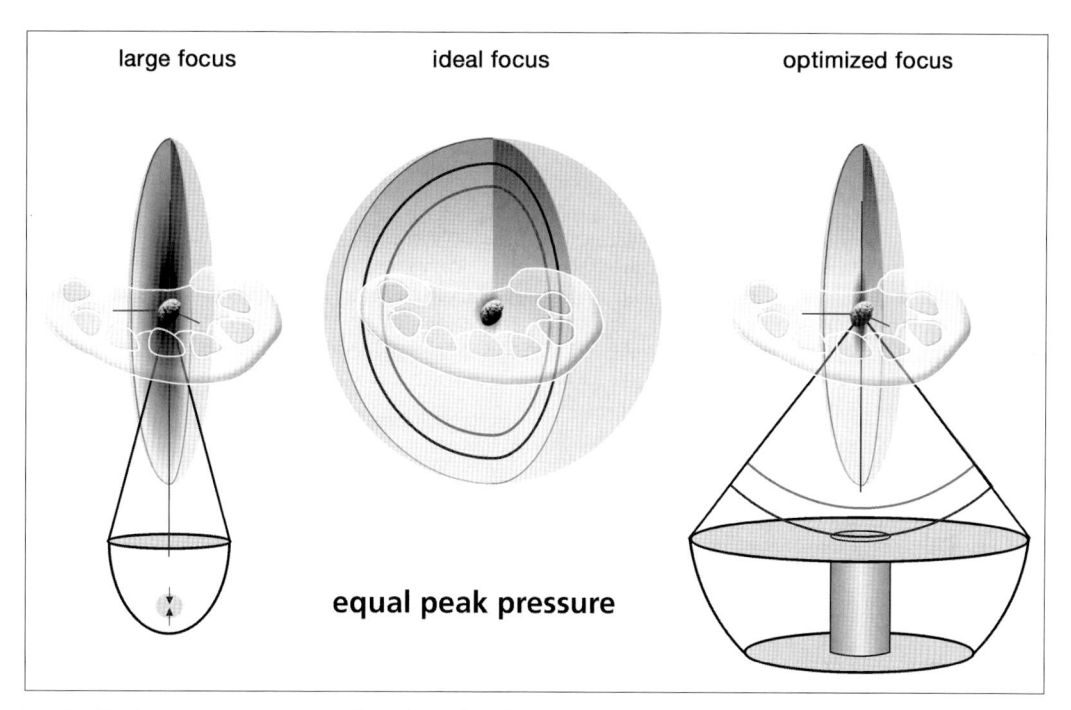

Fig. 6 Gentle treatment strategy utilizing limited peak pressure.

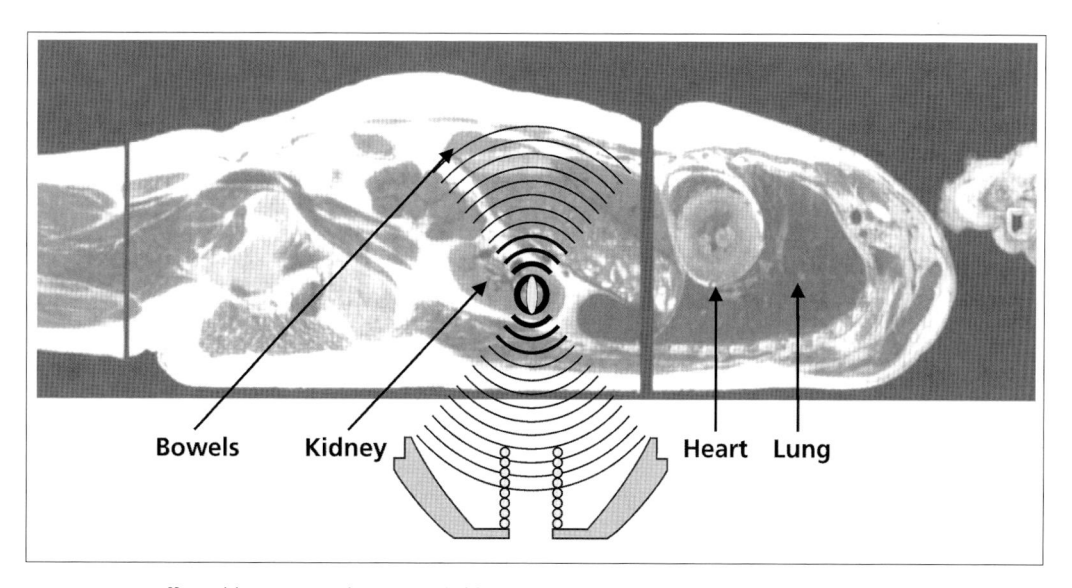

Fig. 7 Tissue affected by optimized pressure field of a cylinder/paraboloid configuration. Due to the aperture of 84° skin stress is significantly reduced. Usually shock wave load to critical organs such as heart and lung can be reliably prevented.

Clinical Aspects

Clinical routine confirms anesthesia requirements as being significantly reduced compared to conventional electrohydraulic techniques. General or peridural anesthesia is performed only in very specific cases, in children and if pretreatment ureteral manipulations are required. Perirenal and subcapsular hematoma occur in the range of 1% as known and experienced in all other techniques. Skin bleeding, superficial petechia, and other side effects are almost completely eliminated by this type of wide aperture generator. This is due to the fact of rapidly decreasing energy values in front of and behind the focal zone.

A relatively short axial dimension of the pressure distribution also reduces the need of ECG-triggering significantly. Usually free running modes with up to 2 pulses per second may be selected without shock wave interference with cardiac cycles. Depending on stone location and applied energy level, ECG monitoring is considered mandatory.

Clinical routine conditions of reduced anesthesia requirements, however, may result in increased mobility of the patient treated. Due to respiratory movement of kidney stones, pain-related patient shift etc., precise targeting may become more difficult. These reasons may favor a larger focal zone in order to increase the hit rate. No doubt, under controlled fragmentation conditions, the advantage of a small focus is obvious. However, for practical reasons both options, precise and extended focus, would offer the choice to match individual treatment conditions and compensate for inaccuracies of localization when needed.

Comparison of Different Lithotripters

Optimized focal zones (smaller than HM3, bigger than ideal) can be generated by a cylindrically shaped generator. The cylinder generator is built with an extremely large aperture which matches with the limitations of anatomical access. The focal region features a small cigar-shaped volume avoiding unnecessary side effects while, simultaneously, providing higher energy concentration to the region of interest.

For comparison, the left system (Fig. 8) is shown with a peak pressure of 100 MPa whereas

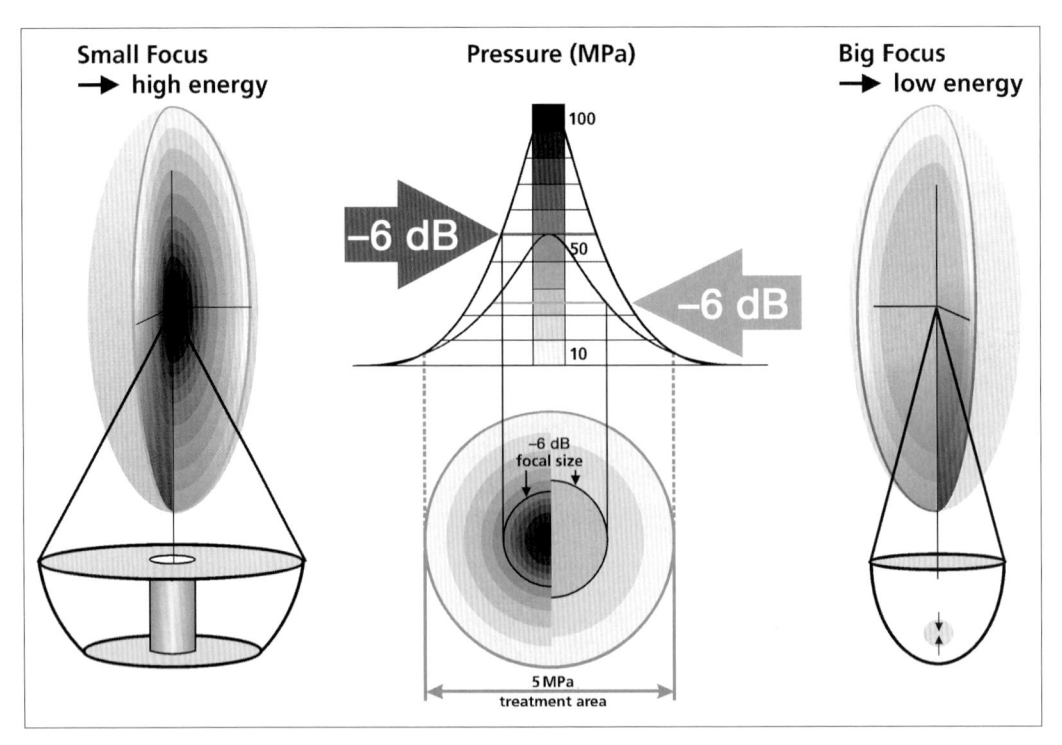

Fig. 8 Focus and treatment zones of different devices.

Device	HM3 unmodified	Modulith SLX
Peak pressure	32 MPa (320 bar)	100 MPa (1000 bar)
50% (–6 dB value)	16 MPa (160 bar)	50 MPa (500 bar)
Axial focus extension	100 mm	28 mm
Lateral focus extension	16 mm	6 mm

Table 1 Comparison of –6 dB zones

Device	HM3 unmodified	Modulith SLX
16 MPa (160 bar) limit (–6 dB-zone HM3) axial	100 mm	110 mm
16 MPa (160 bar) limit (–6 dB-zone HM3) lateral	16 mm	18.5 mm

Table 2 Comparison of equal pressure limits (16 MPa)

the right system features a smaller peak pressure of only 50 MPa. At any position within the focus area the left system provides higher pressure values than the right system as shown by the pressure curves. Therefore, the left system clearly contains more energy than the right system although the right system has a bigger –6 dB-focal zone according to definition.

The above stated relation of small and large focal zones holds true also for real lithotripsy systems. Comparison of two specific lithotripters such as the MODULITH SLX (Storz Medical AG, Kreuzlingen/CH) and HM3 (Dornier MedTech, Wesseling/D) can be done on the basis of equal pressure limits or –6 dB-focal zones (Table 1).

From these data, the larger –6 dB-focal zone of the HM3 is obvious (Fig. 9). However, we have to keep in mind the definition of the –6 dB-focal zone. For the HM3 the area of pressure values above 160 bars is displayed whereas for the Modulith only values above 500 bars are depicted. Obviously, the HM3 does not feature values of 500 bars at all.

Taking the same pressure limit of 16 MPa (Table 2), both systems feature comparable zones of axial 110 mm (Modulith) vs. 100 mm (HM3) extensions. Also in the lateral dimensions similar extensions are characteristic of both systems 18.5 mm (Modulith) vs. 16 mm (HM3) as shown in Fig. 10.

Although significantly different in –6 dB-focal dimensions, the two systems provide excellent fragmentation efficiency.

These facts are proven by an independent test

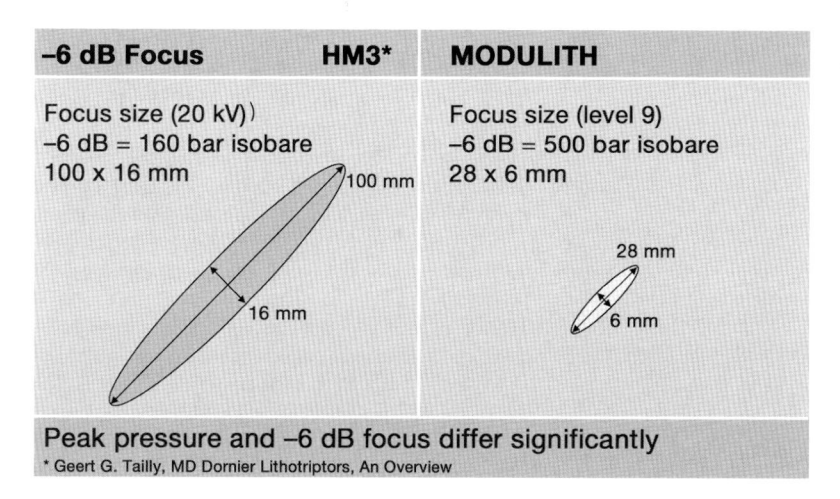

Fig. 9 Comparison of –6 dB-zones.

–6 dB Focus   HM3*   MODULITH

Focus size (20 kV)
–6 dB = 160 bar isobare
100 × 16 mm

100 mm
16 mm

Focus size (level 9)
–6 dB = 500 bar isobare
28 × 6 mm

28 mm
6 mm

Peak pressure and –6 dB focus differ significantly
* Geert G. Tailly, MD Dornier Lithotriptors, An Overview

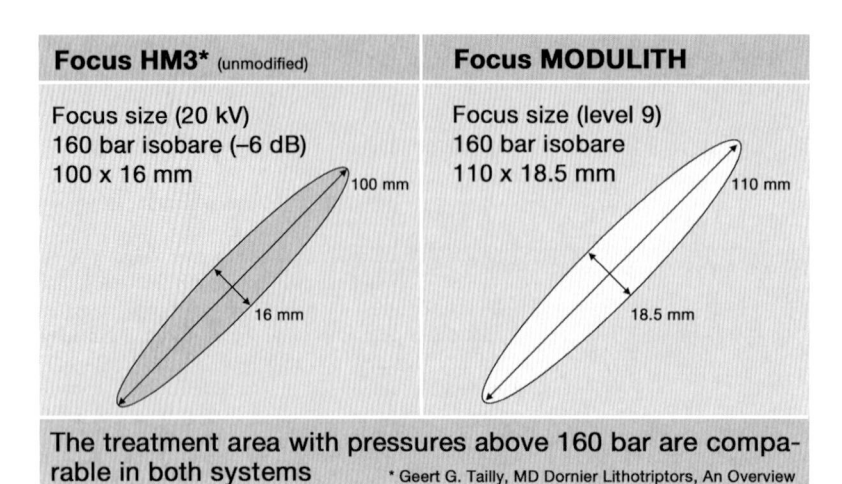

Fig. 10 Comparison of equal (16 MPa) pressure values.

Focus HM3* (unmodified)
Focus size (20 kV)
160 bar isobare (−6 dB)
100 x 16 mm
100 mm
16 mm

Focus MODULITH
Focus size (level 9)
160 bar isobare
110 x 18.5 mm
110 mm
18.5 mm

The treatment area with pressures above 160 bar are comparable in both systems
* Geert G. Tailly, MD Dornier Lithotriptors, An Overview

published by Teichman et al. [10]. Fragmentation experiments with natural stone showed best results for the cylinder generator of the MODULITH SLX when equal numbers of shock waves were applied. The HM3 does not break difficult stones better than the MODULITH SLX with the wide aperture electromagnetic cylinder source. In spite of the high power of fragmentation, the extremely large aperture provides gentle energy transmission, less anesthesia requirement, and reduced extrasystoles when used without ECG-triggering in a free running mode.

Current Developments

Small focal dimensions provide favorable shock wave field parameters but require precise localization. Due to clinical restrictions, lack of continuous fluoroscopic target control, small respiratory movements of kidney stones etc., extension of focal zones may facilitate routine treatment. Whereas extraordinary hard and impacted (ureter) stones may be best treated with precisely confined focal zones, slightly moving stones may be more easily fragmented by larger focal zones.

Following clinical needs, new technical developments offer selectable focal dimensions to match with different treatment conditions. The MODULITH SLX-F2 offers 2 selectable focal zones, precise and extended, with an unchanged large aperture of 300 mm. The favorable gentle energy transmission is preserved while, simultaneously, the focal zone may be selected according to individual treatment conditions to match the hardness and mobility of the target stones.

Conclusion

Comparisons different lithotripsy devices are often based on focal zones without using an appropriate definition of the term "focus." The −6 dB focus, which is usually taken for comparison, does not provide relevant data to judge the performance of different machines. The criterion "large focus" or "small focus" alone does not characterize the performance of a lithotriptor. The 5 MPa treatment zone and the 10 MPa fragmentation zone introduced by the *German Society of Shock Wave Lithotripsy* [9] provide parameters appropriate for realistic comparisons.

Additional parameters such as aperture size, confined area of high energy concentration, and stability of shock wave delivery are important measures to increase fragmentation performance and simultaneous reduction of tissue stress.

All these comparisons are in favor of modern large aperture systems such as electromagnetic cylinder sources. This type of shock wave generator features at least equal or even better performance than the "old gold standard" HM3. Simultaneously, the ratio of fragmentation efficiency vs. out of focus side effects such as petechia and anesthesia requirements is optimized.

In spite of the described benefits of precise focal zones, clinical routine procedures may be facilitated by larger focal zones for ease of localization. New developments in lithotripsy provide both options: precise focusing with highest possible energy density for hard and impacted stones as well as (selectable) larger focal zones with lower pressure to tolerate small target movements and small shifts of target positions.

References

[1] Chaussy C, Brendel W, Schmiedt E. Extracorporeally induced destruction of kidney stones by shock waves. Lancet 1980; 2: 1265

[2] Chaussy C, Schmiedt E, Jocham D. Extracorporeal shock wave lithotripsy (ESWL) for treatment of urolithiasis. Urology 1984; 23: 59–66

[3] Lingeman JE. Shock Wave Lithotripsy: Innovation and future directions. Urolithiasis 2000. Proceedings of the 9th International Symposium on Urolithiasis, University of Cape Town, 2000, pp 717–726

[4] Cass AS, Broker W, Duthoy E et al. Clinically diagnosed renal hemorrhage after ESWL with Dornier HM3 and Medstone lithotripters. J Endourol 1992; 6: 413

[5] Knapp PM, Kulb TB, Lingeman JE, Newman DM, Mertz JH, Mosbaugh PG, Steele RE. Extracorporeal shock wave induced perirenal hematomas. J Urol 1987; 137: 700

[6] Chaussy C, Schuller J, Schmiedt E, Brandl H, Jocham D, Liedl B. Extracorporeal shock wave lithotripsy for treatment of urolithiasis. Urology 1984; 23: 59

[7] Rubin JI, Arger PH, Pollack HM, Banner MP, Coleman BG, Mintz MC, Van Arsdalen KN. Kidney changes after extracorporeal shock wave lithotripsy: CT evaluation. Radiology 1987; 162: 21

[8] Kaude JV, Williams CM, Millner MR, Scott KN, Finlayson B. Renal morphology and function immediately after extracorporeal shock wave lithotripsy. AJR Am J Roentgenol 1985; 145: 305

[9] Wess O, Ueberle F, Dührßen R-N, Hilcken D, Krauß W, Reuner Th, Schultheiß R, Staudenraus J, Rattner M, Haaks W, Granz B. In: Working Group Technical Developments – Consensus Report, in: High Energy Shock Waves in Medicine, (Chaussy C, Eisenberger F, Jocham D, Wilbert D, eds), Thieme Verlag, Stuttgart, 1997, pp 59–71.

[10] Teichman JMH, Portis AJ, Cecconi PP, Bub WL, Endicott RC, Denes B, Pearle MS, Clayman R. In vitro comparison of shock wave lithotripsy machines. J Urol 2000; 164:

Treatment of Urinary Stones

Consensus

K. U. Köhrmann (Chairman), R. Hofmann, T. Knoll, D. Neisius, C. Türk, G. Haupt

Principle of Treatment Decision

The first step for optimal treatment is to decide about the indication out of the different treatment options for the specific patient. This should be performed according the flow-sheet in Fig. 1.

For the individual patient there will usually be different treatment options according to the state of scientific knowledge. In most institutions, however, not all of them will be provided with the same high degree of expertise. Therefore, the patient should be informed about all of the scientifically proven options and about those which can be optimally performed in the specific institution. Based on the patient's preference and the institutional circumstances, the decision is then drawn or the number of options is reduced. When there is a remaining range of options additional criteria, e. g., economic aspects, can be respected.

For the different stone situations, usually different treatment options can be recommended. For this short summary, location and size of the stone are used for characterization of the stone situation. For the final treatment decision, further criteria, e. g., co-morbidity, and preferences of the individual patient have to be respected. In the following a healthy, adult patient is taken as the example.

Principally all stones in the kidney can be treated by ESWL, ureterorenoscopy (including flexible URS) or PCNL (including percutaneous antegrade lithotripsy of ureter stones), but the location and size of the stone decide about primary, secondary, or third choice procedures. PCNL is, when performed by experienced urologists, a procedure with very high immediate stone-free rate and is safe. Flexible URS is usually safe but the efficacy is dependent on a long learning curve. Running costs of the flexible URS, including maintenance of the endoscope and disposable tools (nitinol baskets, laser fibers, access sheaths) should not be underestimated.

The actual development in the management of urinary stone disease with the intention of effec-

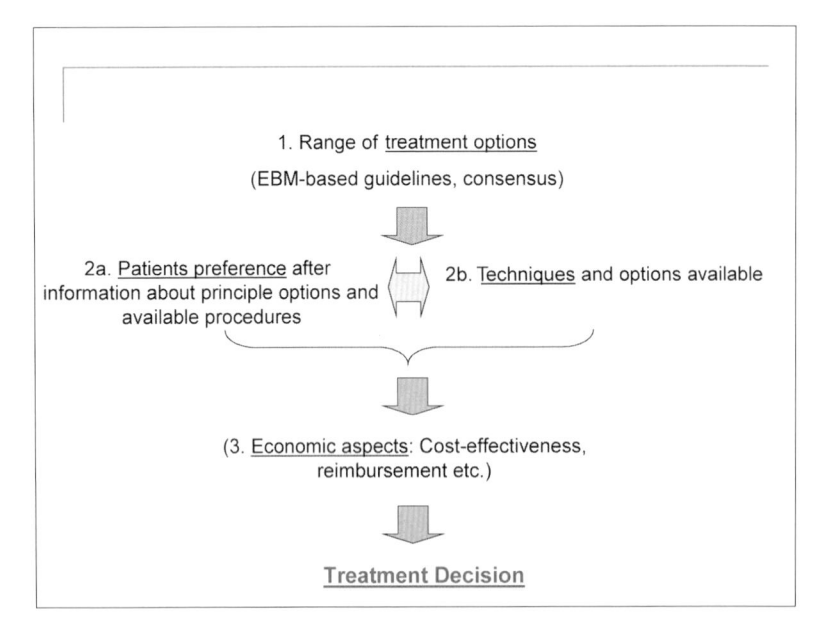

Fig. 1 Criteria and procedure for treatment decision.

1. Range of treatment options
(EBM-based guidelines, consensus)

2a. Patients preference after information about principle options and available procedures

2b. Techniques and options available

(3. Economic aspects: Cost-effectiveness, reimbursement etc.)

Treatment Decision

Table 1 Treatment options for staghorn stones

Stone size, anatomy	ESWL	PCNL (+/− ESWL)	Open surgery
No dilatation	1	1	–
Complicated (e. g., dilatation)	2	1	3
Large peripheral stone mass	–	1	2

tive and economic treatment trends towards a faster and complete stone removal. Additionally, on the one hand, the technical developments have improved endoscopes significantly in terms of smaller diameter, improved irrigation and optical systems, wider range of tools for disintegration and removal of the stone. This has resulted in increased efficacy, a wider range of indications, and reduced invasiveness. On the other hand, lithotripter technology has not been able to reach higher disintegration or stone-free rates using the third generation lithotripters compared to the classical Dornier HM3. The consequence is a tendency to a more frequent use of endoscopic procedures and a limited indication for ESWL. This is justified despite the situation that the available literature (evidence-based) sometimes leads to recommendations to the contrary. Therefore, in the following "consensus recommendations" the new technical and economical developments, which are not completely represented in the literature, are also respected. They were established after intensive panel discussion of the literature reviews given in the book chapters about the special stone situations.

Stones in the Renal Pelvis and Calices (Lower Calyx Excluded)

Stones < 10 mm and 10–20 mm should primarily be treated by ESWL, for stones < 10 mm flexible URS and for stones > 15–20 mm PCNL are the secondary options. For stones > 10 mm ESWL should be performed after insertion of a stent to reduce the risk of complication due to the passage of fragments. For staghorn stones see Table 1.

Lower Calyx Stones

Stones in the lower calyx represent a special stone situation since fragments after ESWL of these stones tend to pass less frequently than from other locations in the kidney (Table 2). A small uretero-caliceal angle, a long calyx, and a narrow caliceal nack seem to predict a smaller stone-free rate of ESWL. Therefore endoscopic procedures with immediate stone removal should be respected for lower calyx stones: flexible URS for stones < 1 cm and PCNL for stones > 1 cm, when different negative factors predict limited ESWL success. The patient has to be informed about the higher success rate but also about the slightly higher complication rate of PCNL.

Proximal Ureter Stones

The probability to remove a stone from the proximal ureter by ESWL within a reasonable time period and with few interventions (re-treatments, auxiliary procedures) decreases with the size of the stone (Table 3). Therefore ESWL is univocally the primary choice for stones up to a diameter of 1 cm. For larger stones URS is more effective, but also more invasive with the risk of ureteral lesions. Antegrade URS (PCNL via the middle or upper calyx) should be reserved for very large stones in the ureteropelvic junction and the upper part of the proximal ureter.

Table 2 Treatment options for lower calyx stones

Stone size	ESWL	PCNL	flex. URS
< 10 mm	1	3	2
10–20 mm	1	2	3
> 20 mm	2	1	–

Table 3 Treatment options for proximal ureter stones

Stone size	ESWL	URS	push–/+bang
< 10 mm	1	2	3
> 10 mm	2	1	–

Distal Ureter Stones

The most important decision for the stones in the distal ureter is "to treat or not to treat." Most of the distal ureter stones can pass spontaneously. For stones larger than 4–6 mm the likelihood that the stone passes without significant symptoms in a reasonable time decreases distinctly and recommends active intervention. But the differential indication between watchful waiting and intervention (URS, ESWL, stent) depends on different factors beside the stone size:
- willingness of the patient to accept the risk of unpredictable complications (colic, fever, renal impairment), not calculable duration and efficacy of the conservative treatment,
- willingness of the patient to accept anesthesia and the very low, but remaining risk of a severe complication by endoscopic procedures,
- equipment and experience of the institution, and
- economic aspects for the patient (including time period of "not fit for work") and for the institution (costs, refunding).

After this decision for stones ≤ 10 mm URS and ESWL are estimated to be equivalent despite different profile for efficacy and risk (Table 4). URS has a nearly 100% success rate but also a risk for severe complications (perforation, sepsis, irritation). ESWL has a reduced stone-free rate of 85% with nearly no significant complication rate. A stent can be used as monotherapy to dilate the ureter, but is recommended to be used as an auxiliary measure for URS or ESWL.

Table 4 Treatment options for distal ureter stones

Stone size	ESWL	URS
< 10 mm	1	1
> 10 mm	2	1

Lower Pole Stones

D. Neisius

Introduction

For most symptomatic renal stones ESWL is the first choice of treatment due to its non-invasive procedure and high level of patient and physician acceptance. But the stone-free rates following ESWL — especially for lower pole calices — are problematic compared with the good results of other techniques like PNL or flexible URS. Since the publication of a meta-analysis by Lingeman [1] on the results of ESWL for lower pole stones in 1994, a number of additional studies showed a reduced value of ESWL for this purpose.

Incidence

While the meta-analysis of Lingeman [1] showed the percentage of kidney stones in the lower pole on ESWL had increased steadily from 2% in 1984 to 48% in 1992, two other studies showed a relatively similar portion of lower caliceal stones compared with other localized kidney stones of about 30% to 35% [2]. The Lithotripters Incorporation examined 47,303 stones following ESWL treatment by 1,000 urologists in private practice from 1989 to 1995. An essentially constant incidence of lower pole stones was found from 28% in 1990 to 30% in 1995. At the Midwest Urologic Stone Unit 9,357 stones were treated with ESWL by 200 urologists in private practice from 1987 to 1995 and this sample showed a relatively constant incidence from 30% in 1987 to 36% in 1995. The incidence of lower pole stones has remained stable from 1990.

Guidelines

There are no special guidelines for the therapy of lower caliceal stones. According to the guidelines of the German Urological Association (1999) ESWL is the treatment of choice for symptomatic caliceal stones. The success rate depends on stone localization: lower calyx 60%, middle and upper calyx 70% to 80%. For kidney stones >2 cm in diameter (caliceal stones >2 cm are also included) ESWL monotherapy, PNL monotherapy, or the combination of both are recommended. Very seldom open surgery is needed. The EAU guidelines (2001 [3]) recommend treatments according to stone size and composition: radiopaque kidney stones ≤20 mm (1) ESWL, (2) PNL; stones ≥20 mm (1) PNL, (2) ESWL, (3) PNL + ESWL.

For infected stones, uric acid stones and cystine stones, ESWL and PNL are recommended combined with oral chemolysis and antibiotics. Residual fragments, so-called clinically insignificant fragments, are common after ESWL treatment of stones in the kidney. Lower calix fragments are more commonly seen when there is an infundibulopelvic angle according Elbahnasy [4] of less than 90°. Elbahnasy et al. determine the lower pole infundibulopelvic angle as a line connecting the central point of the pelvis opposite the margins of the superior and inferior renal situs to the central point of the ureter opposite the lower kidney pole. There are no AUA guidelines for lower pole stones, but there are recommendations for ureteral stones (08/1997) and staghorn stones (2004).

Stone-Free Rate Following ESWL

Calculi in the lower pole treated by ESWL are less likely to clear from the collecting system than stones in other calices [1, 5–9]. Although the role of ESWL for lower pole stones has been questioned in some studies [1, 10, 11], many have suggested it as the primary treatment modality for lower stones less than 2 cm [11–14]. Öbek [15] showed in comparison with different caliceal stones following ESWL treatment an overall stone-free rate of 66% for stones < 20 mm^2, and of 63%, 73%, and 71% for lower, middle, and upper caliceal stones, respectively. For the group with stones >20 mm^2 the overall stone-free rate decreased to 49%, and 53%, 60% and 23% in lower, middle, and upper caliceal locations, respectively. Similar results have been published in comparable literature [6, 14, 16–19]. Only Psihramis [20] reported about a higher success

Table 1 Stone clearance of lower pole stones following ESWL stratified to stone size, EBM: 2a, 2c

Author	Stone size [mm]		
	< 10	10–20	> 20
Lingeman (1994)	74%	56%	33%
Öbek (2001)	70%	57%	53%
May (1998)	76%	74%	33%
Netto (1991)	78%	85%	50%

rate for lower caliceal stones of 53% vs. 43% for middle and 45% for upper caliceal stones. Lingeman [1] showed in a critical analysis of 13 reviewed publications about ESWL of lower pole stones a stone-free rate of 25% to 85%, on average 60%. When stratified according to stone size, the stone-free rates for those less than 10, 10–20 mm and greater than 20 mm were reported to be 74%, 56%, and 33%, respectively (Table 1). May and Chandhoke [11] reported stone-free rates of 75%, 74%, and 33% for a single session in solitary lower pole stones less than 10, 10–20, and greater than 20 mm, respectively; Öbek [15] gave 70%, 57%, and 53%, respectively, while Netto [12] mentioned 78%, 85%, and 50%, respectively.

Reasons for Reduced Stone-Free Rates

Disintegration efficacy is not significantly different in lower caliceal stones compared with those localized in the middle and upper calices. But an inverse relationship between stone burden and stone-free rate has been observed. Also other factors may interfere and provide as reasons for a reduced stone-free rate of lower pole stones following ESWL. Sampaio and Aragao [21] first described the spatial anatomy of the lower pole as a possible factor in stone passage. Three anatomical features may have a role in the stone clearance: the angle between the lower pole infundibulum and the renal pelvis, the diameter of the lower pole infundibulum, and the spatial distribution of the calices. They suggested that a lower pole infundibulopelvic angle less than 90°, lower pole infundibulum diameter less than 4 mm and multiple lower pole calices may decrease the stone clearance [22]. In this prospective study they found that 72% of patients became stone-free when the lower pole infundibulopelvic angle was greater than 90° while only 23% of patients were stone-free when the angle was less than 90°.

Several retrospective studies further investigated the interference of lower pole anatomy on stone clearance [22–24]. Patients with favorable factors had post-shock wave lithotripsy clearance rates of 70% or greater, whereas those with unfavorable factors had a clearance rate of less than 20%. In a retrospective study Poulakis et al. [25] investigated the prediction of lower pole stone clearance after shock wave lithotripsy using an artificial neural network (ANNA). Stone-free rates following sufficient disintegration by ESWL are better in patients with a normal body mass index, a physiological urinary transport system, an infundibulum diameter of ≥ 5 mm, and an infundibulopelvic angle of $\geq 45°$ as measured by the method of Elbahnasy [4]. Stone size and stone composition are not significant predictors for the stone-free rate.

Improvement of ESWL Results

In a prospective randomized trial, 69 patients with residual lower caliceal fragments 3 months after shock wave lithotripsy received either mechanical percussion and inversion or observation for 1 month [26].

The mechanical percussion and inversion group had a substantially higher stone-free rate than the observation group (40% versus 3%, respectively, $p < 0.001$). This fact has been described by other retrospective studies using either mechanical percussion or inversion, diuresis, or a combination of these methods [12, 27–29]. The recent years have shown tendentious improvements of stone clearance from the lower pole following ESWL.

This may be explained by the relatively higher retreatment rates of the second and third generation lithotripters. May and Netto and Öbek [11, 12, 15] achieved stone-free rates of about 10% greater for lower pole stones with second generation lithotripters than the authors listed in the Lingman study [1] using the HM3 device.

The highest retreatment rate for lower pole stones is found for the "Piezolith Group" of Poulakis et al. [25] with 4.4 treatments for stones of 15.7 mm diameter on average, but with a stone-free rate of 70.7%. Fast and short repeated treatments with the anesthesia-free piezoelectric procedure should improve the result, so-called "stir up" [30].

Author	No. lower pole stones	Stone size [~ mm]	Stone free after 1 treatment [%]
Elashry (1996)	37	8.5	94
Gould (1998)	30	not available	83
Grasso (1998)	48	15.4	73
Fabrizio (1998)	63	10	77
Menezes (1999)	14	12	80
Tawfiek (1999)	23	8	87
Grasso (1999)	90	15	82
Schuster (2002)	95	10.3	in situ 77; displaced 89
Mariani (2004)	9	> 20	77

Table 2 Flexible URS for the treatment of lower pole stones, EBM: 2c, 3a, 3b

Alternative Management of Lower Pole Stones

Albala et al. [31] performed a prospective randomized, multicenter trial comparing shock wave lithotripsy and percutaneous stone removal for symptomatic lower pole stones of 30 mm or less. 58 patients with a mean stone size of 14.4 mm were randomized to PNL, 60 patients with a mean stone size of 14.0 mm to ESWL. The 3-month overall postoperative stone-free rates were 95% for PNL versus 37% for ESWL (p < 0.001). While the PNL results were independent of stone size, they found for all stones larger than 10 mm after ESWL a significantly lower stone-free rate of only 21%. For percutaneous stone removal, which preceded shock wave lithotripsy by several years, early techniques and technologies were crude, experience was limited, and significant complications were frequent [32–34]. Although the outcomes produced with percutaneous removal were good [35–37] the non-invasive ESWL procedure rapidly became the standard for the majority of non-staghorn renal calculi [38, 39]. Reduction of complications by improved PNL techniques and more effective endoscopic lithotripter systems (e.g., holmium laser, Lithoclast Master) increased the value of PNL although only for renal calculi less than 20 mm, especially for those with reduced stone-free rates following ESWL like lower pole stones.

Flexible URS with its low morbidity can be seen as an optional therapy for lower pole stones, especially in relation to the higher complication rates of PNL [40–46]. Very thin, flexible ureteroscopes now range between 7.4 and 8.6 F with a 1.2 mm channel. Together with new grasping devices and laser lithotripters, excellent results can be achieved for lower calix stones with stone-free rates of 94% after one treatment (Table 2; [41, 44, 47–53]).

Discussion and Conclusions

The high efficiency of PNL and URS divides lower pole stones into those amenable for PNL (≥ 20 mm) and those suitable for flexible URS (≤ 10 mm). But is the complication rate for PNL comparable to the complication rate after ESWL as Albala [31] reported: 23% following PNL and 12% after ESWL? The list of ESWL complications contains urinary tract infection, obstruction, colic, hematoma, and steinstrasse. The list of PNL complications comprises urinary tract infection, ileus, sepsis, hematoma, obstruction, perforation, transfusion, and AV fistula. Although the authors found no statistically significant difference in the frequency of complications, the lists hardly appear comparable. Only one AV fistula counterbalances all ESWL complications.

In recent years, some investigators have reported about good results with flexible URS in the treatment of caliceal stones. Stone clearance is very high and the morbidity very low, comparable to the morbidity of ESWL. But the technical procedure, operation time, and expertise of the surgeon are reasons that the flexible URS is today not the first choice of treatment for lower pole stones. Helpful for the decision could be the prediction of stone clearance after ESWL with respect to the anatomic situation of the lower calix

with or without an artificial neural network. Further prospective, randomized trials are necessary to evaluate therapeutic modalities like ESWL, PNL, and flexible URS for the treatment of lower caliceal stones. Technical developments will give further impulses in the one or the other direction. Today we would recommend the following guidelines for the treatment of lower caliceal stones:
- for stones up to 10 mm (1) ESWL, (2) flexible URS, (3) PNL;
- for stones 10–20 mm (1) ESWL, (2) PNL, (3) flexible URS;
- for stones larger than 20 mm (1) PNL, (2) ESWL.

References

[1] Lingemann JE, Siegel YI, Steele B. et al. Management of lower pole nephrolithiasis: a critical analysis. J Urol 1994; 151: 663

[2] Cass AS, Grine WB, Jenkins JM et al. The incidence of lower-pole nephrolithiasis-increasing or not? Br J Urol 1998; 82: 12

[3] Tiselius HG, Ackermann D, Alken P, Buck C, Conort P, Gallucci M. Guidelines on urolithiasis. European Association of Urology. Eur Urol 2001, 40: 362

[4] Elbahnasy AM, Shalhav AL, Hoenig DM, Elashry OM, Smith DS, McDougall EM et al: Lower caliceal stone clearance after shock wave lithotripsy or ureteroscopy: the impact of lower pole radiographic anatomy. J Urol 1998; 159: 676

[5] Politis G, Griffith DP. ESWL: stone-free efficacy based upon stone size and location. World J Urol 1987; 5: 255

[6] Graff J, Diederichs W, Schulze H. Long-term follow-up in 1,003 extracorporeal shock wave lithotripsy patients. J Urol 1988; 140: 479

[7] McCullough DL. Re: Extracorporeal shock wave lithotripsy and residual stone fragments in lower calices (letter to the editor). J Urol 1989; 141: 140

[8] McDougall EM, Denstedt JD, Brown RD et al. Comparison of extracorporeal shock wave lithotripsy and percutaneous nephrolithotomy for the treatment of renal calculi in lower pole calyces. J Endourol 1989; 3: 265

[9] Tolon M, Miroglu C, Erol H et al. A report on extracorporeal shock wave lithotripsy results on 1,569 renal units in an outpatient clinic. J Urol 1991; 145: 695

[10] Drach GW, Dretler S, Fair W et al. Report of the United States cooperative study of extracorporeal shock wave lithotripsy. J Urol 1986; 135: 1127

[11] May DJ, Chandhoke PS. Efficacy and cost-effectiveness of extracorporeal shock wave lithotripsy for solitary lower pole renal calculi. J Urol 1998; 159: 24

[12] Netto RN Jr, Claro JF, Lemos GC et al. Renal calculi in lower pole calices: what is the best method of treatment? J Urol 1991; 146: 721

[13] Chen RN, Streem SB. Extracorporeal shock wave lithotripsy for lower pole calculi: long-term radiographic and clinical outcome. J Urol 1996; 156: 1572

[14] Talic RF, El Faqih SR. Extracorporeal shock wave lithotripsy for lower pole nephrolithiasis: efficacy and variables that influence treatment outcome. Urology 1998; 51: 544

[15] Öbek C, Önal B, Kantay K, Kalkan M, Yalcin V, Öner A, Solok V, Tansu N. The efficacy of extracorporeal shock wave lithotripsy for isolated lower pole calculi compared with isolated middle and upper caliceal calculi. J Urol 2001; 166: 2081

[16] Keeley FX, Moussa SA, Smith G et al. Clearance of lower pole stones following shock wave lithotripsy: effect of the infundibulopelvic angle. Eur Urol 1999; 36: 371

[17] Kupeli B, Biri H, Sinik Z et al. Extracorporeal shock wave lithotripsy for lower calyceal calculi. Eur Urol 1998; 34: 203

[18] Havel D, Saussine C, Fath C et al. Single stones of the lower pole of the kidney. Eur Urol 1998; 33: 396

[19] El-Damanhoury H, Schärfe T, Rüth J et al. Extracorporeal shock wave lithotripsy of urinary calculi: experience in treatment of 3,278 patients using the Siemens Lithostar and Lithostar Plus. J Urol 1991; 145: 484

[20] Psihramis KE, Jewett MA, Bombardier C at al. Lithostar extracorporeal shock wave lithotripsy: the first 1.000 patients. Toronto Lithotripsy Associates. J Urol 1992; 147: 1006

[21] Sampaio FJ, Aragao AHM. Limitations of extracorporeal shock wave lithotripsy for lower calyceal stones: anatomic insight. J Endourol 1994; 8: 241

[22] Sampaio FJ, D'Anunciacao AL, Silva EC. Comparative follow-up of patients with acute and obtuse infundibulopelvic angle submitted to extracorporeal shock wave lithotripsy for lower calyceal stones: preliminary report and proposed study design. J Endourol 1997; 11: 157

[23] Elbahnasy AM, Clayman RV, Shalhav AL et al. Lower pole calyceal stone clearance after shock wave lithotripsy, percutaneous nephrolithotomy, and flexible ureteroscopy: impact of radiographic spatial anatomy. J Endourol 1998; 12: 113

[24] Gupta NP, Singh DV, Hemal AK et al. Infundibulopelvic anatomy and clearance of inferior caliceal calculi with shock wave lithotripsy. J Urol 2000; 163: 24

[25] Poulakis V, Dahm P, Witzsch U, De Vries R, Remplik J, Becht E. Prediction of lower pole stone clearance after shock wave lithotripsy using an artificial neural network. J Urol 2003; 169: 1250

[26] Pace KT, Tariq N, Dyer SJ, Weir MJ, D'a Honey RJ. Mechanical percussion, inversion and diuresis for residual lower fragments after shock wave lithotripsy: a prospective, single blind, randomized controlled trial. J Urol 2001; 166: 2065

[27] Brownlee N, Foster M, Griffith DP et al. Controlled inversion therapy: an adjunct to the elimination of gravity-dependent fragments following extracorporeal shock wave lithotripsy. J Urol 1990; 143: 1096

[28] D'a Honey RJ, Luymes J, Weir MJ et al. Mechanical percussion inversion can result in relocation of lower pole stone fragments after shock wave lithotripsy. Urology 2000; 55: 204

[29] Netto NR Jr, Claro JF, Cortado PL et al. Adjunct controlled inversion therapy following extracorporeal shock wave lithotripsy for lower pole caliceal stones. J Urol 1991; 146: 953

[30] Krings F, Tuerk C, Steinkogler I, Marberger M. Extracorporeal shock wave lithotripsy retreatment (stir-up) promotes discharge of persistent caliceal stone fragments after primary extracorporeal shock wave lithotripsy. J Urol 1992; 148: 1040

[31] Albala DM, Assimos DG, Clayman RV, Denstedt JD, Grasso M, Gutierrez-Aceves J, Kahn RI, Leveillee RJ, Lingman JE, Macaluso JN Jr, Munch LC, Nakada StY, Newman RC, Pearle MS, Preminger GM, Teichman J, Woods JR. Lower pole I: a prospective randomized trial of extracorporeal shock wave lithotripsy and percutaneous nephrostolithotomy for lower pole nephrolithiasis – initial results. J Urol 2001; 166: 2072

[32] Patterson DE, Segura JW, LeRoy AJ et al. The etiology and treatment of delayed bleeding following percutaneous lithotripsy. J Urol 1985; 133: 447

[33] Lee W, Smith A, Cubell V et al. Complications of percutaneous nephrolithotomy. Am J Roentgenol 1987; 148: 177

[34] Branner GE, Bush WH. Complications and morbidity of endourology. AUA Update Series 1985; 4: 2

[35] White EC, Smith AD. Percutaneous stone extraction from 200 patients. J Urol 1984; 132: 437

[36] Segura JW, Petterson DE, LeRoy AJ et al. Percutaneous removal of kidney stones: review of 1,000 cases. J Urol 1985; 134: 1077

[37] Marberger M, Stack W, Mruby W. Percutaneous lithopaxy of renal calculi with ultrasound. Eur Urol 1982; 8: 236

[38] Chaussy C, Schmiedt E, Jocham D. et al. First clinical experience with extracorporeally induced destruction of kidney stones by shock waves. J Urol 1982; 125: 417

[39] Chaussy C, Schmiedt E. Shock wave treatment for stones in the upper urinary tract. Urol Clin North Am 1983; 10: 743

[40] Grasso M, Loisides P, Beaghler M et al. The case for primary endoscopic management of upper urinary tract calculi: a critical review of 121 extracorporeal shock wave lithotripsy failures. Urology 1995; 45: 363

[41] Fabrizio MD, Behari A, Bagley DH. Ureteroscopic management of inrarenal calculi. J Urol 1998; 159: 1139

[42] Yowell CW, Delvechio FC, Preminger GM et al: Ureteroscopic management of lower pole renal calculi. J Urol 1999; 161: 370

[43] Grasso M, Conlin M, Bagley D. Retrograde ureteropyeloscopic treatment of 2 cm or greater upper urinary tract and minor Staghorn calculi. J Urol 1998; 160: 346

[44] Grasso M, Ficazzola M. Retrograde ureteropyeloscopy for lower pole caliceal calculi. J Urol 1999; 162: 1904

[45] Hollenbeck BK, Schuster TG, Faerber GJ, Wolf JS. Flexible ureteroscopy in conjunction with in situ lithotripsy for lower pole calculi. Urology 2001; 58: 859

[46] Kourambas J, Delvecchio FC, Munver R, Preminger GM. Nitinol stone retrieval assisted ureteroscopic management of lower pole renal calculi. Urology 2001; 56: 935

[47] Elashry OM, DiMeglio RB, Nakada SY et al. Intracorporeal electrohydraulic lithotripsy of ureteral and renal calculi using small caliber (1.9 Fr) electrohydraulic lithotripsy probes. J Urol 1996; 156: 1581

[48] Gould DL. Holmium:YAG laser and its use in the treatment of urolithiasis: our first 160 cases. J Endourol 1998; 12: 23

[49] Grasso M, Chalik Y. Principles and applications of laser lithotripsy: experience with the holmium laser lithotripter. J Clin Laser Med Surg 1998; 16: 3

[50] Menezes P, Dickinson A, Timoney AG. Flexible ureterorenoscopy for the treatment of refractory upper urinary tract stones. BJU Int 1999; 84: 257

[51] Tawfiek ER, Bagley DH. Management of upper urinary tract calculi with ureteroscopic techniques. Urology 1999; 53: 25

[52] Schuster TG, Hollenbeck BK, Faerber GJ, Wolf JSt Jr. Ureteroscopic treatment of lower pole calculi: comparison of lithotripsy in situ and after displacement. J Urol 2002; 168: 43

[53] Mariani AJ. Combined electrohydraulic and holmium:YAG laser ureteroscopic nephrolithotripsy for 20 to 40 mm renal calculi. J Urol 2004; 172: 170

Proximal Ureteral Stones

P. Olbert, R. Hofmann

Epidemiology and Definitions

In Western Europe and North America, urolithiasis has the status of a major public health issue. 1–5% of the total population of industrialized countries are affected. The life time risk to experience at least one episode of urolithiasis is about 20% in men and 5–10% in women. In Calcium Oxalate stones recurrence rates are up to 50% within 10 years after initial diagnosis. All publications providing consistent, reliable data are referring to urolithiasis of the complete upper urinary tract, to the best of our knowledge there is no epidemiological publication addressing upper ureteral stones in particular.

Anatomically, the proximal ureter is defined by the following landmarks: the cranial border is the pyeloureteral junction. Caudally, the proximal ureter ends at the level of the pelvic brim or the cranial margin of the iliosacral joint as defined on a plain KUB X-ray.

For the different therapeutic modalities that will be discussed, we chose stone-free rates ≥ 90% 4 weeks after therapy as a measure of acceptable therapeutic efficacy.

EBM — System and Data Sources

Approaching a clinical problem or question according to EBM criteria, 2 systems of evaluation have to be considered. The quality of all publications available for the question of interest is judged by levels of evidence as defined by the Oxford Centre of Evidence-Based Medicine:
- Levels of evidence:
  - 1a: systematic review or meta-analysis of randomized clinical trials (RCT);
  - 1b: single RCT with narrow confidence interval;
  - 2a: systematic review or meta-analysis of cohort studies;
  - 2b: single cohort study or low quality RCT (e.g. >80% follow-up);
  - 2c: outcomes research;
  - 3a: systematic review or meta-analysis of case-control studies;
  - 3b: individual case-control study;
  - 4: case series or "low quality" cohort studies or case control studies;
  - 5: expert opinions.

After categorizing the available citations according to these criteria, a recommendation can be made. The quality or reliability of this recommendation depends on the level of evidence evaluated before:
- Grade of recommendation:
  - A: consistent level 1 trials;
  - B: consistent level 2 or 3 trials or extrapolations of level 1 trials;
  - C: level 4 trials or extrapolations of level 2 or 3 trials;
  - D: level 5 evidence or inconsistent or inconclusive trials or case series.

Data research was performed primarily in Cochrane library databases (Cochrane Reviews and Cochrane central directory of controlled trials). In the case of a negative search result, the MedLine database (PUBMED) was searched using the same key words. If possible, only level 1–3 studies were considered for evaluation. Level 4 studies were accepted if case numbers were high enough. Level 5 citations were excluded from evaluation. The literature of the past 5 years was used preferentially to provide adequate topicality of the conclusions drawn in this comment.

The following specific problems in the therapy of proximal ureteric stones have been addressed:
- Is it possible to give an evidence-based recommendation for ESWL or endoscopic modalities as first-line therapy for proximal ureteral stones?
- Which of the available disintegration technologies is supported by the qualitatively best data in terms of efficacy, complication rates, and cost efficiency?

Extracorporeal Shock Wave Lithotripsy (ESWL) of Proximal Ureteric Stones

For proximal ureteral stones, ESWL, a non-invasive technique of stone disintegration that is usually performed without anesthesia nowadays, reaches stone-free rates between 62 and 100%. The probably largest case series of almost 20,000 patients by Mobley et al. revealed stone-free rates of 89–89,5% for the proximal ureter [1] (EBM 4/C). These figures do not differentiate whether auxiliary interventions were used or not but the same group found that the use of internal stents does not affect treatment outcome [2] (EBM 2c/B). These data were confirmed by Chen et al. in a prospectively randomized trial for the entire ureter [3] (EBM 1b/B). The results of these really impressive databases probably render ESWL the principal option for the therapy of proximal ureteral stones, because localization in the proximal ureter seems to be a favorable prognosticator for stone clearance [4] (EBM 2c/B). Arrabal-Martin et al. reviewed the results of 734 proximal ureteral calculi and concluded that ESWL provides high stone-free rates and low complication rates in the absence of criteria for urinary diversion and might thus be the primary therapeutic option for these cases [5] (EBM 4/C). The plenty of smaller and predominantly retrospective case series or small case-control studies dating back to the early 1990s or 1980s are not mentioned here and do not add any useful data for the implementation of a therapeutic guideline.

Adhering to stringent EBM criteria, only level 4 evidence with a grade C recommendation can be documented for ESWL in the therapy for proximal ureteral calculi as far as stone-free rates are concerned. There is a lack of prospectively randomized or at least controlled data comparing ESWL with alternative therapeutic modalities. Another problem in evaluating ESWL in general, and in proximal ureteral stones in particular, is the use of different SWL generators with often quite diverging characteristics. There are recent experimental studies comparing different SWL technologies in artificial stones or in animal models, but to the best of our knowledge there are no valid clinical data on this subject. Another difficulty is the fact that most authors do not comment in detail on the presence of auxiliary interventions in their patient cohorts. There is only one group who compared ESWL on proximal ureteral stones with and without push-back in a prospectively randomized fashion and found no differences between their groups [6] (EBM 1b/B). Thus, homogenization of the available data for a reasonable meta-analysis or a systematic review seems almost impossible.

In conclusion, ESWL of the proximal ureteral stone is an efficient, non-invasive therapeutic option that is available almost everywhere and that can be done on an outpatient basis. Its quality is most probably much better than it seems after evaluation by the stringent EBM pattern. There is good evidence against the routine use of stents and against routinely performed push-back.

Endoscopic (Ureterorenoscopic) Therapy of Proximal Ureteral Stones

Laser lithotripsy

All citations reviewed for the present comment confirmed stone-free rates of ≥ 90% for Ho:YAG laser lithotripsy of proximal ureteral stones. One controlled, prospective case-control study could show a ≥ 90% stone-free efficacy [7] (EBM 3b/C). Wu et al. showed significantly higher stone-free rates for laser lithotripsy after a single treatment session in comparison to ESWL in impacted proximal ureteral stones (92 vs. 60%). This prospective trial convincingly shows the efficacy of laser lithotripsy. However, this is not a randomized comparison and so the results have to be considered carefully due to selection bias. One large prospective cohort study confirmed laser efficacy for upper ureteric stones [8] (EBM 2b/B). Laser lithotripsy is judged to be more cost-effective than ESWL as well [7]. Lam et al. retrospectively compared the results of ESWL and Ho:YAG laser lithotripsy in proximal ureteric stones. Despite higher initial stone-free rates of laser lithotripsy (90–100%), efficiency quotients of both treatment modalities were not significantly different [9] (EBM 3b/C). Especially for smaller stones ESWL is rated as first-line therapy by these authors. In comparison to electrohydraulic lithotripsy, stone-free rates directly after therapy were significantly better for Ho:YAG laser lithotripsy (65 vs. 97%) [10] (EBM 3b/C). Stone-free rates are probably not different in flexible and semi-rigid instruments but there are no data evaluating a direct comparison. Summarizing these data, we can conclude that laser lithotripsy is a highly efficient technique for stone disintegration, however, there are no precise data to prove its superiority to ESWL, especially as first line therapy.

Ballistic/pneumatic lithotripsy

The data to evaluate ballistic lithotripsy in the proximal ureter according to EBM criteria in terms of efficacy and complications are close to insufficient. Case numbers are small and the number of randomized or at least prospectively controlled studies is limited. There is one prospectively randomized trial comparing 2 different ballistic lithotripters for endoscopic ureterolithotripsy [11]. 38 patients were randomized to either a Swiss LithoClast® or an Olympus® Electrokinetic Lithotriptor treatment, however, only 17 had stones of the mid or proximal ureter. Stone-free rates were 90% for both devices and for all patients (EBM 2b/C), upper ureteral stones were not evaluated separately. Stone migration rates were 15–25%. Another nicely conducted, prospectively randomized trial by Hofbauer et al. compared EHL and pneumatic disintegration of ureteral stones unsuitable for SWL [12]. They found equivalent efficacy (85 and 89% stone-free, respectively), however, complication rates in EHL were significantly higher (EBM 1b/B). As far as the objective of this comment is concerned, the major drawback of this study is once more that proximal stones have not been evaluated separately. Thus, EBM-based recommendations based on these randomized data cannot be made for upper ureteral calculi.

There are 2 larger case series reporting on the efficacy and push-back rates of ballistic lithotripsy [13, 14]. Aghamir et al. evaluated the outcome of ballistic lithotripsy in 340 patients, 32% of whom had upper ureteral stones. Complete fragmentation was achieved in 73% of these patients with a migration rate of 17%. Robert et al. reported on the results of 150 ballistic lithotripsies (54% in the upper ureter). Although all patients in whom fragmentation was completed were rendered stone free, they criticize a quite high migration rate of 48% in this subgroup of patients (EBM 4/C). Yagisawa et al. were able to show high efficacy of pneumatic lithotripsy in 22 cases of impacted ureteral stones, with the majority located proximally. The 1 month stone-free rate was 91%. Major complications did not occur and the migration rate in this preselected patient cohort was only 5% [15] (EBM 4/C).

In summary, for proximal ureteral stones the EBM level for an acceptable stone-free rate is not better than 4/C due to the poor quality of the reviewed studies, although the available data are consistent. Proximal stone migration seems to be higher than in other modalities, but there are no controlled, comparative data supporting this adequately. All authors emphasize the cost effectiveness of ballistic lithotripsy because of reusable components and moderate capital costs.

Ultrasonic lithotripsy

There are neither controlled prospective data nor even a larger case series to support ultrasonic stone disintegration in the proximal ureter in an adequate quality for an EBM-based recommendation.

Electrohydraulic lithotripsy

Electrohydraulic lithotripsy in the ureter is an effective means of stone disintegration with stone-free rates in the range of 90%. However, there are almost no high quality data to support EHL use in upper ureteral stones. One case series by Yang et al. [16] (EBM 4/C) shows an 84% success rate that rises to 98% after adjuvant SWL. Menezes et al. presented another series in 1999 and showed a 93% stone-free rate after flexible ureteroscopy and EHL in refractory ureteric stones [17] (EBM 4/C). Older reports that confirm the excellent disintegration efficacy of EHL do even less fulfill the criteria for a critical EBM-based review. The literature of the last 5 years almost completely neglects EHL for the disintegration of ureteral stones. This may be due to the introduction of the other intracorporeal technologies for stone disintegration that seem to be at least equally effective but have a much more favorable complication profile. The high complication rate of EHL in the ureter is nicely demonstrated by Hofbauer et al. in a prospectively randomized comparison of EHL and pneumatic disintegration (17.6 vs. 2.6%) [12] (EBM 1b/B). Piergiovanni et al. showed the traumatic potential of EHL on the experimental level [18]. Briefly, the role of EHL for the treatment of upper ureteral stones is questionable in a modern endourological setting because equally effective and less traumatic options are available. However, the level of evidence for these recommendations is moderate.

Open surgery

Considering the multitude of effective non- and minimally invasive therapeutic modalities for upper ureteric stones, the role of open surgery is clearly limited. Ather et al. reviewed a large, single-center case series of more than 1000 patients and found an indication for open surgery in 20% of cases in a Pakistani referral population [19] (EBM 4/C). However, the rate of open surgery has decreased from around 40 to 15% over the last decade. The authors state that the indication for open surgery is limited to high risk patients with large stones requiring definitive therapy in one session or with contraindications to lithotomy positioning. Other groups showed high success rates for mini-access ureterolithotomy [20] in a retrospective analysis (EBM 4/C) or for retroperitoneoscopic ureterolithotomy [21] in a prospective, non-randomized trial (EBM 3b/B). However, all authors clearly define the restricted indications for open surgery in ureteric stones: Only patients with endoscopic failure of stone disintegration or removal are candidates for open or laparoscopic surgery.

Conclusions and Recommendations

The intention of this comment was to give an evidence-based guideline for the therapy of proximal ureteral stones. In reviewing the literature on the topic, the authors had to face several problems:
- The body of literature on the therapy of ureteral stones predominantly consists of retrospective case series and personal experiences. The number of randomized trials or at least well conducted prospective cohort studies is very small.
- Most publications on ureteral stones do not differentially comment on the results in upper ureteral calculi. Papers dealing explicitly with proximal stones are rare.
- Especially in ESWL, it seems almost impossible to achieve homogeneity in patient-, stone-, and lithotriptor-related factors when comparing different publications.

Despite these drawbacks we tried to summarize those papers giving valuable information on modern therapy for proximal ureteral stones and we think that it actually is possible to make a suggestion for a clinical guideline.

ESWL still is the therapy of choice for proximal ureteral stones. Although initial stone-free rates and efficiency quotient seem to be slightly lower than in the endourological alternatives, it has some inherent advantages: it is noninvasive and repeatable, can be performed on an outpatient basis, and stone location in the proximal ureter probably is a prognostically favorable factor. There are no convincing prospectively randomized data giving enough evidence to displace ESWL as first line therapy for the proximal ureteral stone.

Endourological stone disintegration and removal can be performed with high success and low complication rates by Ho:YAG laser lithotripsy and pneumatic lithotripsy after ESWL failure or if it is the patient's and surgeon's preference to achieve a definitive therapeutic solution in one session. In experienced hands, both devices are probably equally successful. Migration of stones or stone fragments seems to be seen more frequently in ballistic lithotripsy. Again, there are no precise comparative data to support one of these two endourological options in terms of an EBM-based recommendation. EHL is probably equally effective, but there are experimental data and at least one prospectively randomized trial to confirm a significantly higher complication rate in the ureter.

Routine stenting is unnecessary in ESWL and in uncomplicated ureteroscopy for proximal ureteral stones.

Open surgery nowadays should be limited to stones refractory to ESWL or endoscopic therapy or to highly selected patient subgroups displaying contraindications to the above-mentioned procedures.

One the one hand, the existing literature leaves enough room for any kind of prospective study to compare different treatment modalities for proximal ureteral stones. On the other hand, we feel that success rates of 90% or higher for each therapeutic option will require very high patient numbers and accurate study design to guarantee patient homogeneity and to find significant differences in parameters of therapeutic success or failure.

Issues to be addressed more intensely in the future are cost-effectiveness and complication rates.

References

1. Mobley TB, Myers DA, Grine WB, Jenkins JM, Jordan WR. Low energy lithotripsy with the Lithostar: treatment results with 19962 renal and ureteral calculi. J Urol 1993; 149: 1419–1424
2. Mobley TB, Myers DA, Jenkins JM, Grine WB, Jordan WR. Effect of stents on lithotripsy of ureteral calculi: treatment results with 18,825 calculi using the Lithostar lithotripter. J Urol 1994; 152: 66–67
3. Chen YT, Chen J, Wong WY, Yang SS, Hsieh CH, Wang CC. Is ureteral stenting necessary after uncomplicated ureteroscopic lithotripsy? A prospective, randomized controlled trial. J Urol 2002; 167: 1977–1980
4. Abdel-Khalek M, Sheir KZ, Elsobky E, Showkey S, Kenawy M. Prognostic factors for extracorporeal shock-wave lithotripsy of ureteric stones. A multivariate analysis study. Scand J Urol Nephrol 2003; 37: 413–418
5. Arrabal-Martin M, Pareja Vilches M, Gutierrez-Terrejo F, Miján-Ortiz JL, Palao-Yago F, Zuluaga-Gómez A. Therapeutic options in lithiasis of the lumbar ureter. Eur Urol 2003; 43: 556–563
6. Danuser H, Ackermann DK, Marth DC, Studer UE, Zingg E. Extracorporeal shock wave lithotripsy in situ or after push up for upper ureteral calculi: a prospective randomized trial. J Urol 1993; 150: 824–826
7. Wu CF, Shee JJ, Lin WY, Lin CL, Chen CS. Comparison between extracorporeal shock wave lithotripsy and semirigid ureterorenoscope with holmium:YAG laser lithotripsy for treating large proximal ureteral stones. J Urol 2004; 172: 1899–1902
8. Sofer M, Watterson JD, Wollin TA, Nott L, Razvi H, Denstedt JD. Holmium:YAG laser lithotripsy for upper urinary tract calculi in 598 patients. J Urol 2002; 167: 31–34
9. Lam JS, Greene TD, Gupta M. Treatment of proximal ureteral calculi: holmium:YAG laser ureterolithotripsy versus extracorporeal shock wave lithotripsy. J Urol 2002; 167: 1972–1976
10. Teichman JM, Rao RD, Rogenes VJ, Harris JM. Ureteroscopic management of ureteral calculi: electrohydraulic vs. holmium:YAG lithotripsy. J Urol 1997; 158: 1357–1361
11. De Sio M, Autorino R, Damiano R, Oliva A, Perdonà S, D'Armiento M. Comparing two different ballistic intracorporeal lithotripters in the management of ureteral stones. Urol Int 2004; 72: 52–54
12. Hofbauer J, Hobarth K, Marberger M. Electrohydraulic versus pneumatic disintegration in the treatment of ureteral stones: a randomized, prospective trial. J Urol 1995; 153: 623–625
13. Aghamir SK, Mohseni MG, Ardestani A. Treatment of ureteral calculi with ballistic lithotripsy. J Endourol 2003; 17: 887–890
14. Robert M, Bennani A, Guiter J, Averous M, Grasset D. Treatment of 150 ureteric calculi with the LithoClast®. Eur Urol 1994; 26: 212–215
15. Yagisawa T, Kobayashi C, Ishikawa N, Kobayashi H, Toma H. Benefits of ureteroscopic pneumatic lithotripsy for the treatment of impacted ureteral stones. J Endourol 2001; 15: 697–699
16. Yang SS, Hong JS. Electrohydraulic lithotripsy of upper ureteral calculi with semirigid ureteroscope. J Endourol 1996; 10: 27–30
17. Menezes P, Dickinson A, Timoney AG. Flexible ureterorenoscopy for the treatment of refractory upper urinary tract stones. BJU Int 1999; 84: 561–562
18. Piergiovanni M, Desgrandchamps F, Cochand-Priollet B, Janssen T, Colomer S, Teillac P, LeDuc A. Ureteral and bladder lesions after ballistic, ultrasonic, electrohydraulic or laser lithotripsy. J Endourol 1994; 8: 293–299
19. Ather MH, Paryani J, Memon A, Sulaiman MN. A 10-year experience of managing ureteric calculi: changing trends towards endourological intervention — is there a role for open surgery? BJU Int 2001; 88: 173–177
20. Sharma DM, Maharaj D, Naraynsingh V. Open mini access ureterolithotomy: the treatment of choice for the refractory ureteric stone? BJU Int 2003; 92: 814–816
21. Goel A, Hemal AK. Upper and mid ureteric stones: a prospective unrandomized comparison of retroperitoneoscopic and open ureterolithotomy. BJU Int 2001; 88: 679–682

Distal Ureteral Stones

C. Türk

Introduction

Based on a systematic review of the published literature from 1997 to January 2005, specific aspects of the management of distal ureteral stones are described in this chapter. The outcomes of the individual treatment modalities are enumerated on the basis of the available prospective randomized studies and meta-analyses related to this subject. Publications with evidence level 1a and 1b (*grade of recommendation A*) are marked; those of lower levels are not categorized.

Definition

In clinical urology the distal ureter is defined as that portion of the ureter that lies below the lower margin of the sacroiliac joint. Occasionally, the margin between the middle and the caudal ureter is drawn at the point of crossing between the ureter and the iliac vessels. In anatomy the pelvic part (pars pelvina) of the ureter is defined as the portion below the linea terminalis. A ureteral calculus confirmed diagnostically in this section may be managed either conservatively until passage of the stone, or by *in situ* ESWL, endourological procedures with stone extraction or in combination with intracorporeal lithotripsy. A further alternative is ureterolithotomy as an open procedure or as a laparoscopic/retroperitoneoscopic intervention. The main determinants of treatment selection are the size and position of the stone, specific anatomic features, the ability to visualize the stone, concomitant urological or non-urological diseases, the symptoms, the patient's medical history, and the patient's personal preferences. The local availability or accessibility of technical equipment and expertise are also important criteria for selection of the treatment procedure.

Conservative Therapy

The likelihood of a ureteral stone passing without intervention is rated differently. It depends on the size and location of the stone at its initial manifestation, and on previous episodes of stones occurring on the same side. Calculi diagnosed primarily in the distal ureter are more likely to pass spontaneously under conservative non-interventional therapy than proximal ureteral stones of the same size [1]. Distal ureteral stones less than 5 mm in size pass spontaneously under conservative treatment in 71% to 98% of cases, while larger stones up to 1 cm in size pass spontaneously in 25% to 53% of cases [2] *(evidence levels T1a)*. Extended medication treatment with steroids, antibiotics, Ca-antagonists or high doses of acetaminophen (paracetamol) are known to accelerate the passage of stones [3] *(evidence level T1b/A)*. The addition of tamsulosin also appears to be beneficial for the clearance of lower ureteral stones [4, 5] *(evidence levels T1b)* [6–8].

ESWL (Extracorporeal Shock Wave Lithotripsy)

At the beginning of the ESWL era, ureteral calculi, particularly those in the distal portion of the ureter, did not belong to the domain of *in situ* ESWL. With the Dornier HM3, the first series-produced model of an ESWL, the patient was positioned in a "bath-tub" by means of a hydraulic device. This made it difficult to localize stones in the distal portion of the ureter. The effects of X-ray radiation during the localization procedure and the impact of the shock wave on the adjacent organs, particularly in women of reproductive age, were not fully known. Seven years after the introduction of the first ESWL for humans, Chaussy and Fuchs still questioned the value of ESWL for distal ureteral stones [9]. Following the introduction of ESWL devices of the second and third generations, the positioning of the patient was significantly improved by the use of flat treatment tables as well as X-ray- and ultrasound-guided localization.

Analgesia

ESWL was initially performed under general anesthesia. As the technique became more refined, general anesthesia was replaced by spinal anesthesia and sedoanalgesia. Piezoelectric shock wave devices require no analgesia; they are also marked by a smaller focal zone and a lower energy density [10]. Currently, ESWL is frequently performed either as a day-case procedure or on an outpatient basis.

Results

The mean duration of ESWL treatment is approximately 60 minutes. Stone-free rates based on the available high-evidenced literature are shown in Table **1**. Treatment parameters and further clinical data in Table **2** provide more information about the clinical outcome and also an impression of the invasive nature of each therapeutic modality (*both tables are based solely on evidence level 1a and 1b publications*). In sum-

Table **1** Stone-free rates

Author	Observation/Medical therapy			ESWL			URS		
	<5 mm	5–10 mm	>10 mm	<5 mm	5–10 mm	>10 mm	<5 mm	5–10 mm	>10 mm
Segura et al. (1a)	71–98%	25–53%	–	85%		74%	89% (82–95)		73% (63–82)
Peschel et al. (Observ. 43 days) (1b)	–	–	–	85%; 15% re-treatment	95%; 5% re-treatment		100%	100%	100%
Pearle et al. (1b)	–	–	–	0–7 mm, 100%	>7 mm, 100%		0–7 mm, 100%		>7 mm, 100%
Lotan et al. (1b)	45% (36–71)			82–89% (59–97), Depends on lithotripter			95% (86–100)		
Cooper et al. (1b — comparing different medical strategies)	54–86%	–	–	–	–	–	–	–	–
(in parentheses: evidence level)	*(in parentheses: 95% confidence interval)*			*(in parentheses: 95% confidence interval)*			*(in parentheses: 95% confidence interval)*		

Table **2** Invasiveness

Author	Operating Time (min)		Analgesia		Postoperative ancillary measures		Postoperative Complications		Retreatment	
	ESWL	URS	ESWL	URS	ESWL	URS	ESWL	URS	ESWL	URS
Segura et al. *(1a)*	–	–	–	–	10%	7%	significant: 4% less signif.: 9%	significant: 9% less signif.: 1% + 1% long-term complications	21%	4%
Peschel et al. *(1b)*	57	23	epidural/general		10%	100% (URS) (routine stents)	0	0	10%	0
Pearle et al. *(1b)*	34	65	sedation/local 67% 34% general anesthesia 31% 66%		–	91% (stents)	severe 0 minor 9%	severe 10% minor 25%	–	–

mary, the mean stone-free rate ranges from 74% to 100%, postoperative ancillary measures are required in 10%, re-treatments in 10% to 21%, and significant complications occur in 0% to 4%.

Studies published after the above-mentioned systematic comprehensive literature review show further improvements in the outcome of in situ ESWL. In 2003 Hochreiter et al. reported a stone-free rate of 97% at three months after in situ ESWL [11]; only 9% of these patients required multiple treatments. Adjunctive medical therapy with nifedipine and deflazacort after ESWL may increase the success rate [12][12]. If one accepts the effort of multiple ESWL treatments, even large ureteral stones can be resolved in situ [13]. In situ ESWL for distal ureteral stones can be applied successfully even in children [14, 15]; ESWL devices with ultrasound-guided localization and a small focus are given preference in this setting. Forced diuresis during ESWL appears to improve the outcome of the treatment [16] (evidence level T1b). While the female genital system obviously remains unaffected by ESWL treatment of distal ureteral stones [17], transient alterations of the semen are reported in men, including microscopic hemospermia, decline in sperm density, mobility, and vitality; however, these return to normal within 12 weeks after ESWL [18, 19].

Ureteroscopy (URS)

URS in the distal ureter is usually performed with a 6.5 F to 9.5 F semi-rigid ureteroscope. Thus, compared to the tools used in the past, we now have much thinner instruments with a sufficiently capacious working channel. With thicker instruments intracorporeal lithotripsy can be performed with ultrasound. However, electrohydraulic, electropneumatic and laser devices can be used with thinner working channels [20]. The stone-free rate after laser lithotripsy using the Ho:YAG laser (holmium-yttrium-aluminum-garnet laser) is reported to be higher than that after electrohydraulic lithotripsy, as the fragments created by this procedure are very small [21].

Analgesia

Ureteroscopy is usually performed under general anesthesia or spinal anesthesia. A few authors have used sedoanalgesia for URS in selected patients with distal ureteral stones less than 5 mm in diameter, who were unlikely to require intracorporeal lithotripsy. In some cases the treatment can be performed as a day-case procedure or on an outpatient basis [22, 23]; however, as a rule the patient needs to be hospitalized.

Results

Results are shown in Tables **1** and **2**. Peschel et al. report a mean operating time of 18.8 minutes (range: 12–25 minutes) for the removal of distal ureter stones less than 5 mm in size by ureteroscopy, and 28 minutes (range: 20–43 minutes) for larger stones. No complications were encountered [24] (evidence level 1b). Pearle et al. report a mean operating time of 65 minutes, serious postoperative complications in 10%, and mild postoperative complications in 25% of cases [25] (evidence level 1b). In a meta-analysis Segura et al. report significant complications in 9% and less significant complications in 1% [2] (evidence level 1a). Other authors registered primary success rates of 93% to 100% for URS of distal ureteral stones, the actual rate being mainly dependent on stone size [26, 27]. A repeat URS after failure of the initial intervention was required in 0% to 4% of cases [2, 24, 28].

The occurrence of a postoperative obstruction due to missed residual fragments or due to ureteral stenosis depends on stone size, stone impaction, and the duration of impaction prior to URS. Obstructions have been reported in up to 12% of cases for unselected ureteral stones and in 24% of cases for impacted stones [29, 30]. However, Stackl registered no stenosis following URS with the use of 10 F to 11.5 F ureteroscopes after a mean follow-up period of 14 months [31]. Segura reports complications by way of ureteral strictures in 1% of cases. Obstructions may develop without overt symptoms (reported in 3%); therefore, postoperative imaging should be performed at least 3 months after URS.

Routine ureteral stenting after URS has been considered the standard of care. However, in recent times there have been numerous reports about the benefits of no stenting, particularly in the treatment of distal ureteral stones. Unstented patients after uncomplicated URS of distal ureteral calculi have less pain, fewer urinary symptoms, and require less analgesics [32] (evidence level T1b) [33].

ESWL or URS as Primary Therapy?

ESWL and URS are the most common treatment modalities for distal ureter stones requiring therapy. However, as far as the preferred technique is concerned, the authors of the two previously mentioned, prospective randomized studies [24, 25] have drawn diverse conclusions. While the group in the USA (Pearle et al.) gives preference to ESWL, the Austrian group (Peschel et al.) favors ureteroscopy. The outcomes of the two forms of treatment are similar in regard to stone-free rates and complications. The most remarkable differences concern operating times. The Austrian group reports a markedly shorter operating time for ureteroscopy than the group from the USA. One reason could be the large number of surgeons involved in the multicenter US study. ESWL, on the other hand, was performed with different devices in the two countries. This explains the shorter duration of the ESWL treatments and the lower re-treatment rate in the USA, where all ESWL therapies were performed with a Dornier HM3.

Tables **1** and **2** show that the number of re-treatments and ancillary measures were higher in the ESWL group if one excludes the several ureteral stents placed routinely after URS. The results also depend on the size of the calculi. The outcome of ESWL is poorer in cases of stones larger than 1 cm in size. This was confirmed in a study from the Netherlands which registered a stone-free rate of 73% for distal + medial ureteral stones less than 1 cm in size treated by ESWL, and a low stone-free rate of 17% for calculi larger than 1 cm. The corresponding rates for primary URS are 85% and 75%, respectively.

The time to achievement of a stone-free state after URS is markedly shorter than that after primary ESWL.

General anesthesia or spinal anesthesia is needed much more frequently in the URS group. Serious complications also occur more frequently in the URS group than in the ESWL group (Table **2**: 9–10% vs. 0–4%, respectively).

Thus, the choice between the two most common modalities for distal ureteral calculi requiring treatment depends on stone size, the surgeon's expertise, the lithotripter used, and the availability or accessibility of technical equipment. On account of the invasive nature of, and the need for sedation with URS, the patient's comorbidities – in addition to the patient's preference – also must be taken into account. ESWL serves best in ureteral stones smaller than 10 mm in size and may obviate the need for more invasive treatment. Given the minimal differences in results, the invasive nature of URS should be weighed against the longer time needed to achieve a stone-free state after ESWL.

The costs cannot be compared because of differences in the public health systems and the different importance assigned to this parameter.

In regard to treatment selection, highly obese patients constitute an exception to the rule. Positioning the patient and focusing on the calculus may be rendered impossible by obesity. In these cases ureteroscopy undoubtedly is superior to ESWL [34].

Other Therapy Alternatives

Open surgery

Open ureterolithotomy is not a first-choice procedure for distal ureteral stones. It may be used in exceptional situations or in cases of simultaneous open surgery for an additional purpose (e.g., distal ureteral stone + RPE) [2, 35, 36].

Laparascopy/retroperitoneoscopy

Laparoscopy is of equally negligible importance in the distal ureter as in other portions of the ureter. The indication is similar to that for open surgery. Laparoscopy may be used as a salvage procedure in cases of ureteral calculi after failed ESWL and/or URS. Laparoscopy may also be discussed as a first-line therapy in selected cases of very large, impacted or multiple ureteral stones, particularly in patients with a single kidney [37].

Gaur et al. favor the retroperitoneal access even in cases of distal ureteral stones, whereas Türk et al. use the transperitoneal access for the distal ureter [38]. The authors report mean operating times of 79 and 90 minutes, respectively. Only two of the 15 cases of distal ureteral stones reported by Türk required conversion to open surgery because the location of the calculi could not be established with certainty; both authors were able to achieve successful outcomes by the primary procedure in all other cases.

Loop, blind basket extraction

In earlier times blind basket extraction (Zeiss' loop) was frequently used for the management of distal ureteral stones. At the time, open ureterolithotomy was the only available modality for active treatment. In view of the complications and discomfort of blind basket extraction and the availability of the above-mentioned therapy alternatives, blind basket extraction is no longer regarded as a viable treatment option [2].

Stent

Ureteral stents are frequently used prior to definitive treatment of ureteral stones. The indications include ureteral calculi with simultaneous urinary infection, frequent colic attacks, or a symptomatic ureteral stone in a pregnant woman. Stones are more likely to pass spontaneously after stent extraction [39].

References

[1] Miller OF, Kane, CJ. Time to stone passage for observed ureteral calculi: a guide for patient education. J Urol 1999; 162: 688
[2] Segura JW, Preminger GM, Assimos DG et al. Ureteral Stones Clinical Guidelines Panel summary report on the management of ureteral calculi. The American Urological Association. J Urol 1997; 158: 1915
[3] Cooper JT, Stack GM, Cooper TP. Intensive medical management of ureteral calculi. Urology 2000; 56: 575
[4] Kupeli B, Irkilata L, Gurocak S et al. Does tamsulosin enhance lower ureteral stone clearance with or without shock wave lithotripsy? Urology 2004; 64: 1111
[5] Porpiglia F, Ghignone G, Fiori C et al. Nifedipine versus tamsulosin for the management of lower ureteral stones. J Urol 2004; 172: 568
[6] Cervenakov I, Fillo J, Mardiak J et al. Speedy elimination of ureterolithiasis in lower part of ureters with the alpha 1-blocker – Tamsulosin. Int Urol Nephrol 2002; 34: 25
[7] Dellabella M, Milanese G, Muzzonigro G. Efficacy of tamsulosin in the medical management of juxtavesical ureteral stones. J Urol 2003; 170: 2202
[8] Sigala S, Dellabella M, Milanese G et al. Evidence for the presence of alpha(1) adrenoceptor subtypes in the human ureter. Neurourol Urodyn 2005; 24: 142
[9] Chaussy C, Fuchs G. Extracorporeal shock-wave lithotripsy of distal-ureteral calculi: Is it worthwhile? J Endourol 1987; 1: 1
[10] Marberger M, Turk C, Steinkogler I. Painless piezoelectric extracorporeal lithotripsy. J Urol 1988; 139: 695
[11] Hochreiter WW, Danuser H, Perrig M et al. Extracorporeal shock wave lithotripsy for distal ureteral calculi: what a powerful machine can achieve. J Urol 2003; 169: 878
[12] Porpiglia F, Destefanis P, Fiori C et al. Role of adjunctive medical therapy with nifedipine and deflazacort after extracorporeal shock wave lithotripsy of ureteral stones. Urology 2002; 59: 835
[13] Ghobish A. In situ extracorporeal shock wave lithotripsy of middle and lower ureteral stones: a boosted, stentless, ventral technique. Eur Urol 1998; 34: 93
[14] al Busaidy SS, Prem AR, Medhat M et al. Paediatric ureteric calculi: efficacy of primary in situ extracorporeal shock wave lithotripsy. Br J Urol 82: 90, 1998
[15] Marberger M, Turk C, Steinkogler I. Piezoelectric extracorporeal shock wave lithotripsy in children. J Urol 1989; 142: 349
[16] Azm TA, Higazy H. Effect of diuresis on extracorporeal shock wave lithotripsy treatment of ureteric calculi. Scand J Urol Nephrol 2002; 36: 209
[17] Vieweg J, Weber HM, Miller K et al. Female fertility following extracorporeal shock wave lithotripsy of distal ureteral calculi. J Urol 1992; 148: 1007
[18] Andreessen R, Fedel M, Sudhoff F et al. Quality of semen after extracorporeal shock wave lithotripsy for lower urethral stones. J Urol 1996; 155: 1281
[19] Martinez Portillo FJ, Heidenreich A, Schwarzer U et al. Microscopic and biochemical fertility characteristics of semen after shock wave lithotripsy of distal ureteral calculi. J Endourol 2001; 15: 781
[20] Grasso M III. Ureteroscopic lithotripsy. Curr Opin Urol 1999; 9: 329
[21] Teichman JM, Rao RD, Rogenes VJ et al. Ureteroscopic management of ureteral calculi: electrohydraulic versus holmium:YAG lithotripsy. J Urol 1997; 158: 1357
[22] Hosking DH, Bard RJ. Ureteroscopy with intravenous sedation for treatment of distal ureteral calculi: a safe and effective alternative to shock wave lithotripsy. J Urol 1996; 156: 899
[23] Wills TE, Burns JR. Ureteroscopy: an outpatient procedure? J Urol 1994; 151: 1185
[24] Peschel R, Janetschek G, Bartsch G. Extracorporeal shock wave lithotripsy versus ureteroscopy for distal ureteral calculi: a prospective randomized study. J Urol 1999; 162: 1909
[25] Pearle MS, Nadler R, Bercowsky E et al. Prospective randomized trial comparing shock wave lithotripsy and ureteroscopy for management of distal ureteral calculi. J Urol 2001; 166: 1255
[26] Hamano S, Nomura H, Kinsui H et al. Experience with ureteral stone management in 1,082 patients using semirigid ureteroscopes. Urol Int 2000; 65: 106

[27] Strohmaier WL, Schubert G, Rosenkranz T. et al. Comparison of extracorporeal shock wave lithotripsy and ureteroscopy in the treatment of ureteral calculi: a prospective study. Eur Urol 1999; 36: 376

[28] Eden CG, Mark IR, Gupta RR et al. Intracorporeal or extracorporeal lithotripsy for distal ureteral calculi? Effect of stone size and multiplicity on success rates. J Endourol 1998; 12: 307

[29] Weizer AZ, Auge BK, Silverstein AD et al. Routine postoperative imaging is important after ureteroscopic stone manipulation. J Urol 2002; 168: 46

[30] Roberts WW, Cadeddu JA, Micali S et al. Ureteral stricture formation after removal of impacted calculi. J Urol 1998; 159: 723

[31] Stackl W, Marberger M. Late sequelae of the management of ureteral calculi with the ureterorenoscope. J Urol 1986; 136: 386

[32] Borboroglu PG, Amling CL, Schenkman NS et al. Ureteral stenting after ureteroscopy for distal ureteral calculi: a multi-institutional prospective randomized controlled study assessing pain, outcomes and complications. J Urol 2001; 166: 1651

[33] Hosking DH, McColm SE, Smith, WE. Is stenting following ureteroscopy for removal of distal ureteral calculi necessary? J Urol 1999; 161: 48

[34] Nguyen TA, Belis JA. Endoscopic management of urolithiasis in the morbidly obese patient. J Endourol 1998; 12: 33

[35] Kane CJ, Bolton DM, Stoller ML. Current indications for open stone surgery in an endourology center. Urology 1995; 45: 218

[36] Bichler KH, Lahme S, Strohmaier WL. Indications for open stone removal of urinary calculi. Urol Int 1997; 59: 102

[37] Gaur DD, Trivedi S, Prabhudesai MR et al. Laparoscopic ureterolithotomy: technical considerations and long-term follow-up. BJU Int 2002; 89: 339

[38] Turk I, Deger S, Roigas J et al. Laparoscopic ureterolithotomy. Tech Urol 1998; 4: 29

[39] Deliveliotis C, Giannakopoulos S, Louras G. et al. Double-pigtail stents for distal ureteral calculi: an alternative form of definitive treatment. Urol Int 1996; 57: 224

Endourological Techniques — Clinical Pathways

T. Knoll, P. Honeck

Introduction

The aim of this chapter is to give an overview about the endourological techniques SWL, PNL, and URS with respect to common indications and contraindications, underlying techniques, clinical performance, and potential complications. Differential indications and results of the particular treatment will be discussed elsewhere.

Extracorporeal Shock Wave Lithotripsy (SWL)

Indications

Principally, SWL can be used for all sorts of stones in the upper urinary tract (kidney, ureter) as long as the following conditions are fulfilled (evidence level V):
- *Disintegration of the stone:* Depending on the stone composition; cystine, calcium oxalate monohydrate and brushite have lower disintegration rates. However, a reliable prognosis about the composition of the stone is mostly impossible. Non-contrast spiral computed tomography (CT) is utilized for distinguishing stone compositions through determination of the Hounsfield unit values by many authors. Although the data are still conflicting, discrimination between uric acid- and calcium-containing calculi seems to be possible [1–3] (evidence level IIc).
- *Ability of fragments to pass the ureter:* Risk of steinstrasse with gross stone mass (>2 cm), outlet obstruction like ureter stenosis, stone in lower calyx with narrow/steep caliceal infundibulum [4].
- *Localization of the stone by ultrasound/fluoroscopy:* Radio-opaque stones, sonographic localization, adipositas, or orthopedic deformations may interfere with stone focusing.

Technique

Extracorporeal lithotripsy machines today are based on electrohydraulic, electromagnetic, or piezoelectric shock wave generation. Acoustic lens systems or autofocusing geometry are used for focusing. These techniques will be discussed in detail elsewhere.

One of the most important factors for SWL treatment is the coupling of the shock wave generator to the patient. The ideal method is the placement of the patient in degassed water (water-bath). However, this method has been abandoned because of high costs, need for space, and the lack of possibility to integrate a shock wave source into multifunctional treatment benches. The water-bath was replaced by water cushions, filled with degassed water, and coupling gel.

Treatment

The following examinations are necessary to evaluate the size and localization of the stone, the anatomy of the urinary tract, renal function, and to exclude contraindications (evidence level V):
- patient's history, physical examination;
- discontinuation of thrombocyte-aggregation-inhibitors/anticoagulation treatment (ASA 7 days, clopidogrel [Plavix®/Iscover®] 10 days, coumarins until Quick >75%);
- plain X-ray, intravenous urography in case of ureter stones (not necessarily in case of renal stones); retrograde pyelography if necessary (contraindications against intravenous contrast agents, persistent renal colic);
- alternative: helical CT scan [5];
- ultrasound;
- serum creatinine, coagulation status (Quick, PTT, thrombocytes), inflammatory parameters (white blood count/CRP);
- urinary dip stick analysis, if necessary urine culture and antibiotic pre-treatment according to antibiogram;
- written informed consent: colic, obstruction,

fever, sepsis, skin hematoma, renal bleeding, loss of kidney (<0.1%), supportive treatment (indwelling ureter stent, percutaneous nephrostomy, re-SWL), failure of treatment (alteration to alternative therapies).

During SWL monitoring of vital functions should be done according to the patient's history, at least pulse oxymetry in case of analgosedation (evidence level V).

Analgosedation usually is sufficient when using modern lithotripters. Especially with piezoelectric SW sources analgesia is often unnecessary. Children and non-cooperative patients are treated under general anesthesia. For analgosedation predefined applications are used, i. e., Piritramid/Midazolam (7.5 mg/2 mg intravenously), with increasing dosage if needed.

The position of the patient depends on the actual lithotripter and localization of the stone: in general a supine position for renal and proximal ureter stones, a prone position for middle (superposition of os ileum/os sacrum) and distal ureter stones. Loss of energy due to shock wave passage through intestines containing air leads to reduced efficiency.

The localization of the stone is performed in 3 planes and has to be checked during treatment at regular intervals. A preoperatively inserted ureter stent can simplify the localization of poorly radio-opaque stones, but may interfere with the application of shock waves resulting in reduced efficacy [6]. The focus should be positioned at the point the stone rests the longest during breathing.

The amount and energy level of the applied shock waves depends on the device. Generally a lower amount of total energy is applied to renal stones than to ureter stones.

Treatment should be stopped ahead of schedule if imaging shows adequate disintegration or side effects occur (pain despite of sufficient analgesia, hypertension, extrasystoles).

With increasing *shock wave frequency* the efficiency of disintegration decreases and tissue trauma may occur [7] (evidence level Ib).

Plain X-ray and ultrasound should ideally be performed on the following day to evaluate treatment success and possible complications. Generally accepted criteria for treatment success are stone-free patients or persistent fragments which can pass the ureter spontaneously (≤ 4 mm). However, it should be kept in mind that also such small fragments can grow to new stones when persisting within the collecting system [8, 9] (evidence level IIc).

Patients with fragments which can pass the ureter spontaneously should receive NSAIDs (i. e., Diclofenac) for spasmoanalgesia. Recently, improved passage of distal stones could be demonstrated by administration of alpha-receptor-antagonists (e. g., Tamsulosin) [10, 11] (evidence level Ib). Urine should be filtered until stone loss to acquire fragments for stone analysis. Supportive measures to increase the rate of stone loss are movement, head-down position, and Vibrax treatment [12]. Increased diuresis may further support stone expulsion [13] (evidence level IIc). The application of alkali citrates in case of calcium stones is discussed [14] (evidence level IIc).

If adequate disintegration is not achieved after one SWL treatment, the procedure can be repeated one or more times. Alternatively, auxiliary measures like URS or PNL may be considered. While repeated SWL for lower proximal and distal ureter stones can be performed the day after the first treatment, upper proximal ureter stones and renal stones require an interval of 1–2 days to avoid renal tissue injury, depending on the lithotripter used and co-morbidity (evidence level V). Generally not more than 2 treatments within 7 days should be performed in case of renal stones (evidence level V).

Complications

Side effects like hemospermia and hematuria have to be distinguished from *complications*.

Complications caused by shock waves are (peri-) renal hematoma, impaired renal function, lesions in surrounding tissues (pleura, lung, vessels, intestines, ovaries).

Risk factors for renal hematoma after SWL: anticoagulation (coumarins, thrombocyte-aggregation inhibitors), congenital or acquired coagulopathies, arteriosclerosis, untreated arterial hypertension, and diabetes mellitus [15] (evidence level V). SWL during pregnancy is contraindicated. Presence of *impaired renal function* increases the risk for further impairment through SWL. Unfortunately, most available data reporting side effects of SWL were obtained from first generation lithotripsy machines. A significantly lower complication rate of second and third generation generators may be assumed.

Complications caused by passing fragments: colic, hydronephrosis, fever, sepsis, inadequate renal function. The risk rises with increasing stone mass, proximal location of fragments, and obstruction of the urinary tract. The preoperative insertion of a ureter stent may reduce that risk (evidence level V).

Percutaneous Nephrolithotomy (PNL)

Indications

Main indications for PNL are by large stone masses with diameters of 1.5–2 cm or more. Smaller stones can be treated with PNL if successful SWL or URS seems unlikely (especially for stones in the lower calyx, obstruction within the upper urinary tract, caliceal diverticulum). Some stone compositions (cystine stones, calcium oxalate monohydrate, brushite) show limited disintegration through SWL. In these cases PNL may be the better therapeutic option even for smaller stones. Rapid growing struvite stones require complete elimination and are therefore adequately treated by PNL.

The use of flexible nephroscopes reduces the necessity of multiple percutaneous accesses, as they allow visualization of most localizations.

Due to the excellent results of SWL in the treatment of children, PNL is an exceptional indication [16] (evidence level IIa). Anatomic anomalies like horse-shoe kidneys are generally accessible for PNL but need careful imaging for planning the optimal access and the identification of blood vessels.

Contraindications for PNL are untreated coagulopathies, pregnancy, and untreated urinary tract infections. Apart from that, skeletal (i. e., distinctive scoliosis) or renal anomalies (i. e., renal malrotation) can act as specific contraindications preventing a safe access to the stone.

Technique

Renal stones are disintegrated and removed endoscopically through a percutaneously applied and dilated *nephrostomy tract*. The puncture is performed under sonographic and/or fluoroscopic control. For *dilatation* of the nephrostomy tract, metal, plastic, or balloon dilatators are available. After dilatation, the tract is kept open through a working shaft (plastic/metal shaft or endoscope shaft). Rigid (24–28 Ch.) and flexible nephroscopes (~15 Ch.) are used. The calculi are usually disintegrated by *ultrasound or pneumatic lithotripsy systems*, the resulting fragments are removed by forceps or baskets. For flexible nephroscopy *laser lithotripsy* (e. g., holmium:YAG laser) is primarily used today. The available systems for intracorporeal lithotripsy will be demonstrated in detail in the URS section.

Treatment

The following *examinations* are required (evidence level V):
- patient's history, physical examination;
- discontinuation of thrombocyte aggregation inhibitors/anticoagulation treatment (ASA 7 days, clopidogrel [Plavix®/Iscover®] 10 days, coumarins until Quick >75%);
- plain X-ray and intravenous urography;
- retrograde pyelography if required or, respectively, non-contrast helical CT;
- ultrasound;
- serum creatinine, coagulation (Quick, PTT, thrombocytes), inflammatory parameters (white blood count/CRP);
- urinary dip stick analysis, if necessary urine culture and antibiotic treatment according to antibiogram;
- informed consent: infection, fever, bleeding/transfusion (HIV, hepatitis), influx of irrigation fluid, lesions in surrounding tissues (pleura, lung, vessels, intestine, liver, spleen), UPJ obstruction, AV fistula, aneurysm, open surgical revision/selective angiography, loss of kidney (very rare), ureter catheter, persisting fragments with necessity for ancillary treatments.

Prophylactic antibiotics are administered preoperatively by most urologists (evidence level V).

The procedure is usually performed under *general anesthesia* in the *prone position*.

Retrograde insertion of a *(balloon) ureter catheter* and retrograde injection of contrast medium and, respectively, methylene blue may simplify the puncture by dilating and contrasting the renal pelvis and calices. For PNL the calices are punctured under *fluoroscopic, ultrasound, or combined control*. The puncture through the *dorsal calyx* of the lower pole minimizes the risk of bleeding because of the ventral path of the caudal branch of the arteria segmentalis inferior, which supplies the lower renal pole. Via this access most intrarenal localizations are accessible. The primary access through the upper calices (supracostal approach) is also described, but includes a higher risk of complications [17] (evidence level IV).

After puncture, the access tract is dilated to 18 to 30 Fr. The nephrostomy tract is held open by the *working shaft* (Amplatz or nephroscope shaft). The collecting tract is then inspected under continuous flow and the stone is disintegrated. During the whole procedure a low pressure system within the pelvis should be assured to prevent influx. Fragments are washed out, exhausted or extracted with forceps or basket. The use of a flexible scope may be necessary to reach peripheral stones. It is inserted over the working shaft and can also be used to extract proximal ureter stones.

A stone-free state at the end of the procedure is confirmed by endoscopy and fluoroscopy. If residual fragments are hard to reach or if complications occur, the termination of the procedure and a subsequent SWL or re-PNL can be indicated. Usually, a nephrostomy is placed until macrohematuria has stopped, a stone-free condition is proved, and adequate urine outlet through the ureter is ensured. After uncomplicated PNL without any fragments left, the procedure may be completed tubeless [18, 19] (evidence level Ib). In case of a supracostal access, a chest X-ray has to rule out accidental injury of pleura or lung.

Complications

The *rate of complications* depends on stone size and localization as well as its composition, the number of nephrostomy tracts, previous renal surgery, and the surgeon's experience (evidence level V). The most frequent complication is bleeding, in the literature transfusion rates of 10% are reported. Fever after PNL is seen in up to 30%, in case of urinary tract infection and insufficient urine drainage the risk of urosepsis is increased. Solely radiographic-guided punctures are at higher risk of injury to neighboring organs. Hydrothorax is a specific complication after a supracostal access (< 1%) [20].

Bleeding after PNL can often be stopped by temporary clamping of the PCN. If the bleeding persists, arterial injury is likely that should be treated by selective angiography. Open surgery and nephrectomy are rarely necessary to treat PNL complications.

Mini-PNL

Mini-PNL is mostly used in children, where the nephrostomy tract is dilated only to 18–21 Fr (conventional PNL 26–30 Fr) [21, 22] (evidence level IV). A reduced renal trauma compared to conventional PNL is discussed even in adults, but complications and clinical value must still be confirmed by prospective studies.

Ureterorenoscopy (URS)

Indications

Ureter stones: SWL and URS show comparable stone-free rates for distal ureter stones [23–26] (evidence level Ib). While the advantage of SWL is its noninvasiveness, the advantage of URS is the immediate stone removal [13]. For stones in the middle part of the ureter SWL shows reduced disintegration rates due to bone and intestine superposition, which is why URS could be beneficial in these cases [27, 28]. Proximal ureter stones had been treated primarily with SWL for a long time, but newer studies indicate that URS in combination with the Ho:YAG laser may be advantageous, particularly for stones > 10 mm [29–32] (evidence level IIc).

Renal stones: Renal stones up to 15–20 mm can be treated using semi-rigid or flexible URS [4, 30, 33] (evidence level IV). As SWL shows good results for such stones, it should be used primarily because of its lower invasiveness. Large pelvic and staghorn stones (> 20 mm) should be treated with PNL primarily [4, 20], flexible URS can be applied afterwards to extract residual fragments [34, 35] (evidence level IV).

Flexible URS is ideal for the removal of caliceal stones [35]. Due to often inadequate stone-free rates of SWL for lower pole stones, flexible URS is an excellent option [36–40].

Technique

Endoscopes

Semi-rigid URS: The semi-rigid ureterorenoscope consists of a stainless steel shaft and fiberoptic bundles as well as a working channel for irrigation and insertion of working instruments. Because of the use of glass fiber, a limited flexion of the "semi-rigid" endoscope of approximately 20° is possible. Modern semi-rigid ureterorenoscopes with external diameters of 6–10.5 Fr. allow access to the upper urinary tract, mostly without separate dilatation of the ureter [41, 42] (evidence level V). Instruments with larger diameters are associated with a higher risk for ureter injury due to the stronger dilatation.

Flexible URS: Flexible ureterorenoscopes with shaft diameters of 6.5–9 Fr. also allow easy access to the upper urinary tract in most cases without previous dilatation [43]. Flexible ureterorenoscopes should not be used in the distal ureter, where semi-rigid instruments are a lot easier to handle.

Intracorporeal lithotripsy

Endoscopic, intracorporeal lithotripsy is usually necessary before extraction of larger fragments. Electrohydraulic, pneumatic, ultrasound, and laser probes are available.

Electrohydraulic: Flexible electrohydraulic lithotripsy probes (EHL) are available in different sizes for semi-rigid and flexible ureterorenoscopes. Technical principle: An electric spark is generated at the tip by electric current. The resulting heat creates a cavitation bubble which generates a shock wave. Generally, EHL can be used to disintegrate all stones (even cystine or hard stones like calcium oxalate monohydrate). However, the heat spreading in all directions often causes damage to surrounding tissues why EHL is not recommended for intracorporeal lithotripsy anymore [44] (evidence level V).

Pneumatic: Pneumatic or ballistic lithotripters are often used with 2.4 Fr. probes for semi-rigid ureterorenoscopy. The achieved disintegration rates reach > 90%. The main advantages are high cost-efficiency through low purchase costs and safe application [45–48] (evidence level V). A frequently seen problem, however, is proximal stone migration [48, 49]. By inserting a dormia basket or special tools like the stone cone this side effect can be inhibited [48, 50] (evidence level IV). Flexible probes are available but cause a significant restriction of flexion [36, 51].

Ultrasound: Ultrasound-based lithotripsy probes induce a high frequent swinging of the handle through a piezoceramic element which transforms electric energy into ultrasound (23,000–27,000 Hz). This ultrasound is passed along the metal probe to the tip and induces a vibration. Contact with the stone causes disintegration. Recently, probes are available that combine ultrasound and pneumatic lithotripsy and can be used for semi-rigid URS as well as for PNL [52, 53].

Laser-based systems: Today *neodymium:yttrium-aluminum-garnet* (Nd:YAG; frequency-doubled [FREDDY, 532 and 1064 nm]) and *holmium:YAG* (Ho:YAG; 2100 nm) lasers are established systems for intracorporeal lithotripsy. For both lasers, fibers with different diameters are available (mostly 365 µm for semi-rigid ureterorenoscopy and 220 µm fibers for flexible URS) [36]. The FREDDY laser has limited efficacy for hard stones (e.g., calcium oxalate monohydrate) and cannot disintegrate cystine stones [54] (evidence level IV), but is less expensive than the Ho:YAG laser [55], which disintegrates stones of all compositions [56]. The Ho:YAG laser with the 220 µm fiber seems to be the first choice for flexible URS [30, 32, 57, 58] (evidence level IV). Compared to the Nd:YAG laser, the minimal tissue penetration of < 0.5 mm reduces thermal damage. Therefore contact to the stone is mandatory for disintegration. While perforation of the ureter or renal pelvis may occur accidentally, an increased incidence for strictures could not be verified so far [29].

Stone extraction (basket, forceps)

Stone manipulation within the ureter: Small fragments can often be extracted primarily or after disintegration using a forceps. Baskets can also be used to extract fragments quickly, although there is a higher risk of getting stuck within the ureter [23, 59, 60].

Stone manipulation within the kidney: Especially for flexible ureterorenoscopy, baskets made of Nitinol (nickel-titanium alloy) are suitable for stone extraction because of their high flexibility and minimal risk of tissue injury. This applies especially for so-called "tipless" baskets.

The use of stone extraction and disintegration tools reduces the maximal tip deflection to a variable amount [34, 36]. These factors have to be known preoperatively to be able to plan and perform a successful therapy.

Treatment

The following *examinations* are required (evidence level V):
– patient's history, physical examination;
– anatomic variants may complicate or prevent retrograde stone manipulation (prostate adenoma, ureter implantation, ureterocele, ureter strictures, urinary diversion (conduit, neobladder, pouch, ureterointestinal implantation);

- discontinuation of thrombocyte aggregation inhibitors/anticoagulation treatment should be aspired, but is not obligatory. Normal coagulation status (Quick/INR, PTT) reduces the rate of complications after URS [61]. In case of limited coagulation ability, URS shows a minor probability for complications compared to SWL and should therefore be preferred [61] (evidence level IV);
- plain X-ray and intravenous urography;
- retrograde pyelography or, respectively, non-contrast helical CT scan;
- sonography;
- serum creatinine, coagulation (Quick, PTT, thrombocytes);
- urinary dip stick analysis, if necessary urine culture and antibiotic treatment according to antibiogram [4, 23];
- informed consent: infection, hematuria, colic, fever, sepsis, pigtail catheter, PCN, injury of urethra/ureter and stenosis, perforation of bladder or ureter, open surgical revision, loss of kidney (very rare), administration of contrast medium, hypersensitivity to contrast medium.

Basically no intervention should be performed during pregnancy. However, URS seems to be a safe technique if treatment is absolutely necessary [62] (evidence level IV).

Most interventions are performed with *general anesthesia*. Due to the miniaturization of the instruments a comparable outcome can be achieved by intravenous sedation [63] (evidence level IV). This approach is especially suitable for female patients with distal ureter stones (evidence level V).

Patients are placed in the lithotomy position. An abduction of the contralateral leg allows more elbow-room for the surgeon. A slight head-down position (Trendelenburg) will inhibit mobilization of fragments into lower calices (evidence level V).

The procedure starts with a cystoscopy, a retrograde pyelography and the insertion of a safety wire/guide wire. The *insertion of a safety wire* should always be performed as it allows insertion of an ureter stent even after ureter perforation.

The use of a thin ureterorenoscope allows intubation of the ostium without previous dilatation in most cases. If primary intubation is not possible, pigtail insertion and delayed URS after 7–14 days offers an appropriate alternative to dilatation. If dilatation is necessary, balloon and plastic dilators are available. If insertion of a flexible urterorenoscope is difficult, prior semi-rigid ureteroscopy can be helpful in the sense of optical dilatation (evidence level V).

Semi-rigid endoscopes are usually inserted without using a guide wire. If direct intubation of the orifice is difficult, the insertion of a second wire through the working channel can be supportive.

Flexible endoscopes have to be inserted via a guide wire in most cases. New generation ureterorenoscopes are equipped with enhanced shafts which principally allow a direct (= free) intubation of the orifice [34, 64].

Access sheaths, which are available in different calibers, can be inserted via a guide wire into the ureter and allow easy repeated access to the proximal ureter and the renal pelvis/calices. Especially in patients with large stone masses requiring multiple ureter passages, the procedure is significantly simplified [65]. In most cases though successful treatment will be possible without using such sheaths [66].

Stone extraction: Small fragments are extracted by forceps or basket. Larger fragments are disintegrated before extraction. The aim of *stone disintegration* should be to achieve fragment sizes that can be extracted easily. When using a holmium laser, very small fragments ("dust") may occur. Such fragments have a high probability of passing spontaneously and can be left in place. Disintegration of stones in the lower calices may be easier after prior relocation into the pelvis or upper calices.

Stenting after URS: Ureter catheters themselves have a significant morbidity. Therefore stenting after URS should not be performed routinely. Insertion of a ureter stent is only necessary in the following cases [67–69] (evidence level Ib): significant residual fragments, ureter injury (perforation, mucosa lesions), prolonged performance time, edematous stone bed. The time of stent treatment conforms with the indication, normally 7–14 days are sufficient.

Complications

The rate of significant complications after URS is stated with 9–11% in literature [23, 42]. Today, ureter stricture in the sense of a long-term complication is rare (< 1%), previous perforations are the most important risk factor. The most serious complication after URS is an avulsion trauma of the ureter [70].

References

1. Thoeny HC, Hoppe H. Unenhanced spiral CT in urolithiasis: indication, performance and interpretation. Röfo 2003; 175: 904
2. Motley G, Dalrymple N, Keesling C et al. Hounsfield unit density in the determination of urinary stone composition. Urology 2001; 58: 170
3. Sheir KZ, Mansour O, Madbouly K et al. Determination of the chemical composition of urinary calculi by noncontrast spiral computerized tomography. Urol Res 2005; in press
4. Tiselius HG, Ackermann D, Alken P et al. Guidelines on urolithiasis. Eur Urol 2001; 40: 362
5. Lang EK, Macchia RJ, Thomas R et al. Improved detection of renal pathologic features on multiphasic helical CT compared with IVU in patients presenting with microscopic hematuria. Urology 2003; 61: 528
6. Abdel-Khalek M, Sheir K, Elsobky E et al. Prognostic factors for extracorporeal shock-wave lithotripsy of ureteric stones – a multivariate analysis study. Scand J Urol Nephrol, 2003; 37: 413
7. Madbouly K, El Tiraifi AM, Seida M et al. Slow versus fast shock wave lithotripsy rate for urolithiasis: a prospective randomized study. J Urol 2005; 173: 127
8. Beck EM, Riehle RA Jr. The fate of residual fragments after extracorporeal shock wave lithotripsy monotherapy of infection stones. J Urol 1991; 145: 6
9. Khaitan A, Gupta NP, Hemal AK et al. Post-ESWL, clinically insignificant residual stones: reality or myth? Urology 2002; 59: 20
10. Dellabella M, Milanese G, Muzzonigro G. Efficacy of tamsulosin in the medical management of juxtavesical ureteral stones. J Urol 2003; 170: 2202
11. Porpiglia F, Ghignone G, Fiori C et al. Nifedipine versus tamsulosin for the management of lower ureteral stones. J Urol 2004; 172: 568
12. Kosar A, Ozturk A, Serel TA et al. Effect of vibration massage therapy after extracorporeal shock wave lithotripsy in patients with lower caliceal stones. J Endourol 1999; 13: 705
13. Pace KT, Weir MJ, Tariq N et al. Low success rate of repeat shock wave lithotripsy for ureteral stones after failed initial treatment. J Urol 2000; 164: 1905
14. Cicerello E, Merlo F, Gambaro G et al. Effect of alkaline citrate therapy on clearance of residual renal stone fragments after extracorporeal shock wave lithotripsy in sterile calcium and infection nephrolithiasis patients. J Urol 1994; 151: 5
15. Kostakopoulos A, Stavropoulos NJ, Macrychoritis C et al. Subcapsular hematoma due to ESWL: risk factors. A study of 4,247 patients. Urol Int 1995; 55: 21
16. Muslumanoglu AY, Tefekli A, Sarilar O et al. Extracorporeal shock wave lithotripsy as first line treatment alternative for urinary tract stones in children: a large scale retrospective analysis. J Urol 2003; 170: 2405
17. Aron M, Goel R, Kesarwani PK et al. Upper pole access for complex lower pole renal calculi. BJU Int 2004; 94: 849
18. Desai MR, Kukreja RA, Desai MM et al. A prospective randomized comparison of type of nephrostomy drainage following percutaneous nephrostolithotomy: large bore versus small bore versus tubeless. J Urol 2004; 172: 565
19. Karami H, Gholamrezaie HR. Totally tubeless percutaneous nephrolithotomy in selected patients. J Endourol 2004; 18: 475
20. Segura JW, Preminger GM, Assimos DG et al. Nephrolithiasis Clinical Guidelines Panel summary report on the management of staghorn calculi. The American Urological Association Nephrolithiasis Clinical Guidelines Panel. J Urol 1994; 151: 1648
21. Lahme S, Bichler KH, Strohmaier WL et al. Minimally invasive PCNL in patients with renal pelvic and calyceal stones. Eur Urol 2001; 40: 619
22. Jackman SV, Hedican SP, Peters CA et al. Percutaneous nephrolithotomy in infants and preschool age children: experience with a new technique. Urology 1998; 52: 697
23. Segura JW, Preminger GM, Assimos DG et al. Ureteral Stones Clinical Guidelines Panel summary report on the management of ureteral calculi. The American Urological Association. J Urol 1997; 158: 1915
24. Pearle MS, Nadler R, Bercowsky E et al. Prospective randomized trial comparing shock wave lithotripsy and ureteroscopy for management of distal ureteral calculi. J Urol 2001; 166: 1255
25. Peschel R, Janetschek G, Bartsch G. Extracorporeal shock wave lithotripsy versus ureteroscopy for distal ureteral calculi: a prospective randomized study. J Urol 1999; 162: 1909
26. Turk TM, Jenkins AD. A comparison of ureteroscopy to in situ extracorporeal shock wave lithotripsy for the treatment of distal ureteral calculi. J Urol 1999; 161: 45
27. Wu CF, Shee JJ, Lin WY et al. Comparison between extracorporeal shock wave lithotripsy and semirigid ureterorenoscope with holmium:YAG laser lithotripsy for treating large proximal ureteral stones. J Urol 2004; 172: 1899
28. Arrabal-Martin M, Pareja-Vilches M, Gutierrez-Tejero F et al. Therapeutic options in lithiasis of the lumbar ureter. Eur Urol 2003; 43: 556
29. Teichman JM, Rao RD, Rogenes VJ et al. Ureteroscopic management of ureteral calculi: electrohydraulic versus holmium:YAG lithotripsy. J Urol 1997; 158: 1357
30. Bagley DH. Expanding role of ureteroscopy and laser lithotripsy for treatment of proximal ureteral and intrarenal calculi. Curr Opin Urol 2002; 12: 277
31. Dogan HS, Tekgul S, Akdogan B. et al. Use of the

holmium:YAG laser for ureterolithotripsy in children. BJU Int 2004; 94: 131
32. Sofer M, Watterson JD, Wollin TA et al. Holmium:YAG laser lithotripsy for upper urinary tract calculi in 598 patients. J Urol 2000; 167: 31
33. Stav K, Cooper A, Zisman A et al. Retrograde intrarenal lithotripsy outcome after failure of shock wave lithotripsy. J Urol 2003; 170: 2198
34. Troy AJ, Anagnostou T, Tolley DA. Flexible upper tract endoscopy. BJU Int 2004; 93: 671
35. Menezes P, Dickinson A, Timoney AG. Flexible ureterorenoscopy for the treatment of refractory upper urinary tract stones. BJU Int 1999; 84: 257
36. Michel MS, Knoll T, Ptaschnyk T et al. Flexible ureterorenoscopy for the treatment of lower pole calyx stones: influence of different lithotripsy probes and stone extraction tools on scope deflection and irrigation flow. Eur Urol 2002; 41: 312
37. Schuster TG, Hollenbeck BK, Faerber GJ et al. Ureteroscopic treatment of lower pole calculi: comparison of lithotripsy in situ and after displacement. J Urol 2002; 168: 43
38. Albala DM, Assimos DG, Clayman RV et al. Lower pole I: a prospective randomized trial of extracorporeal shock wave lithotripsy and percutaneous nephrostolithotomy for lower pole nephrolithiasis-initial results. J Urol 2001; 166: 2072
39. Hollenbeck BK, Schuster TG, Faerber GJ et al. Flexible ureteroscopy in conjunction with in situ lithotripsy for lower pole calculi. Urology 2001; 58: 859
40. Grasso M, Ficazzola M. Retrograde ureteropyeloscopy for lower pole caliceal calculi. J Urol 1999; 162: 1904
41. Dretler SP, Cho G. Semirigid ureteroscopy: a new genre. J Urol 1989; 141: 1314
42. Yaycioglu O, Guvel S, Kilinc F et al. Results with 7.5 F versus 10 F rigid ureteroscopes in treatment of ureteral calculi. Urology 2004; 64: 643
43. Elashry OM, Elbahnasy AM, Rao GS et al. Flexible ureteroscopy: Washington University experience with the 9.3 F and 7.5 F flexible ureteroscopes. J Urol 1997; 157: 2074
44. Zheng W, Denstedt JD. Intracorporeal lithotripsy. Update on technology. Urol Clin North Am 2000; 27: 301
45. Puppo P, Ricciotti G, Bozzo W et al. Primary endoscopic treatment of ureteric calculi. A review of 378 cases. Eur Urol 1999; 36: 48
46. Schock J, Barsky RI, Pietras JR. Urolithiasis update: clinical experience with the Swiss LithoClast. J Am Osteopath Assoc 2001; 101: 437
47. Delvecchio FC, Kuo RL, Preminger GM. Clinical efficacy of combined lithoclast and lithovac stone removal during ureteroscopy. J Urol 2000; 164: 40
48. Tan PK, Tan SM, Consigliere D. Ureteroscopic lithoclast lithotripsy: a cost-effective option. J Endourol 1998; 12: 341
49. Robert M, Bennani A, Guiter J et al. Treatment of 150 ureteric calculi with the Lithoclast. Eur Urol 1994; 26: 212
50. Desai MR, Patel SB, Desai MM et al. The Dretler stone cone: a device to prevent ureteral stone migration — the initial clinical experience. J Urol 2002; 167: 1985
51. Zhu S, Kourambas J, Munver R et al. Quantification of the tip movement of lithotripsy flexible pneumatic probes. J Urol 2000; 164: 1735
52. Kuo RL, Paterson RF, Siqueira TM, Jr et al. In vitro assessment of lithoclast ultra intracorporeal lithotripter. J Endourol 2004; 18: 153
53. Auge BK, Lallas CD, Pietrow PK et al. In vitro comparison of standard ultrasound and pneumatic lithotrites with a new combination intracorporeal lithotripsy device. Urology 2002; 60: 28
54. Delvecchio FC, Auge BK, Brizuela RM et al. In vitro analysis of stone fragmentation ability of the FREDDY laser. J Endourol 2003; 17: 177
55. Ebert A, Stangl J, Kuhn R et al. The frequency-doubled double-pulse neodymium:YAG laser lithotripter (FREDDY) in lithotripsy of urinary stones. First clinical experience. Urologe A 2003; 42: 825
56. Teichman JM, Vassar GJ, Glickman RD. Holmium:yttrium-aluminum-garnet lithotripsy efficiency varies with stone composition. Urology 1998; 52: 392
57. Delvecchio FC, Preminger GM. Endoscopic management of urologic disease with the holmium laser. Curr Opin Urol 2000; 10: 233
58. Grasso M, Chalik Y. Principles and applications of laser lithotripsy: experience with the holmium laser lithotrite. J Clin Laser Med Surg 1998; 16: 3
59. Bagley DH, Kuo RL, Zeltser IS. An update on ureteroscopic instrumentation for the treatment of urolithiasis. Curr Opin Urol 2004; 14: 99
60. Anagnostou T, Tolley D. Management of ureteric stones. Eur Urol 2004; 45: 714
61. Klingler HC, Kramer G, Lodde M et al. Stone treatment and coagulopathy. Eur Urol 2003; 43: 75
62. Lifshitz DA, Lingeman JE. Ureteroscopy as a first-line intervention for ureteral calculi in pregnancy. J Endourol 2002; 16: 19
63. Cybulski PA, Joo H, Honey RJ. Ureteroscopy: anesthetic considerations. Urol Clin North Am 2004; 31: 43
64. Chiu KY, Cai Y, Marcovich R et al. Are new-generation flexible ureteroscopes better than their predecessors? BJU Int 2004; 93: 115
65. Vanlangendonck R, Landman J. Ureteral access strategies: pro-access sheath. Urol Clin North Am 2004; 31: 71
66. Abrahams HM, Stoller ML. The argument against the routine use of ureteral access sheaths. Urol Clin North Am 2004; 31: 83
67. Knudsen BE, Beiko DT, Denstedt JD. Stenting after ureteroscopy: pros and cons. Urol Clin North Am 2004; 31: 173

[68] Jeong H, Kwak C, Lee SE. Ureteric stenting after ureteroscopy for ureteric stones: a prospective randomized study assessing symptoms and complications. BJU Int 2004; 93: 1032

[69] Srivastava A, Gupta R, Kumar A et al. Routine stenting after ureteroscopy for distal ureteral calculi is unnecessary: results of a randomized controlled trial. J Endourol 2003; 17: 871

[70] Martin X, Ndoye A, Konan PG et al. Hazards of lumbar ureteroscopy: apropos of 4 cases of avulsion of the ureter. Prog Urol 1998; 8: 358

Statement of the "German Society for Shock Wave Lithotripsy" about "Outpatient versus Inpatient" ESWL

K. U. Köhrmann, C. Chaussy

Background

With an increasing frequency, hospitals are asked (e.g., by insurance companies) to perform ESWL as an outpatient procedure with intent to lower costs. In this case the physician has to give medically based arguments to prove the necessity of the inpatient therapy. This discussion is primarily driven by economical interests.

Statement of the "German Society of Shock Wave Lithotripsy" in Cooperation with the "Working Group on Urolithiasis of the Academy of German Urologists":

- The Members of both Societies restrict their recommendations to medical criteria only.
- From the medical standpoint an inpatient performance of a treatment is indicated if a short-term medical supply has to be provided which cannot be given in the outpatient situation.
- This short-term supply can become necessary to avoid severe sequels or complications.
- After ESWL severe complications include colic, fever, sepsis, renal hematoma which can result in life-threatening situations.
- The probability of occurrence depends on different factors of the disease, the course of the treatment, co-morbidity, and other factors of the patients up to the general situation of the patient after dismissal from the treating institution.
- Principally ESWL can be performed as an outpatient procedure when there is a low risk for severe complications.
- Also in an outpatient setting ESWL treatment has to be performed according to a high quality standard which respects standard operating procedures and secure postoperative care (e.g., conditions included in the principles of "ambulantes Operieren" according to § 105 SGB of the German law).
- The guidelines and consensus statements for "diagnosis, treatment and metaphylaxis of urinary stone disease" of the scientific urological societies should provide criteria to support the decision between the possibility of outpatient and the necessity of inpatient ESWL treatment.

Speyer, March 2005

Prof. Kai Uwe Köhrmann
Chairman of the Working Group "Urolithiasis"
of the Academy of the German Urologists

Prof. Christian Chaussy
President of the "German Society
of Shockwave Lithotripsy"

Diagnosis and Metaphylaxis in Urolithiasis

Diagnostic Approach

W. L. Strohmaier

Introduction

In suspected cases of nephrolithiasis, the primary aim of diagnosis is to confirm or exclude urinary stones. The secondary aim is to provide the basis for individual therapeutic strategies.

History

The patient's history reveals relevant signs regarding the possible diagnosis (basically, the differential diagnosis comprises the complete spectrum of causes of acute abdominal pain) and the location of calculus. The development of renal calculi does not cause discomfort. Additionally, quiescent stones in the kidney generally cause no or only few uncharacteristic symptoms (for example, flank pain).

Typical pain, such as renal colic (severe undulating pain) develops when renal stones pass into the ureter. Recent research has shown that renal colic is primarily due to an intraluminal pressure increase (20–50 cm H_2O). There is an increase in peristalsis above the stone and a decrease in peristalsis below it. With increasing duration of obstruction, peristalsis decreases [9, 46].

Affected patients are very agitated and complain of flank pain. Depending on the position of the stone, pain radiates into the middle and lower abdomen, groin, and genital region. Often, the pain is associated with vegetative symptoms (nausea, vomiting, flatulence, reduced intestinal activity). Stones in the vicinity of the ureteropelvic junction cause difficulties during micturition (polyuria) [37].

Renal bladder stones also cause discomfort (for example, polyuria, dysuria). Should the stone pass into the urethra, then urinary obstruction can result. Renal calculi can also cause macrohematuria. Fever indicates additional urinary tract infection.

Previous history

Urinary calculi, urological diseases and operations

Restrictions and contraindications must be regarded when employing imaging techniques: contrast medium allergy or intolerance, thyroid gland disease (hyperactivity, autonomous adenoma), impaired renal function, myeloma and similar diseases, massive proteinuria, concurrent metformin medication, and thyroid gland medication.

Regarding therapeutic options the following are of special interest: blood coagulation abnormalities, concurrent anticoagulation medication (for example, ASA), allergies to medication, ulcer and gastritis history (especially non-steroidal anti-inflammatory agents), and pregnancy.

Family history

Urolithiasis, especially cystinuria.

Physical examination

To effectively differentiate, it is mandatory to examine the complete abdomen and genitals including a digital rectal examination. In the case of renal colic, typically tender renal beds are found on percussion; depending on the position of the stone in the ureter tenderness may be found in the middle and lower abdomen. Typically, bowel sounds are sparse; additionally, meteorism can be present. Furthermore, the body temperature should be measured.

Laboratory Examinations

Urine analysis

Generally, midstream urine samples are adequate, however, in women catheter urine may be required should, for example, leukocyturia be present during menstruation.

The basic examination is performed with a test strip for blood (hemoglobin), leukocytes, pH value, nitrite. The test strip examination is more sensitive than microscopic evaluation, for example sediment [3] (evidence level Ib). 92–95% of all patients with renal stone colic show microhematuria [3, 21, 28] (evidence level Ia).

A urine culture should be taken in the case of positive leukocyte and/or nitrite results and/or clinically suspected urinary tract infection.

The pH value can give a first indication of the type of stone (alkaline urine is often associated with infection stones, acidic urine often with uric acid stones).

Blood

A blood count is mandatory (hemoglobin, erythrocyte, leukocyte, and thrombocyte concentrations). Occasionally, leukocytosis is present in renal colic. Therefore, leukocytosis does not always indicate infection, but can be induced by physical stress with activation of adrenal hormones.

Determination of C-reactive protein (CRP) is more reliable as it is increased in bacterial infection [18, 23]. CRP is not increased in renal colic [12] (evidence level IIb). Serum creatinine is a useful judge of renal function, also regarding possible employment of contrast medium in imaging. With respect to therapeutic options, measurement of plasma coagulation (Quick, PTT) is recommended. Determination of TSH is useful when thyroid dysfunction is suspected.

Imaging Techniques

Imaging techniques are used to exclude or substantiate the diagnoses and to determine the size and location of a stone, including assessment of the consequences of obstruction to the urinary tract and renal function. Knowledge of these parameters is necessary to plan therapy adequately.

Sonography

Sonography can reveal stones in the kidney and in the proximal ureter at approximately the height of the lower renal pole. Calculi in the distal (intramural) ureter can be identified using a transrectal or transvaginal ultrasound probe. Generally, stones in the other ureter segments cannot be visualized (intestinal gases). Dilatation of the pelvicalyceal system is an indirect sign of renal calculus [15]. Sensitivity and specificity of sonographic diagnosis of renal stones are approximately 61–93% and 95–100%, respectively [29, 35] (evidence level Ia).

The value of resistive index (renal arteries) to estimate obstruction and urine propulsion out of the ureteral orifice is controversial [11, 16, 34, 41]. Controversial as well is the so-called twinkling artefact (twinkling sign). The twinkling sign is a rapidly changing color signal behind structures like a stone as it can be observed with color-coded duplex sonography. The appearance of the twinkling artefact is highly dependent on the machine settings. Thus it is not a valid parameter [1–3].

Conventional radiology (plain renal film, excretory urography)

Plain renal film

The plain renal film (without contrast medium) can only reveal radio-opaque calculi. Diagnostic sensitivity and specificity of the plain renal film are 69% and 82%, respectively (evidence level IIb). Examination of the skeleton can provide evidence of other causes of pain (for example, the vertebrae). The radiation dose is approximately 0.5 mSv [7, 10, 40].

Excretory urography

In general, films are taken at least twice within 20 minutes following intravenous contrast medium application. Enhanced parenchymal contrast on early films (for example, 3 minutes after contrast medium administration) can indicate obstruction on the affected side. However, early urogram films are generally not required as sonography will have already been performed, thus, also reducing radiation dose.

To reduce exposure to radiation, further films should not be taken if the first film reveals all relative information. Often, it is adequate to concentrate radiography on the affected side. Delayed contrast medium excretion necessitates late films (for example, after several hours).

The excretion urogram is analyzed regarding renal function, dilatation of renal pelvicalyceal system and ureters, location and area of the renal stone and radiologic opacity. Non-opaque stones (generally uric acid stones) are noticed as contrast medium filling defects. Sensitivity and specificity of excretion urography in the diagnosis of ureteral stones are 92–98% and 59–100%, respectively [2, 22, 30, 40] (evidence level Ia). The radiation dose is approximately 1.4–1.5 mSv [7, 12, 17, 19, 22, 25, 40].

Excretory urography is contraindicated in acute ureteral stone colic (danger of fornix rupture), renal failure (creatinine > 200 µmol/L), myeloma and similar diseases, contrast medium allergy, untreated hyperthyroidism.

Computed tomography

Non-enhanced spiral computed tomography (CT) is the method with the highest sensitivity and specificity (91–100% and 95–100%, respectively) for examining a ureteral stone (evidence level Ia). A prerequisite is utilization of thin layers (< 5 mm) to also detect small concrements. Computed tomography is superior to all other imaging techniques [2, 5, 8, 20, 22, 29, 30, 35, 43, 44]. Additionally, CT addresses to some extent other differential diagnoses. Density measurement (Hounsfield units) also facilitates estimation of the stone's composition. This is important for therapeutic planning [4, 6, 13, 24, 26, 27, 36, 45]. However, native CT overestimates stone size by 30–50% [43]. The radiation dose is approximately 2.8–5.0 mSv [7, 12, 17, 19, 22, 40] and is, therefore, significantly higher than conventional radiology. Recently, examination protocols with lower radiation doses have been developed (so-called ultra-low-dose CT). Using these protocols the radiation dose can be reduced to approximately 1–2.2 mSv [20, 22, 33]. However, resolution also suffers especially in regard to stone composition (measurement of Hounsfield units), thus, compromising therapeutic planning.

Aspects of differential indication of imaging techniques

Sensitivity and specificity are of great importance when comparing imaging methods. In this respect, native computed tomography is superior to all other techniques. Additionally, other criteria must be taken into consideration: radiological protection, side effects, availability, estimation of renal function, follow-up examinations, therapeutic relevance, and cost.

Radiological protection

The 2004 report from the German government ministry for radiological protection describes consistently higher radiological dosages in Germany than in other countries. Radiological doses increased 12% from 1996 to 2001. Increased use of computed tomography was primarily responsible. Indeed, the dosage for this technique is significantly higher than in conventional radiology, even when employing ultra-low-dose protocols. CT methods only offer a relatively small increase in sensitivity and specificity (see above).

Untoward effects

Except for radiological dosage, native CT and plain renal films have no adverse effects. When contrast medium is employed (contrast medium CT and contrast medium infusion urography), contrast medium incidents and renal function deterioration can occur.

Availability

Computed tomography is not widely available, this is especially true for equipment of the latest generation, which is suitable for the diagnosis of ureteral stones. Emergency examinations are problematic in general medical practice. In comparison, sonography and conventional radiology are widely available. This is also demonstrated in a study in the USA in which 203 university clinics and 513 practices were analyzed. Only 44% of the clinics and 13% of practices examined flank pain primarily with computed tomography [1].

Assessment of function

Sonography, plain renal films, and native computed tomography do not assess renal function. Renal function is only evaluated by contrast medium infusion urography and contrast medium tomography.

Follow-up examinations

Principally, it is possible to perform follow-up examinations of ureteral colic with all described imaging techniques. Radiological dose and availability are significantly problematic regarding computed tomography. Often, conventional radiology is performed following initial computed tomography diagnostics. However, comparability often suffers due to the change of method.

Therapeutic relevance

Therapeutic planning is a major aim of imaging techniques. Many interventional methods (extracorporeal shock wave lithotripsy, ureterorenoscopy, percutaneous nephrolithotomy) are managed with conventional radiology. Comparability is definitely at best when the same imaging method is used for diagnosis and therapy. Ultra-low-dose protocols in computed tomography are hampered by reduction of differentiation between non-opaque uric acid stones and other concrements. However, as uric acid stones can be dissolved by medication, this differentiation is of therapeutic relevance.

Costs

Table 1 shows the costs in Euro (€) for various imaging techniques according to the German general fee reference guide (EBM) and the doctors' fee reimbursement guide (GOÄ) (basic factor).

Cost effectiveness

Table 2 shows a semi-quantitative comparison of all described parameter with regard to specific imaging techniques.

Conclusions

Native computed tomography is the method with the greatest accuracy. However, conventional diagnostics are significantly worse in this respect. Radiation dose, costs, and availability promote primarily the use of conventional diagnostics.

Table 1 Costs in Euro (€) for various imaging techniques according to the German general fee reference guide (Einheitlicher Bewertungsmaßstab = EBM) and the doctors' fee reimbursement guide (Gebührenordnung Ärzte = GOÄ) (basic factor)

	EBM	GOÄ
Native CT	101	272
Sonography	14	48
Plain renal film	11	32
Excretory urography including plain renal film	30	63

Other techniques

Magnetic resonance (MR) urogram

Recently, magnetic resonance imaging has been increasingly employed in the diagnosis of obstructive uropathy. Reports have also been published regarding the diagnosis of acute flank pain [31, 32, 38, 39]. However, renal stones are not detected directly but only indirectly by signal loss, and, therefore, cannot be differentiated from blood clots or tumors [31, 38, 39]. Furthermore, smaller stones can resist detection by magnetic resonance [39]. However, indirect signs of stones can indicate calculi (filling defect, non-enhancement following contrast medium administration). Specificity and sensitivity are comparable to those of computed tomography [39] (evidence level IIb).

The major advantage of magnetic resonance is the absence of radiation. Therefore, the method is advantageous in pregnancy. The long examination time, comparatively high costs, and limited availability are disadvantages.

Table 2 Semiquantitative evaluation of imaging techniques

	Sensitivity	Specificity	Radiation dose	Untoward effects	Availability	Function evaluation	Follow-up	Cost	Total
Native CT	+	+	–	+	–	–	–	–	3+
Sonography	(+)	(+)	+	+	+	–	+	+	6+
Plain renal film	–	–	(+)	+	+	–	(+)	+	4+
Excretory urography	(+)	(+)	(+)	–	+	+	–	(+)	4+

Renal function scintigraphy

Renal scintigraphy with determination of MAG3-clearance examines glomerular and tubular function of the individual kidneys. The method plays no role in acute diagnostics of flank pain or urolithiasis. However, it does address therapeutic aspects (for example, renal function of a calculus affected kidney) (evidence level V).

Retrograde (anterograde) ureteropyelography

Contrast medium can be introduced via cystoscopy or nephrostomy into the ureter and the pelvicalyceal system. High contrast density is facilitated independent of renal function and avoiding systemic effects. Compared to native computed tomography, the method is obsolete as a pure diagnostic procedure. However, ureteropyelography can also be performed without prior computed tomography as it is necessary as an imaging technique in ureter catheterization and nephrostomy for renal decompression (for example, febrile infection, postrenal kidney failure, therapeutically refractory pain) (evidence level V).

References

[1] Amis ES Jr. Epitaph for the urogram. Radiology 1999; 213: 639–640
[2] Anfossi E, Eghazarian C, Portier F, Prost J, Ragni E, Daou N, Rossi D. Evaluation of non-enhanced spiral CT in the assessment of renal colic: prospective series of 81 patients. Prog Urol 2003; 13: 29–38
[3] Argyropoulos A, Farmakis A, Doumas K, Lykourinas M. The presence of microscopic hematuria detected by urine dipstick test in the evaluation of patients with renal colic. Urol Res 2004; 32: 294–297
[4] Aytac SK, Ozcan H. Effect of color Doppler system on the twinkling sign associated with urinary tract calculi. J Clin Ultrasound 1999; 27: 433–439
[5] Bellin MF, Renard-Penna R, Conort P, Bissery A, Meric JB, Daudon M, Mallet A, Richard F, Grenier P. Helical CT evaluation of the chemical composition of urinary tract calculi with a discriminant analysis of CT-attenuation values and density. Eur Radiol 2004; 14: 2134–2140
[6] Blandino A, Minutoli F, Scribano E, Vinci S, Magno C, Pergolizzi S, Settineri N, Pandolfo I, Gaeta M. Combined magnetic resonance urography and targeted helical CT in patients with renal colic: A new approach to reduce delivered dose. J Magn Reson Imaging 2004; 20: 264–271
[7] Burgos FJ, Sanchez J, Avila S, Saez JC, Escudero BA. The usefulness of computerized axial tomography (CT) in establishing the composition of calculi. Arch Esp Urol 1993; 46: 383–391
[8] Chateil JF, Rouby C, Brun M, Labessan C, Diard F. Practical measurement of radiation dose in pediatric radiology: use of the dose-area product in digital fluoroscopy and neonatal chest radiographs. J Radiol 2004; 85: 619–625
[9] Chen MY, Zagoria RJ, Saunders HS, Dyer RB. Trends in the use of unenhanced helical CT for acute urinary colic. AJR Am J Roentgenol 1999; 173: 1447–1450
[10] Conkbayir I, Yanik B, Senyucel C, Hekimoglu B. Twinkling artifact in color Doppler ultrasonography: pictorial essay. Tani Girisim Radyol 2003; 9: 407–410
[11] Crowley AR, Byrne JC, Vaughan ED Jr, Marion DN. The effect of acute obstruction on ureteral function. J Urol 1990; 143: 596–599
[12] Dalla PL, Stacul F, Mosconi E, Pozzi MR. Ultrasonography plus direct radiography of the abdomen in the diagnosis of renal colic: still a valid approach? Radiol Med (Torino) 2001; 102: 222–225
[13] de Toledo LS, Martinez-Berganza AT, Cozcolluela CR, Gregorio Ariza MA, Pardina CP, Ripa SL. Doppler-duplex ultrasound in renal colic. Eur J Radiol 1996; 23: 143–148
[14] Denton ER, Mackenzie A, Greenwell T, Popert R, Rankin SC. Unenhanced helical CT for renal colic – is the radiation dose justifiable? Clin Radiol 1999; 54: 444–447
[15] Deveci S, Coskun M, Tekin MI, Peskircioglu L, Tarhan NC, Ozkardes H. Spiral computed tomography: role in determination of chemical compositions of pure and mixed urinary stones – an in vitro study. Urology 2004; 64: 237–240
[16] Eray O, Cubuk MS, Oktay C, Yilmaz S, Cete Y, Ersoy FF. The efficacy of urinalysis, plain films, and spiral CT in ED patients with suspected renal colic. Am J Emerg Med 2003; 21: 152–154
[17] Erwin BC, Carroll BA, Sommer FG. Renal colic: the role of ultrasound in initial evaluation. Radiology 1984; 152: 147–150
[18] Geavlete P, Georgescu D, Cauni V, Nita G. Value of duplex Doppler ultrasonography in renal colic. Eur Urol 2002; 41: 71–78
[19] Greenwell TJ, Woodhams S, Denton ER, Mackenzie A, Rankin SC, Popert R. One year's clinical experience with unenhanced spiral computed tomography for the assessment of acute loin pain suggestive of renal colic. BJU Int 2000; 85: 632–636
[20] Hellerstein S, Duggan E, Welchert E, Mansour F. Serum C-reactive protein and the site of urinary tract infections. J Pediatr 1982; 100: 21–25
[21] Homer JA, Davies-Payne DL, Peddinti BS. Randomized prospective comparison of non-contrast en-

hanced helical computed tomography and intravenous urography in the diagnosis of acute ureteric colic. Australas Radiol 2001; 45: 285–290
22 Kamaya A, Tuthill T, Rubin JM. Twinkling artifact on color Doppler sonography: dependence on machine parameters and underlying cause. AJR Am J Roentgenol 2003; 180: 215–222
23 Knopfle E, Hamm M, Wartenberg S, Bohndorf K. CT in ureterolithiasis with a radiation dose equal to intravenous urography: results in 209 patients. Röfo Fortschr Geb Röntgenstr Neuen Bildgeb Verfahr 2003; 175: 1667–1672
24 Kobayashi T, Nishizawa K, Mitsumori K, Ogura K. Impact of date of onset on the absence of hematuria in patients with acute renal colic. J Urol 2003; 170: 1093–1096
25 Liu W, Esler SJ, Kenny BJ, Goh RH, Rainbow AJ, Stevenson GW. Low-dose non-enhanced helical CT of renal colic: assessment of ureteric stone detection and measurement of effective dose equivalent. Radiology 2000; 215: 51–54
26 Marild S, Wettergren B, Hellstrom M, Jodal U, Lincoln K, Orskov I, Orskov F, Svanborg EC. Bacterial virulence and inflammatory response in infants with febrile urinary tract infection or screening bacteriuria. J Pediatr 1988; 112: 348–354
27 Motley G, Dalrymple N, Keesling C, Fischer J, Harmon W. Hounsfield unit density in the determination of urinary stone composition. Urology 2001; 58: 170–173
28 Muller M, Heicappell R, Steiner U, Merkle E, Aschoff AJ, Miller K. The average dose-area product at intravenous urography in 205 adults. Br J Radiol 1998; 71: 210–212
29 Nakada SY, Hoff DG, Attai S, Heisey D, Blankenbaker D, Pozniak M. Determination of stone composition by non-contrast spiral computed tomography in the clinical setting. Urology 2000; 55: 816–819
30 Newhouse JH, Prien EL, Amis ES Jr, Dretler SP, Pfister RC. Computed tomographic analysis of urinary calculi. AJR Am J Roentgenol 1984; 142: 545–548
31 Paajanen H, Tainio H, Laato M. A chance of misdiagnosis between acute appendicitis and renal colic. Scand J Urol Nephrol 1996; 30: 363–366
32 Patlas M, Farkas A, Fisher D, Zaghal I, Hadas-Halpern I. Ultrasound vs. CT for the detection of ureteric stones in patients with renal colic. Br J Radiol 2001; 74: 901–904
33 Pfister SA, Deckart A, Laschke S, Dellas S, Otto U, Buitrago C, Roth J, Wiesner W, Bongartz G, Gasser TC. Unenhanced helical computed tomography vs. intravenous urography in patients with acute flank pain: accuracy and economic impact in a randomized prospective trial. Eur Radiol 2003; 13: 2513–2520
34 Rao PN. Imaging for kidney stones. World J Urol 2004; 22: 323–327
35 Regan F, Petronis J, Bohlman M, Rodriguez R, Moore R. Perirenal MR high signal – a new and sensitive indicator of acute ureteric obstruction. Clin Radiol 1997; 52: 445–450
36 Rogalla P, Kluner C, Taupitz M. Ultra-low-dose CT to search for stones in kidneys and collecting system. Aktuelle Urol 2004; 35: 307–309
37 Roy C, Tuchmann C, Pfleger D, Guth S, Saussine C, Jacqmin D. Potential role of duplex Doppler sonography in acute renal colic. J Clin Ultrasound 1998; 26: 427–432
38 Sheafor DH, Hertzberg BS, Freed KS, Carroll BA, Keogan MT, Paulson EK, DeLong DM, Nelson RC. Non-enhanced helical CT and US in the emergency evaluation of patients with renal colic: prospective comparison. Radiology 2000; 217: 792–797
39 Sheir KZ, Mansour O, Madbouly K, Elsobky E, Abdel-Khalek M: Determination of the chemical composition of urinary calculi by noncontrast spiral computerized tomography. Urol Res 2005; in press
40 Strohmaier W. Pflege in der Urologie. Stuttgart, W. Kohlhammer, 2002
41 Sudah M, Vanninen R, Partanen K, Heino A, Vainio P, Ala-Opas M. MR urography in evaluation of acute flank pain: T_2-weighted sequences and gadolinium-enhanced three-dimensional FLASH compared with urography. Fast low-angle shot. AJR Am J Roentgenol 2001; 176: 105–112
42 Sudah M, Vanninen RL, Partanen K, Kainulainen S, Malinen A, Heino A, Ala-Opas M. Patients with acute flank pain: comparison of MR urography with unenhanced helical CT. Radiology 2002; 223: 98–105
43 Thomson JM, Glocer J, Abbott C, Maling TM, Mark S. Computed tomography versus intravenous urography in diagnosis of acute flank pain from urolithiasis: a randomized study comparing imaging costs and radiation dose. Australas Radiol 2001; 45: 291–297
44 Tublin ME, Dodd GD III, Verdile VP. Acute renal colic: diagnosis with duplex Doppler US. Radiology 1994; 193: 697–701
45 Van Appledorn S, Ball AJ, Patel VR, Kim S, Leveillee RJ. Limitations of non-contrast CT for measuring ureteral stones. J Endourol 2003; 17: 851–854
46 Wang JH, Lin WC, Wei CJ, Chang CY: Diagnostic value of unenhanced computerized tomography urography in the evaluation of acute renal colic. Kaohsiung J Med Sci 2003; 19: 503–509
47 Yilmaz S, Sindel T, Arslan G, Ozkaynak C, Karaali K, Kabaalioglu A, Luleci E. Renal colic: comparison of spiral CT, US and IVU in the detection of ureteral calculi. Eur Radiol 1998; 8: 212–217
48 Zarse CA, McAteer JA, Tann M, Sommer AJ, Kim SC, Paterson RF, Hatt EK, Lingeman JE, Evan AP, Williams JC Jr. Helical computed tomography accurately reports urinary stone composition using at-

tenuation values: in vitro verification using high-resolution micro-computed tomography calibrated to fourier transform infrared microspectroscopy. Urology 2004; 63: 828–833

[49] Zwergel U, Felgner J, Rombach H, Zwergel T. Current conservative treatment of renal colic: value of prostaglandin synthesis inhibitors. Schmerz 1998; 12: 112–117

Metabolic Evaluation and Metaphylaxis of Stone Disease

M. Straub, A. Hesse

Consensus Statement

Preamble

Worldwide epidemiological data show an increase in prevalence and incidence rates of stone disease. In Germany, for instance, the incidence rate rose during the last decade from 0.54% to 1.47% [34]. In the USA an increase in stone disease of 37% was observed over the last 20 years [76]. The reasons are manifold: lifestyle, dietary habits, and improved medical supply. Today, excellent options for interventional stone therapy, such as ESWL, URS, and PCNL, warrant a comfortable stone management. The new methods are non- or minimally invasive; they can be performed often without general anesthesia in an outpatient setting; only some procedures cause a short hospital stay. It is, therefore, not surprising that stone removal has become more attractive than elaborate metaphylatic measures. In the daily routine, metabolic evaluation and metaphylaxis — which comprises metabolic therapy and secondary prevention of stone disease — have regrettably become less important. On the other hand, we have learned from a lot of other diseases that prevention is superior to intervention. And, in times of financial pressure, it is more cost-effective.

The expert group presents recent concepts in metabolic evaluation of stone disease and metaphylaxis in a consented form. It has to be pointed out that all aspects of the clinical pathways passed the consensus process in the expert group and the plenum of the Speyer Conference and that the paper does not contain any individual opinion. Whenever available evidence from the literature was rated according to the AWMF criteria [49] and included into the concept. Unfortunately, the quality of available references was very inhomogeneous: from double-blinded and randomized trials to case reports. The expert group explicitly regrets the lack of randomized and controlled studies in both the diagnostic and the therapeutic field. Therefore, it is unavoidable that in some cases the given recommendations reflect the opinion of the expert group. The consensus concept considered the EAU Guidelines [79], the results of the 1st International Consultation on Stone Disease (Paris, 2001) and the current literature since 2000. It is at present the most comprehensive and updated review in this field.

Our aim was to compile a concept which is applicable in any clinic or practice. To optimize the acceptance of the recommended diagnostic and therapeutic pathways in the daily routine, a compact program was defined which warrants a high quality standard with a minimum of measures. Deliberately, the expert group excluded such procedures or therapies which represent the expertise of only a few highly specialized stone centers.

Patient selection

Not every patient who passed a stone needs elaborate metaphylactic treatment. More than 50% of all recurrent stone formers have just one recurrence during their lives [78]. In these patients general drinking and nutritional advice is sufficient. If stone disease is highly recurrent and troublesome, specific measures and pharmacological therapy are justified, likewise in patients at high risk (Table **1**). About 10% of the recurrent stone formers develop more than 3 recurrences. The 1st International Consultation on Stone Disease (Paris, 2001) estimated that about 15% of all stone patients require specific metabolic measures for recurrence prevention [26]. In consequence, it is of particular importance to define the risk of stone recurrence in each patient as early as possible.

Consented clinical pathway — diagnostic program

The decision whether a patient needs elaborate metabolic evaluation or not can be facilitated by following the sketched algorithm in Fig. **1**. After stone passage, the patient should be assigned to the low-risk or high-risk group of stone formers.

Table 1 Patients at high risk for recurrent stone disease

Highly recurrent stone formation (≥ 3 stones in 3 years)
Infection stones
Uric acid and urate stones (gout)
Children and teenagers
Genetically determined stones – cystinuria – primary hyperoxaluria – RTA type I – 2,8-dihydroxyadenine – xanthine – cystic fibrosis
Brushite stones
Hyperparathyroidism
Gastrointestinal diseases (Crohn's disease, malabsorption, colitis)
Solitary kidney
Residual stone fragments (3 months after stone therapy)
Nephrocalcinosis
Bilateral vast stone burden
Family history for stone disease

Table 2 The basic evaluation program for stone-formers

Medical history	stone history (former stone events, family history)
	dietary habits
	medication chart
Clinical work-up	physical examination
	ultrasound
Blood analysis	creatinine
	calcium (ionized calcium or total calcium + albumin)
	uric acid
Urine analysis	dipstick test: leukocytes, erythrocytes, nitrite, protein, urine-pH, specific weight
	urine culture

Stone analysis by infrared spectroscopy or X-ray diffraction is an indispensable prerequisite for the correct classification of the patient. Today, stone analysis is a mandatory examination in each stone patient. In a next step the *basic evaluation program* as scheduled in Table **2**

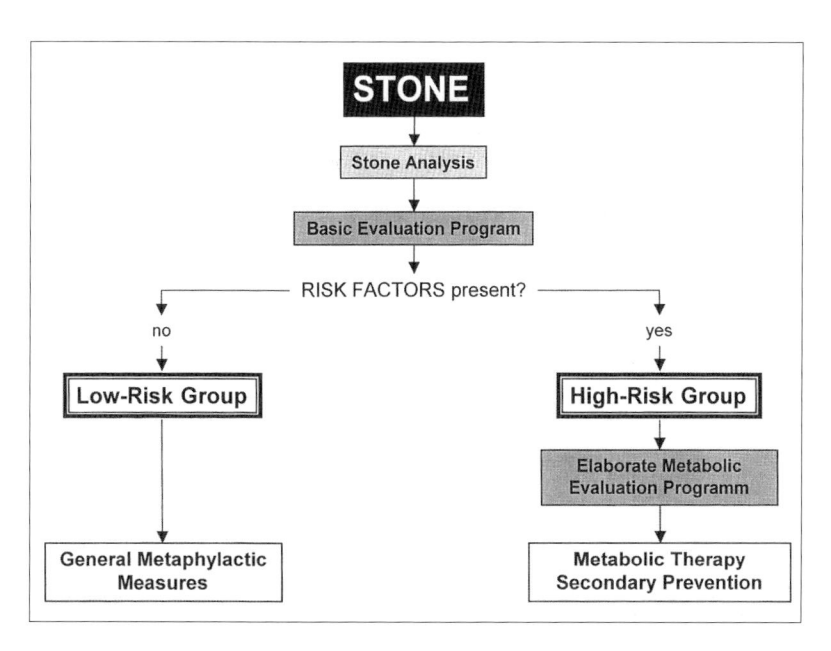

Fig. 1 Current concept (scheme) of the appropriate pathway in metabolic diagnostic and metaphylaxis of stone disease for a patient who passed a stone. If one or more of the risk factors listed in Table **1** is present elaborate metabolic evaluation should be considered.

should be performed to find any severe metabolic risk factors.

Combining the results of the stone analysis and the basic evaluation program, it is possible to detect the high risk stone formers (see Table 1). Only this exactly defined group of patients needs further work-up: the *elaborate metabolic evaluation program*. The recommended diagnostic pathways in the *elaborate metabolic evaluation program* are stone-specific and more complex. This first orientation about the possible causes of stone formation allows us to classify any stone patient
– at low risk or
– at high risk
in regard to the awaited stone recurrence.

Consented clinical pathway — metaphylaxis

All stone-forming patients should be prompted to follow the *general metaphylactic measures* as specified in Table **3,** irrespective to the individual risk state. These measures are targeted basically on the "normalization" of the dietary habits and lifestyle risk factors emerging in the every day life of our western civilizations. To state them in detail: normalization of body weight (BMI), sufficient physical activity, balanced nutrition without excess of any component and sufficient circadian fluid intake would be the appropriate measures to avoid new calculus formation in the majority of stone patients. Anyhow, approximately 15% of the stone formers need additional *specific metaphylactic measures* [26]. An elaborate metabolic evaluation to characterize exactly the metabolic disorder is mandatory to develop an effective custom-made medication regime.

Metabolic Evaluation of a Stone Former

Stone analysis

Stone composition gives information about the potential metabolic disorders behind the "symptom" stone. Thus, it is indispensable to collect the calculi that the patient passed in order to find out the stone components. Generally accepted standard methods in stone analysis are *X-ray diffraction* and *infrared spectroscopy*. Both methods are precise enough to detect stone components in the range of 5–10%. If available, *polarization microscopy* would be the third reliable method, but *de facto* it is performed with expertise only in a few stone centers [33, 35, 39, 52, 67, 72].

Basic evaluation program

The basic evaluation program is a minimum of laboratory investigations to detect severe disorders related with stone formation. Table **2** specifies the program in detail. Exact *medical history* is the first step to discover patients at risk (Table 1) [22]. Then the *clinical work-up* shows, i. e., if the patient is stone-free or not or if her/his urinary tract is obstructed. *Blood analysis* shall find out patients with severe metabolic and organic disorders like renal insufficiency, hyperparathyroidism, or other hypercalcemic states and hyperuricemia. *Urine analysis* at that time will be performed routinely with a dipstick test for demonstration of red cells, white cells, and bacteria (nitrite), and for information on the pH level and specific weight of the urine. In case of signs of infection a urine culture is required.

Table 3 The general metaphylactic measures. Recommendations for stone patients to avoid recurrences

Fluid intake — "drinking advice"	amount: 2.5–3.0 L/day
	circadian drinking
	neutral beverages
	diuresis: 2.0–2.5 L/day
	specific weight of urine < 1.010
Balanced diet — "nutrition advice"	balanced *
	rich in vegetable and fiber
	normal calcium content: 1000–1200 mg/day**
	limited sodium chloride content: 4–5 g/day
	limited animal protein content: 0.8–1.0 g/kg kg/day
Normalized general risk factors — "lifestyle advice"	BMI between 18 and 25 kg/m^2 (target value)
	stress limitation
	adequate physical activity
	balancing of excessive fluid loss

* Avoid excessive consume of vitamin supplements.
** Exception: Patients with absorptive hypercalciuria, calcium excretion ≥ 8 mmol/day.

Elaborate metabolic evaluation program

Preconditions for elaborate laboratory investigations of a stone-former are described in the consensus chapter. Once the necessity for such evaluation is clear, the analytical program depends on the result of the stone analysis. Patients with recurrent stone formation whose calculi were not analyzed require the program "stones with unknown composition" (see Table **12**).

Analytical preconditions

For the analytical work-up the collection of two 24-hour urine samples is the recommended standard, despite other collecting regimes proposed in the literature. The collecting bottles should be either prepared with 5% thymol in isopropyl alcohol (10 mL for a 2-L bottle) or stored at a temperature of 8 °C or less. Immediate urine analysis after completed collection is recommendable to minimize the potential error [39, 59].

Calcium oxalate stones (Table 4)

In case of elevated levels of ionized calcium (or total calcium and albumin), intact parathyroid hormone may confirm the suspected hyperparathyroidism. Constantly acidic values (< pH 6) in the urine pH profile indicate an "acidic arrest" which may promote the co-crystallization of uric acid. Constant alkaline urine (pH > 5.8) in the day profile is a sign of a renal tubular acidosis so far as the urinary tract infection is excluded. The diagnosis of renal tubular acidosis is established with the ammonium chloride loading test. Absorptive hyperoxaluria should be evaluated with the ^{13}C-oxalate absorption test [37, 39, 81, 82].

Calcium phosphate stones (Table 5)

Hyperparathyroidism, renal tubular acidosis, and urinary tract infections must be considered as possible etiology of calcium phosphate stones. Although both minerals contain calcium and phosphate, carbonate apatite and brushite are two totally different stone types. Carbonate apatite crystallization occurs at pH levels ≥ 6.8, it may be infection-associated or form mixed calculi with calcium oxalate. Brushite, however, crystallizes in more acidic and stable urine (opti-

Table **4** Specific evaluation program for calcium oxalate stone-formers

Basic evaluation program +	
Blood analysis	parathyroid hormone (in case of increased calcium levels)
	sodium
	potassium
	chloride
Urine analysis	urine pH profile (measurement after each voiding, minimum 4 times a day)
	24-hour urine sample — 2 collections – volume – urine pH – specific weight – calcium – oxalate – uric acid – citrate – magnesium

Table **5** Specific evaluation program for calcium phosphate stone-formers

Basic evaluation program +	
Blood analysis	parathyroid hormone (in case of increased calcium levels)
	sodium
	potassium
	chloride
Urine analysis	urine pH profile (measurement after each voiding, minimum 4 times a day)
	24-hour urine sample — 2 collections – volume – urine pH – specific weight – calcium – phosphate – citrate

mum pH 6.5–7.2) at high calcium and phosphate concentrations without any relation to urinary tract infections.

Nephrocalcinosis (Table 6)

The causes for nephrocalcinosis are various. Main etiological risk factors are hyperparathyroidism, disorders in vitamin D metabolism, and renal tubular acidosis.

Infection stones (Table 7)

Urinary calculi related with infection are struvite, carbonate apatite, and ammonium urate. Urine culture typically shows infection with urease-producing bacteria, the most important ones are specified in Table **8**. The urease reaction releases bicarbonate and ammonium leading to an alkaline urine pH and facilitating magnesium ammonium phosphate crystallization.

Uric acid and urate stones (Table 9)

Constantly acidic values (< pH 6) in the urine pH profile indicate an "acidic arrest" which promotes the crystallization of uric acid. Hyperuricosuria is the second etiological factor of these stones. Abnormal uric acid excretion occurs in case of dietary excess, endogenous overproduction or catabolic states of the organism. Hyperuricemia may be present, but is not related obliga-

Table 6 Specific evaluation program in patients with nephrocalcinosis

Basic evaluation program +	
Blood analysis	parathyroid hormone (in case of increased calcium levels)
	vitamin D and metabolites
	sodium
	potassium
	chloride
	blood gas analysis
Urine analysis	urine pH profile (measurement after each voiding, minimum 4 times a day)
	24-hour urine sample – 2 collections – volume – urine pH – specific weight – calcium – phosphate – oxalate – uric acid – citrate – magnesium

Table 7 Specific evaluation program for infection stone-formers (struvite)

Basic evaluation program +	
Urine analysis	urine pH profile (measurement after each voiding, minimum 4 times a day)

Table 8 The most important urease-producing (urea-degrading) bacteria

Enterobacter aerogenes
Haemophilus influenzae
Klebsiella
Proteus mirabilis and *P. vulgaris*
Providencia
Pseudomonas
Serratia
Staphylococcus aureus
Ureoplasma urealyticum

Table 9 Specific evaluation program for uric acid- and urate stone-formers

Basic evaluation program +	
Urine analysis	urine pH profile (measurement after each voiding, minimum 4 times a day)
	24-hour urine sample – 2 collections – volume – urine pH – specific weight – uric acid

tory with stone formation. In contrast to uric acid, ammonium urate calculi form in alkaline urine (pH > 6.5). Ammonium urate stones are related with urinary tract infection, malabsorption, and malnutrition.

2,8-Dihydroxyadenine stones and xanthine stones (Table 10)

Both stone types are rare.

2,8-Dihydroxyadenine stones: A genetically determined defect of the adenine phosphoribosyl transferase (APRT) causes a high excretion of poorly soluble 2,8-dihydroxyadenine in urine [36, 85].

Xanthine stones: Markedly decreased levels of serum uric acid are typical for patients forming these stones.

Cystine stones (Table 11)

A genetically determined transport defect for dibasic amino acids leads to an increased excretion of the poorly soluble cystine in urine. Cystine solubility depends strongly on urine pH: at pH 6.0 the limit of solubility amounts to 1.33 mmol/L. In cystineuric patients the daily excretion exceeds 0.8 mmol/day [33, 39].

Stones with unknown composition (Table 12)

Exact *medical history* is the first step to discover risk factors (Table **1**). The *diagnostic imaging* begins with an ultrasound examination of both kidneys to clarify if the patient is stone-free or not. So far as stones are sonographically present, an unenhanced spiral CT should follow to differentiate between calcium-containing and non-calcium calculi based on Houndsfield unit determination. *Blood analysis* shall find out patients with severe metabolic and organic disorders like

Table 10 Specific evaluation program for stone-formers with 2,8-dihydroxyadenine or xanthine calculi.

Basic evaluation program +	
Urine analysis	urine pH profile (measurement after each voiding, minimum 4 times a day)
	24-hour urine sample — 2 collections – volume – urine pH – specific weight – uric acid

Table 11 Specific evaluation program for cystine stone-formers

Basic evaluation program +	
Urine analysis	urine pH profile (measurement after each voiding, minimum 4 times a day)
	24-hour urine sample — 2 collections – volume – urine pH – specific weight – cystine

Table 12 Evaluation program for recurrent stone-formers with unknown stone composition

Medical history	stone history (former stone events, family history)
	dietary habits
	medication chart
Diagnostic imaging	ultrasound
	in case of a suspected stone
	unenhanced helical-CT (including Houndsfield unit determination: information about the possible stone composition)
Blood analysis	creatinine
	calcium (ionized calcium or total calcium + albumin)
	uric acid
Urine analysis	urine pH profile (measurement after each voiding, minimum 4 times a day)
	dipstick test: leukocytes, erythrocytes, nitrite, protein, urine pH, specific weight
	urine culture
	urinary sediment (morning urine)

renal insufficiency, hyperparathyroidism, or other hypercalciemic states and hyperuricemia. *Urine analysis* will be performed routinely with a dipstick test as described above. In case of signs of infection a urine culture is required. Constantly acidic pH values (< pH 6) in the profile indicate an "acidic arrest" which may promote the crystallization of uric acid. Constant alkaline urine (pH > 5.8) in the day profile is a sign of a renal tubular acidosis provided that urinary tract infection is excluded.

Metaphylaxis — Current Concepts

The intention of metaphylaxis is, on the one hand, specific therapy of metabolic disorders and, on the other hand, the prevention of stone recurrence. While the *general metaphylactic measures* are sufficient in low-risk patients, additional stone-specific therapy is needed in the high-risk group.

General metaphylactic measures (see Table 3)

General metaphylaxis targets on the normalization of dietary habits and risk factors due to our modern lifestyle (see consensus section). Optimal urine dilution is very important to avoid crystallization and urines supersaturated with lithogenic substances. The *drinking advice* defines appropriate fluid intake with ≥ 2.5 L/day and urine output with ≥ 2.0 L/day to achieve the goal of sufficient dilution. Circadian drinking is recommended to avoid crucial concentration peaks especially during the night period [11, 20, 23, 31, 56].

The cornerstones of a "stone-neutral" diet are listed in the *nutrition advice*. Particularly, a limited content of sodium chloride and animal protein as well as a normal content of calcium proved to be beneficial. Foods rich in oxalate and purines are disadvantageous [4, 14, 16–18, 21, 38, 41, 53, 56, 74, 83].

Normalization of general risk factors is an important issue in regard of recurrence prevention. Recent studies confirmed that overweight, stress, and inadequate physical activity contribute to the stone risk. Thus in stone-formers a BMI between 18 and 25 kg/m^2 is highly recommended [10, 12, 19, 25, 54, 56, 66, 75].

Stone-specific metaphylaxis

Calcium oxalate stones (Table 13)

Medical management of calcium oxalate stones is complex. For this reason a consequent implementation of the general metaphylactic measures (see Table **3**) in these patients is fundamental. If there is a need for further metabolic correction *alkaline citrates* are the substances of first choice. They exert beneficial effects on hypercalciuric, hyperoxaluric, and hyperuricosuric states. *Thiazides* are the second effective substance class in recurrence prevention of calcium oxalate urolithiasis. But due to the side effects therapy compliance of thiazides in long-term use is moderate. Some patients — those with hyperoxaluria or isolated hypomagesiuria — may benefit from *magnesium* supplementation [1, 6, 13, 27, 28, 40, 43, 44, 46, 48, 58, 62].

Primary hyperoxaluria (Table 14)

The only causal therapy in the management of primary hyperoxaluria remains the simultaneous liver-kidney transplantation. All pharmacological interventions are considered as symptomatic approaches. *Hyperdiuresis*, *alkaline citrates*, and *magnesium* are therapeutic options to avoid the malignant calcium oxalate crystallization process. In some patients *pyridoxine* improves the oxalate levels, but there also exist pyridoxine-resistant forms of the primary hyperoxaluria [2, 15, 45, 50, 51].

Renal tubular acidosis (Table 15)

Despite the alkaline urine, pH alkalization therapy is needed to normalize the metabolic changes (intracellular acidosis) in renal tubular acidosis. In this regard basic therapy is conducted with *alkaline citrates* or *sodium bicarbonate*, respectively. Therapeutic success can be monitored with a venous blood gas analysis. If the excessive calcium excretion (> 8 mmol/day) persists after re-establishing the acid-base equilibrium there is an indication for the additional use of *thiazides* [24, 65, 71].

Table 13 Metaphylaxis of calcium oxalate stones (whewellite, weddellite)

Lithogenic risk factors	Indication for metabolic therapy or specific prevention	Therapeutic or preventive strategy
	General metaphylactic measures	
Hypercalciuria	calcium excretion 5–8 mmol/day	*alkaline citrate* dose: 9–12 g/day alternatively *sodium dicarbonate* dose: 1.5 g 3 × daily
	calcium excretion > 8 mmol/day	*alkaline citrate (primary)* dose: 9–12 g/day *hydrochlorothiazide (secondary)* dose: 25 mg/day initially, up to 50 mg/day
Hypocitraturia	citrate excretion < 2.5 mmol/day	*alkaline citrate* dose: 9–12 g/day
Hyperoxaluria (secondary)	oxalate excretion > 0.5 mmol/day	foods low in oxalate content *calcium* dose: ≥ 500 mg/day with the meals **caution:** calcium excretion! *magnesium* dose: 200–400 mg/d
Hyperuricosuria	uric acid excretion > 4 mmol/day	foods low in purine content *alkaline citrate* dose: 9–12 g/day alternatively *sodium bicarbonate* dose: 1.5 g 3 × daily additionally *allopurinol* dose: 100 mg/day
	hyperuricosuria and hyperuricemia > 380 µmol	*alkaline citrate* additionally *allopurinol* dose: 300 mg/day
Hypomagnesiuria	magnesium excretion < 3.0 mmol/day	*magnesium* dose: 200–400 mg/day **caution:** no magnesium therapy in case of renal insufficiency!

Calcium phosphate stones (Table 16)

Hyperparathyroidism and renal tubular acidosis are common causes of calcium phosphate stone formation. While hyperparathyroidism needs surgical therapy in the majority of cases renal tubular acidosis can be corrected pharmacologically as described above. As far as both disorders are excluded, pharmacotherapy of calcium phosphate calculi is targeted on decreasing effectively urinary calcium levels with *thiazides*. Additionally, there may be an indication for acidification with *L-methionine* if urine pH remains constantly > 6.2. In case of infection-associated calcium phosphate stones the recommendations for "infection stones" should be accessorily considered [8, 30].

80 Metabolic Evaluation and Metaphylaxis of Stone Disease

Table 14 Metaphylaxis of calcium oxalate stones in case of primary hyperoxaluria

Lithogenic risk factors	Indication for metabolic therapy or specific prevention	Therapeutic or preventive strategy
	General metaphylactic measures	
Primary hyperoxaluria (PH)	oxalate excretion > 0.5 mmol/day	urine dilution fluid intake 3–4 L/day *pyridoxine (vitamin B6)* dose: 300 mg/day initially, up to 1 g/day **caution:** regular measurement of urinary oxalate excretion! *alkaline citrate* dose: 9–12 g/day, normal *calcium intake*! *magnesium* dose: 200–400 mg/day **caution:** no magnesium therapy in case of renal insufficiency!

Table 15 Recommended measures to treat renal tubular acidosis type I

Lithogenic risk factors	Indication for metabolic therapy or specific prevention	Therapeutic or preventive strategy
Hypercalciuria	calcium excretion > 8 mmol/day	*alkaline citrate (firstly)* dose: 9–12 g/day alternatively *sodium bicarbonate* dose: 1.5 g 3 × daily *hydrochlorothiazide (secondly)* dose: 25 mg/day initially, up to 50 mg/day
Alkaline urine pH sometimes hyperphosphaturia	balancing of the acid-base equilibrium **caution:** the indication for alkaline citrate therapy is *independent* from urine pH!	

Table 16 Metaphylaxis of calcium phosphate stones* (carbonate apatite, whitlockiter, brushite)

Lithogenic risk factors	Indication for metabolic therapy or specific prevention	Therapeutic or preventive strategy
	Primary exclusion of **renal tubular acidosis** (RTA type I) and **hyperparathyroidism!**	
	General metaphylactic measures	
Alkaline urine pH	urine pH constantly > 6.2	*L-methionine*** dose: 200–500 mg 3 × daily targeted urine pH 5.8–6.2
Hypercalciuria	calcium excretion > 8 mmol/day	*hydrochlorothiazide* dose: 25 mg/day initially, up to 50 mg/day

* Calcium phosphate is a possible component of mixed struvite calculi.
** Caution: In case of renal tubular acidosis L-methionine is contraindicated!

Table 17 Metaphylaxis of infection (struvite) stones*

Lithogenic risk factors	Indication for metabolic therapy or specific prevention	Therapeutic or preventive strategy
	General metaphylactic measures	
Urinary tract infection with urea degrading bacteria	urinary tract infection	adequate *antibiotics*
	urine pH > 7.0	*L-methionine* dose: 200–500 mg 3 × daily targeted urine pH 5.8–6.2

* Struvite calculi can be mixed with carbonate apatite or ammonium urate components.

Table 18 Metaphylaxis of uric acid and ammonium urate stones. Although both calculi contain uric acid the pathogenesis and the therapeutic concepts are totally different

Lithogenic risk factors	Indication for metabolic therapy or specific prevention	Therapeutic or preventive strategy
	Uric acid: general metaphylactic measures	
Urine pH constantly ≤ 6.0	better solubility of uric acid by urine alkalization *metaphylaxis:* targeted urine pH 6.2–6.8 *chemolitholysis:* targeted urine pH 7.0–7.2*	*alkaline citrate* dose: 9–12 g/day alternatively *sodium bicarbonate* dose: 1.5 g 3 × daily
Hyperuricosuria	uric acid excretion > 4 mmol/day	foods low in purine content *Allopurinol* dose: 100 mg/day
	hyperuricosuria und hyperuricemia >380 μmol	*Allopurinol* dose: 300 mg/day **caution:** dose depends on the serum creatinine!
	Ammonium urate****:** general metaphylactic measures	
Urinary tract infection with urea-degrading bacteria	urinary tract infection	adequate *antibiotics*
	urine pH permanently > 6.5	*L-methionine* dose: 200–500 mg 3 × daily targeted urine pH 5.8–6.2
Hyperuricosuria	uric acid excretion > 4 mmol/day	*Allopurinol* dose: 100 mg/day
	hyperuricosuria and hyperuricemia > 380 μmol	*Allopurinol* dose: 300 mg/d **caution:** dose depends on the serum creatinine!

* Chemolitholysis requires high fluid intake for an effective dilution of the urine.
** Causes for the formation of ammonium urate calculi are either urinary tract infections or malabsorption and malnutrition.

Infection stones (Table 17)

Infection stones and urinary tract infections with urease-producing bacteria are a vicious circle. The therapeutic principles to overcome this problem are total stone clearance, appropriate antibiotic therapy, sufficient urine dilution, and the adjustment of an acidic urine pH. Long-term urine acidification seems to be more difficult to achieve than alkalization. Licensed for this indication is only *L-methionine*. The benefit of urease inhibitors like *acetohydroxamic acid* remains controversially discussed, in Germany the substance is not approved [42, 69].

Uric acid and ammonium urate stones (Table 18)

Uric acid crystals form in an acidic urine at high uric acid levels. Therefore, it is important to keep urine pH at alkaline levels between 6.2 and 6.8 for recurrence prevention. Chemolitholysis requires urine pH levels adjusted between 7.0 and 7.2. Either *alkaline citrates* or *sodium bicarbonate* can be used to achieve this goal. *Allopurinol* is helpful to reduce uric acid levels. By inhibiting the xanthine oxidase allopurinol lowers uric acid production [61, 64, 68, 70, 73, 84].

Ammonium urate stones form under totally different conditions. They are frequently associated with infections. Apart from allopurinol, urine acidification with *L-methionine* showed beneficial effects in recurrence prevention [55].

Cystine stones (Table 19)

The main stay of treatment for cystine stones consists of maintaining urine pH above 7.5 to improve cystine solubility and appropriate hydration with a minimum of 3.5 L/day in adults to achieve optimal dilution. Additionally, free cystine concentration can be decreased by reductive substances, splitting the disulfide bonding in the molecule. *Tiopronin* is today the best substance available for this indication. But the side effects and adverse events often lead to a poor patient compliance — especially in long-term use. *Ascorbic acid*, used at cystine excretions < 3 mmol/day, has limited reductive power; its capacity to lower urinary cystine levels is about 20%. Therefore, its effectiveness and use are a matter of debate. The results concerning *Captopril* are controversial: it is perhaps a second line option [3, 5, 7, 9, 29, 32, 47, 57, 60, 63, 77, 80].

Table 19 Metaphylaxis of cystine stones

Lithogenic risk factors	Indication for metabolic therapy or specific prevention	Therapeutic or preventive strategy
	General metaphylactic measures	
pH dependent solubility of cystine	better solubility of cystine by urine alkalization urine pH — optimal 7.5 – 8.5	urine dilution daily fluid intake 3.5–4 L alkaline citrate dose: according to urine pH alternatively: sodium bicarbonate dose: according to urine pH
	cystine excretion < 3.0–3.5 mmol/day	optional: ascorbic acid dose: 3–5 g/d effervescent tablets or Tiopronin dose: 250 mg/d initially, max. 1–2 g/day
	cystine excretion > 3.0–3.5 mmol/day	obligate: Tiopronin dose: 250 mg/d initially, increase to 250 mg 3 × daily, maximal dose 2 g/day **caution:** tachyphylaxy possible!

References

1. Abdulhadi MH, Hall PM, Streem SB. Can citrate therapy prevent nephrolithiasis? Urology 1993; 41: 221–224
2. Allen AR, Thompson EM, Williams G, Watts RW, Pusey CD. Selective renal transplantation in primary hyperoxaluria type 1. Am J Kidney Dis 1996; 27: 891–895
3. Asper R, Schmucki O. Cystinuria therapy by ascorbic acid. Urol Int 1982; 37: 91–109
4. Assimos DG, Holmes RP. Role of diet in the therapy of urolithiasis. Urol Clin North Am 2000; 27: 255–268
5. Barbey F, Joly D, Rieu P, Mejean A, Daudon M, Jungers P. Medical treatment of cystinuria: critical reappraisal of long-term results. J Urol 2000; 163: 1419–1423
6. Barcelo P, Wuhl O, Servitge E, Rousaud A, Pak CY: Randomized double-blind study of potassium citrate in idiopathic hypocitraturic calcium nephrolithiasis. J Urol 1993; 150: 1761–1764
7. Berio A, Piazzi A. Prophylaxis of cystine calculosis by alpha-mercaptopropionyl-glycine administered continuously or every other day. Boll Soc Ital Biol Sper 2001; 77: 35–41
8. Bilobrov VM, Chugaj AV. Physicochemical background for ambiguity of clinical recommendations in treating phosphate nephrolithiasis. Urol Int 1993; 50: 43–46
9. Birwe H, Schneeberger W, Hesse A. Investigations of the efficacy of ascorbic acid therapy in cystinuria. Urol Res 1991; 19: 199–201
10. Blacklock NJ. The pattern of urolithiasis in the Royal Navy in: Proceedings of the stone research symposium. Hodgkinson A, Nordin BE (eds), London, Churchill, 1969, p 33
11. Borghi L, Meschi T, Amato F, Briganti A, Novarini A, Giannini A. Urinary volume, water and recurrences in idiopathic calcium nephrolithiasis: a 5-year randomized prospective study. J Urol 1996; 155: 839–843
12. Borghi L, Meschi T, Amato F, Novarini A, Romanelli A, Cigala F. Hot occupation and nephrolithiasis. J Urol 1993; 150: 1757–1760
13. Borghi L, Meschi T, Guerra A, Novarini A. Randomized prospective study of a nonthiazide diuretic, indapamide, in preventing calcium stone recurrences. J Cardiovasc Pharmacol 1993; 22 (Suppl 6): S78–S86
14. Borghi L, Schianchi T, Meschi T, Guerra A, Allegri F, Maggiore U, Novarini A. Comparison of two diets for the prevention of recurrent stones in idiopathic hypercalciuria. N Engl J Med 2002; 346: 77–84
15. Cochat P, Gaulier JM, Koch Nogueira PC, Feber J, Jamieson NV, Rolland MO, Divry P, Bozon D, Dubourg L. Combined liver-kidney transplantation in primary hyperoxaluria type 1. Eur J Pediatr 1999; 158 (Suppl 2): S75–S80
16. Curhan GC. Dietary calcium, dietary protein, and kidney stone formation. Miner Electrolyte Metab 1997; 23: 261–264
17. Curhan GC, Curhan SG. Dietary factors and kidney stone formation. Compr Ther 1994; 20: 485–489
18. Curhan GC, Willett WC, Knight EL, Stampfer MJ. Dietary factors and the risk of incident kidney stones in younger women: Nurses' Health Study II. Arch Intern Med 2004; 164: 885–891
19. Curhan GC, Willett WC, Rimm EB, Speizer FE, Stampfer MJ. Body size and risk of kidney stones. J Am Soc Nephrol 1998; 9: 1645–1652
20. Curhan GC, Willett WC, Rimm EB, Spiegelman D, Stampfer MJ. Prospective study of beverage use and the risk of kidney stones. Am J Epidemiol 1996; 143: 240–247
21. Curhan GC, Willett WC, Rimm EB, Stampfer MJ. A prospective study of dietary calcium and other nutrients and the risk of symptomatic kidney stones. N Engl J Med 1993; 328: 833–838
22. Curhan GC, Willett WC, Rimm EB, Stampfer MJ. Family history and risk of kidney stones. J Am Soc Nephrol 1997; 8: 1568–1573
23. Curhan GC, Willett WC, Speizer FE, Stampfer MJ. Beverage use and risk for kidney stones in women. Ann Intern Med 1998; 128: 534–540
24. Domrongkitchaiporn S, Khositseth S, Stitchantrakul W, Tapaneya-olarn W, Radinahamed P. Dosage of potassium citrate in the correction of urinary abnormalities in pediatric distal renal tubular acidosis patients. Am J Kidney Dis 2002; 39: 383–391
25. Ekeruo WO, Tan YH, Young MD, Dahm P, Maloney ME, Mathias BJ, Albala DM, Preminger GM. Metabolic risk factors and the impact of medical therapy on the management of nephrolithiasis in obese patients. J Urol 2004; 172: 159–163
26. Esen T, Marshall VR, Rao N, Ettinger B. Medical Management of Urolithiasis. In: Stone Disease, 1st ed. Segura JW, Conort P, Khoury S, Pak CY, Preminger GM, Tolley D (eds), Paris, Health Publications, 2003, chap. 4, pp 133–149
27. Ettinger B, Citron JT, Livermore B, Dolman LI. Chlorthalidone reduces calcium oxalate calculous recurrence but magnesium hydroxide does not. J Urol 1988; 139: 679–684
28. Ettinger B, Pak CY, Citron JT, Thomas C, Adams-Huet B, Vangessel A. Potassium-magnesium citrate is an effective prophylaxis against recurrent calcium oxalate nephrolithiasis. J Urol 1997; 158: 2069–2073
29. Fjellstedt E, Denneberg T, Jeppsson JO, Tiselius HG. A comparison of the effects of potassium citrate and sodium bicarbonate in the alkalinization of urine in homozygous cystinuria. Urol Res 2001; 29: 295–302
30. Gault MH, Parfrey PS, Robertson WG. Idiopathic calcium phosphate nephrolithiasis. Nephron 1988; 48: 265–273

Pediatric Aspects of Nephrolithiasis and Nephrocalcinosis

B. Beck, B. Hoppe

Introduction

Different incidence and etiological factors were reported in children with urolithiasis, reflecting differences in geographic, genetic and socio-economic background as well as source of the series and study design. The incidence of urolithiasis in childhood is believed to be roughly 10% of that in adults, although a significant part of the patients remains un- or misdiagnosed (incidental discovery reported in 15–40%), therefore figures should be interpreted with caution. About 40% of children with urolithiasis have a positive family history of kidney stones.

Pediatric nephrolithiasis differs substantially with regard to etiological factors, symptoms, imaging techniques, and treatment from that in adults. Any physician involved in the management of pediatric stone disease should be familiar with these aspects.

Metabolic abnormalities account for 25–86% in recent pediatric nephrolithiasis series [3], having surpassed infective causes. Urolithiasis in children after renal transplantation is increasingly reported and more frequent than in adult kidney recipients. Stones can develop as early as the neonatal period and there is good reason for every child with nephrolithiasis to undergo a full metabolic screening.

The term nephrocalcinosis (NC) refers to an increased crystal deposition within the cortex or medulla of the kidney. NC occurs either alone or in combination with calculi. The true incidence of NC is unknown. The diagnosis is made by renal ultrasound. Cortical NC (e.g., in acute cortical necrosis, chronic glomerulonephritis, and chronic graft rejection) and focal NC (e.g., in tuberculosis, abnormal vasculature, and tumors like nephroblastoma) are rarely seen in children. Speaking of NC in childhood usually refers to medullary or diffuse nephrocalcinosis. Medullary NC is well described in preterm neonates with a reported incidence rate of 10–65% and has to be differentiated from physiologically increased echogenicity of the preterm kidney (see Figs. **1a–e**). Risk factors include low birth weight, diuretic therapy, corticosteroids, and parental nutrition. Almost all preterm infants show a marked hypocitraturia within the first weeks of life, an important risk factor often disregarded. NC apart from prematurity is usually a consequence of metabolic disorders like renal tubular acidosis, primary hyperoxaluria, idiopathic hypercalciuria, and other genetic disorders including Dent's disease and Bartter's syndrome (see Table **3** for details).

Obtaining a thorough medical history followed by a careful physical examination seems to have become a lost art but is indispensable for early and correct diagnosis. Always obtain information on family history of renal (stones, renal failure, hematuria) and metabolic diseases (draw a pedigree). Pay particular attention to nutrition, fluid intake, medications (vitamin D/A, steroids, diuretics, etc.), and mineral supplementation. Children with chronic bowel disease (e.g., Crohn's disease, cystic fibrosis, s.p. bowel resection), neurological disorders (anticonvulsant drugs, low fluid intake), and anomalies of the urinary tract predisposing to urine stasis and UTI (neurogenic bladder, ileal loops, megaureter) are at special risk for stone formation.

Presentation

Surprisingly about half of the children with stones do not have pain or it is not the presenting feature. The younger the child the less specific can be the clinical manifestation compared with the more uniform presentation of colicky loin pain in older children and adults. Symptoms ranging from only slight abdominal discomfort to diffuse abdominal pain with nausea and vomiting or frank colic are observed. Therefore urolithiasis is more frequently found than suspected in younger children.

Although urinary tract infections (UTI) account for up to 40% of stones, a past history of UTI does not necessarily mean the calculi are of an infective nature. A history of recurrent UTI or hematuria, however, should always raise suspicion of possible stone disease and warrants further evaluation.

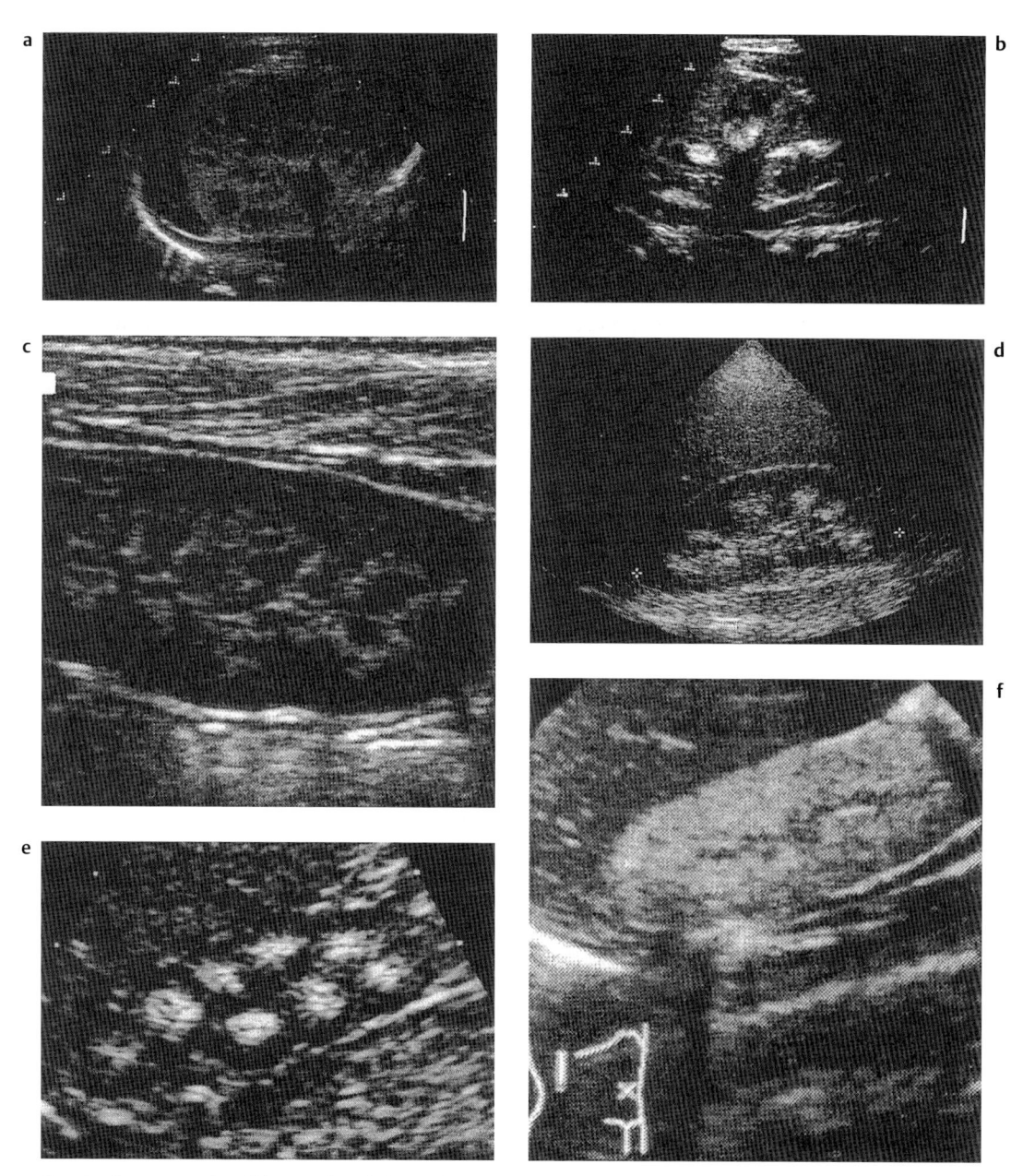

Figs. 1a–f a Normal, still hyperechoic kidney of a preterm infant. b Tamm-Horsefall kidney. c Medullary nephrocalcinosis (NC) grade I (mild echogenicity ↑ around pyramidal border. d Medullary NC grade II (mild echogenicity ↑ whole pyramid). e Medullary NC grade III (more severe echogenicity entire pyramid). f Diffuse corticomedullary NC.

Sole nephrocalcinosis is usually asymptomatic and sometimes reported as an incidental finding. An underlying metabolic disorder should be suspected when polydypsia, polyuria, bone pain, metabolic acidosis or alkalosis, rickets, growth or developmental retardation, hypertension, and chronic renal insufficiency are obvious.

Imaging

Ultrasound (US) imaging represents the method of choice for presumed or known urolithiasis. If no calculi can be detected ultrasound examination should be repeated under better hydration (infravesical stone) and, if needed, bowel preparation. Performed with dedication, sonography allows visualization of renal, ureteral, and bladder stones down to 2 mm in size in most cases. Additionally, it allows detection of present NC or pyelonephritis, gives valuable information about the anatomy and function of the genitourinary tract, and identifies non-urologic pathology within the abdomen mimicking stone disease. For lower radiation exposure abdominal flat plate (KUB) X-ray is preferred over IVP and CT despite its known limitations (non-opaque uric acid, xanthine and less opaque cystine stones).

Although popular among urologists intravenous pyelography (IVP) is rarely needed and considered obsolete as a routine investigation in children. It usually provides little additional information even for the operative management compared with state of the art US.

CT scans of the abdomen seem to provide the best sensitivity and specificity for detection of stones, but series comparing CT to ultrasonography performed by pediatric radiologists are lacking. Supposed superiority is a poor excuse for exposing children to unnecessary radiation hazards and sonography must not be routinely substituted by CT. Also keep in mind that small children require sedation even for short examination times.

Low-dose non-enhanced helical CT is an option for older children with presumed symptomatic stone disease if ultrasound analysis is inconclusive.

Initial Metabolic Evaluation

Capture stone for stone analysis and culture. Perform urinalysis with pH day profile (pH meter), urine culture and sediment (crystals?). If applicable analyze 24-h urine for calcium, oxalate, citrate, uric acid, sodium, phosphorus, magnesium, cystine, creatinine, volume, specific weight, osmolality, protein, and, if positive, tubular proteinuria (e. g., retinol-binding protein).

Serum: Complete blood count, electrolytes, calcium, BUN, creatinine, uric acid, calcium,

Table 1 Normal values for 24-h urine collection (container needs to be preserved with either thymol 5 % in isopropyl alcohol or 2 N HCl). Repeat collection after stone has been captured, as ongoing stone formation may diminish lithogenic excretion parameters. Check urine volume and creatinine excretion (2 mg/kg ± 0.8 mg) to ensure adequate collection [1]

Parameter	Age	Normal Value	Remarks
Calcium	All ages	< 4 mg/kg/day (< 0.1 mmol/kg/day)	see Table 3
Oxalate	< 10 years > 10 years	< 0.37 mmol (< 33 mg)/1.73 m^2/day < 0.50 mmol (< 45 mg)/1.73 m^2/day	consider PH I/II for constant excessive elevation, see below
Citrate	male female	> 1.9 mmol (> 3300 mg)/ 1.73 m^2/day > 1.6 mmol (> 2800 mg)/ 1.73 m^2/day	hypocitraturia: metabolic acidosis, hypokalemia, calcineurin inhibitors
Uric acid	all ages	< 0.12 mmol (< 20 mg)/kg/day	hyperuricosuria = check diet, medication, tumor lysis, inborn errors of metabolism
Magnesium		0.07 ± 0.03 mmol (1.6 ± 0.8 mg)/kg/day	consider FFHNC with hypomagnesemia and elevated FE$_{Mg}$
Phosphorus		12–38 mmol/1.73 m^2/day	
Cystine	<10 years > 10 years adults	< 55 µmol (13 mg)/1.73 m^2/d < 200 µmol (48 mg) < 250 µmol (60 mg)	enhance cystine dissolution by adjusting urine pH > 7.5; check morning urine for hexagonal crystals

phosphorus, intact PTH, alkaline phosphatase, venous blood gases.

Therapy

The basic principles for acute treatment of uncomplicated stones (hydration, analgesia) and complicated stones (de-obstruction of the urinary tract, i.v. antibiotics) apply to all age groups, but successful management of pediatric stone disease requires one to rock the boat and move the stones. Always think of "non-urologic" diseases in children presenting with (recurrent) calculi and/or nephrocalcinosis and look for sometimes subtle clinical clues (failure to thrive, mental retardation, chronic renal insufficiency, cataracts, and relevant electrolyte disturbance etc. can never be explained by urolithiasis alone). Keep in mind that the patient and his parents like many physicians may not be aware of the linkage between stones and metabolic or genetic disorders. Consult with a pediatric nephrologist urgently before signs of chronic failure are present. Early diagnosis of inborn errors of metabolism is of paramount importance and makes all the difference between excellent and disastrous patient care. Use a stepwise approach with patient/parent education and dietary modification (diet/dietary restrictions, fluid intake) as the backbone of therapy. Only the well informed patient will comply with your therapy and avoid episodes of dehydration. With inadequate hydration most of your pharmacological therapy will be useless. Initiate pharmacological intervention directly for severe stone disease (e. g., primary hyperoxaluria type I) or add on later in case of refractory milder disease. Treatment plans should be tailored to the underlying disease, identified individual risk factors, and patient needs (age, comorbid conditions), respectively. A detailed discussion on therapeutic interventions is beyond the scope of this chapter, please refer to [1, 2] for details.

Resist the temptation to apply extracorporeal

Table 2 Normal values for spot urine samples: creatinine ratios (solute/creatinine). Ratios are more error-prone than timed samples. Interpret with respect to daytime, relation to meals, diet, medication, and age [1]

Parameter	Age	Ratio solute/creatinine		Remarks
		mol/mol	mg/mg	
Calcium	< 12 months	< 2	0.15–0.81	ratio↑ after meals up to 40%; higher Ca excretion with breast milk feeding; diuretics, immobilization, corticosteroids
	1–3 years	< 1.5	0.53	
	1–5 years	< 1.1	0.39	
	5–7 years	< 0.8	0.28	
	> 7 years	< 0.6	0.21	
		mmol/mol	mg/g	
Oxalate	0–6 months	< 325–360	288–260	consider PH I/II for constant excessive elevation; check also urinary glycolate, L-glycerate, and plasma oxalate; higher oxalate excretion with formula feeding
	7–24 months	< 132–174	110–139	
	2–5 years	< 98–101	80	
	5–14 years	< 70–82	60–65	
	> 16 years	< 40	32	
		mol/mol	g/g	
Citrate	0–5 years	> 0.25	0.42	low with tubular dysfunction: RTA, prematurity, hypokalemia, renal transplantation
	> 5 years	> 0.15	0.25	
		mg/dL per GFR		
Uric acid	> 2 years	< 0.56 (ratio × plasma creatinine)		excretion substantially higher throughout childhood than in adults; < 2 years: no reliable data

Table 3 Disorders of special interest to the general urologist presenting with urolithiasis and/or nephrocalcinosis

Disorder (defect if known)	Characteristics/hallmark
Idiopathic hypercalcuria, genetic (renal)/environmental (absorptive)	most common cause of normocalcemic hypercalciuria; not influenced/influenced by Ca intake; considerable overlap
Hypercalcemic hypercalcuria	hyperparathyroidism, malignancy, hypervitaminosis D/A, hypophosphatasia, immobilization, hyperthyroidism, sarcoidosis, adrenal insufficiency, corticosteroid excess
Normocalcemic hypercalciuria	renal tubular acidosis, furosemide, hyperalimentation, juvenile rheumatoid arthritis, hypophosphatemia, FFHNC
Primary hyperoxaluria type I (PH I) (AGT; autosomal recessive)	urinary oxalate + glycolate ↑, plasma oxalate ↑; infantile type: early nephrocalcinosis and rapid renal failure childhood type: recurrent urolithiasis and renal failure even siblings with identical mutations may be clinically heterogeneous
Primary hyperoxaluria type II (PH II) (GRHPR; autosomal recessive)	urinary oxalate + L-glycerate ↑, plasma oxalate ↑; phenotype less severe and less common than PH I; present in second to third decade of life with recurrent urolithiasis, renal failure in about 12%; pyridoxine is ineffective in (proven) PH II
Secondary (enteric) hyperoxaluria in malabsorption syndromes	inflammatory bowel disease (e. g., Crohn's disease), cystic fibrosis, resection of small bowel, malabsorption of fat and bile acids (e. g., a-betalipoproteinemia), calcium restricted diets
Renal tubular acidosis (RTA) (rule out secondary causes: hepatic/metabolic/autoimmune disorders)	distal RTA (type I) metabolic acidosis, inability to acidify urine below pH 6.1, hypokalemia, failure to thrive nephrolithiasis/nephrocalcinosis; proximal RTA (type II) metabolic acidosis and urinary bicarbonate wasting, nephrocalcinosis; correct acidosis with alkali citrate (Shohl's solution)
Dent's disease (CLCN5; X-linked)	Fanconi syndrome (hypercalcuria, LMW-proteinuria, glycosuria, aminoaciduria, phosphaturia), nephrocalcinosis may progress to renal failure
Cystinuria (autosomal recessive)	urinary cystine (and other dibasic amino acids) excretion ↑ urine microscopy hexagonal cystine crystals
– type A (SLC3A1)	
– type B (SLC7A1)	cystine stones are poorly fragmented by ESWL
type AB (SLC3A1/SLC7A1)	
Bartter's syndrome (NKCC2, ROMK, CLCNKB)	hypokalemia with hypochloremic metabolic alkalosis, hypercalciuria, nephrocalcinosis
Williams-Beuren syndrome	mental retardation, "happy party manner," aortic stenosis, "Elfin faces," nephrocalcinosis, hypercalcemia
Premature neonate	nephrocalcinosis, hypocitraturia nephrocalcinosis persists in 15–50% beyond infancy
Hyperuricosuria	serum uric acid ↑ secondary to excessive protein intake, ketogenic diet (for seizure control), myeloproliferative disorders, inborn errors of metabolism (type I glycogen storage disease, Lesch-Nyhan syndrome), cystic fibrosis and pancreatic enzyme supplementation, secondary to uricosuric drugs, high-dose aspirin/vitamin C (?)
Xanthinuria (xanthine oxidase)	urinary xanthine ↑, 50% show stone formation in childhood, normal to low plasma urate level; neonatal seizures in combination with other defective molybdenum-dependent enzymes; urine sediment of orange/brown color
Familial hypomagnesemia and hypercalciuria syndrome (FFHNC) (paracellin-I; autosomal recessive)	hypercalciuria, low serum magnesium and increased fractional excretion of Mg (FE_{Mg}); nephrocalcinosis may progress to renal failure
Adenine-phosphoribosyl-transferase (APRT) deficiency	urinary 2,8-dihydroxyadenine ↑; recurrent crystalluria (round + brown), urolithiasis, rarely renal failure from crystal nephropathy

shock wave lithotripsy (ESWL) to patients with nephrocalcinosis with or without present calculi, it may prove harmful.

References

1. Leumann E, Hoppe B. Urolithiasis in childhood. In: Therapeutic Strategies in Children with Renal Disease, Proesmanns W (ed), Bailliere's Clinical Pediatrics, London, Vol 5, 1997, pp 655–674
2. Stapleton FB. Clinical approach to children with urolithiasis. Seminars in Nephrology 1996; 3: 116–124
3. Van't Hoff WG. Aetiological factors in paediatric urolithiasis. Nephron Clin Pract 2004; 98: c45–c48

Energy Application for Non-Surgical Urological Therapies

Consensus

S. Thüroff (Chairman), R. Berges, A. Blana, M. Braun, B. Brehmer, A. Häcker, R. Muschter, S. Neubauer, S. Thüroff, U. Witzsch, Ch. Chaussy

Comment

The working group faced a large number of therapeutic applications in urology for different therapeutic goals and different organs (Section VIII), typically treated by urologists. The variety of different energies, applications, and organs did not allow in the predetermined time a differentiated analysis of each current application, its special technical progress, and its validity within all other applications for each disease or its general acceptance in urology. The working group decided initially as consensus to analyze in this session the current status of "alternative energies/techniques" in Germany (Section I), to present systematically the common characteristics in development of new technologies, to present an outlook to the future development (Section V) of these technologies and to conclude with the formulation of a consensus statement (Section VI). It was obvious and it is typical that especially new technologies take an individual development and have a different recognition in different countries (Section IV). It was not possible to analyze the situation of these technologies in other countries. The statements of this working group are formulated by German urologists and are based on their experience with the technologies (Section VI). As the status of development within the individual technologies in a country depends much on reimbursement and activities of single companies within that country the individual foreign situation seems to be too different to be analyzed and evaluated by a German group. As most of the participants have experience in more than one of these technologies (Section VII), their special input for the technology used within the last five years was considered to be integrated in the discussion. Furthermore, most participants prepared articles on selected topics which show the current status, side effects and results of the individual technology in their hands. For technologies which are already out of the experimental single center application (Section V: **/***) the experts were given more space to report — in regard to public interest — their experiences.

(I) General Indications in Different Pathologies for the Application of "Alternative Technologies"

Prostate cancer

Indications

Cases not suitable for surgery because of high risk, comorbidity, psychological/religious reasons. Localized, palliative or recurrent prostate cancer, or prostatic TCC.

Technique

- **HIFU** all not surgical cases — standardized
- **LDR Brachy** all not surgical cases — standardized
- **CRYO** localized low Gleason + low vol Pca — standardized
- **HDR Brachy** only in combination with external radiation — standardized
- **PDT laser** — experimental
- **Thermo lase** — obsolete

Kidney cancer

Indications

Surgical organ preservation difficult/risky (fear of dialysis): patients preference. Treatment of organ metastasis.

Technique

- TCC
    - Cryo (only 3rd generation,
      Sono + template guided)   not standardized
    - RFA (~ 300 treatments
      have been done)   not standardized
    - HIFU   experimental
    - Thermo laser   experimental
    - Microwave/magnetic rods   experimental
- RCC
    - Thermo laser   experimental

Prostate adenoma

Indications

Alternative to permanent oral medication, LUTS, bladder neck obstruction, high-risk patients with wish for catheter withdrawal, non-bacterial prostatitis.

Technique

- **PLFT/Prostalund®**   standardized
- **TUNA**   standardized
- Laser
    - PVP/green light   still not standardized
    - ILC/Nd:YAG/Ho:YAG/
      Diode/Hol:FP   not standardized
    - VLAP/contact VAP   obsolete
    - E-VAP/WIT/Hyperthermia/
      HIFU/Cryo /LE-TUMT   obsolete

(II) Criteria for the General Distribution and Application of a New Technology

- CE marked technology.
- Standardization of application and teaching (knowledge transfer).
- Reproducibility of results and side effects.

(III) Quality Criteria for New Technologies

- Independence of reimbursement.
- External quality control (university/annual meetings).
- Transparent development and definition of therapy goal.
- Transparent follow-up, registration and publication of data.
- Benchmarking with other technique users (via www).
- Unselected publication and reporting (avoiding of spind-doctors).

(IV) Common Problems for Introduction and/or Development of New Technologies/Therapies

- Borderline detection between treated/untreated tissue.
- Missing optical marker for targeting and control.
- Technology's name "once for ever" connected to initial problems in application, side effects, or results.
- Development phase is misunderstood as "applicative learning curve".
- Conservative monopolistic thinking of opinion leaders do not encourage it.
- Borderline between established and "unserious" medicine.
- Carrier contraproductive: long R&D time.
- Unclear recognition process, not a standardized procedure in Germany.
- High costs for R&D, company and clinicians (no reimbursement under R&D).
- Dilemma between patient's wish and reimbursement.
- Integrated economy (costs/diagnosis/lifetime) still not considered today.
- No standardization of clinical development (parallel actions) and positive selection of published data.

(V) Future of Current Technologies

- Low-dose Brachy (LDR)
    - prostate cancer   ***
    - kidney cancer   o
    - prostate adenoma   o
- High-dose Brachy (HDR)
    - prostate cancer   **
    - kidney cancer   o
    - prostate adenoma   o
- Thermo rods
    - prostate cancer   *
    - kidney cancer   o
    - prostate adenoma   o
- Cryotherapy
    - prostate cancer   ***
    - kidney cancer   *
    - prostate adenoma   o
- Focused Ultrasound (HIFU)
    - prostate cancer   ***
    - kidney cancer   *
    - prostate adenoma   o

- Microwave therapy (TUMT)
  - prostate cancer °
  - kidney cancer °
  - prostate adenoma **
- Radiofrequency (RFA) b
  - prostate cancer °
  - kidney cancer *
  - prostate adenoma °
- Laser therapy
  - prostate cancer *
  - kidney cancer °
  - prostate adenoma **

Key: ° = No future; * = experimental, future development possible but uncertain; ** = proven efficacy, question of market; *** = high potential, "alternative" to classical therapies.

(VI) Consensus Statements

- Established treatment modalities are surgical or radiological interventions.
- "Alternative" treatment modalities are using alternatively applied and controlled energies (hand-guided scalpel versus computer-guided new technologies).
- "Alternative therapies" do not yet have a profound study base to be named even "alternative" in the sense of equi-effectiveness by their results.
- The status of "experimental work" in some mentioned new technologies – which have been in clinical use in some cases since more than 10 years – has already been left behind, some others are not standardized or are still experimental.
- Treatment goal for new technologies is to close therapeutic gaps between "established therapies" or to treat with equi-effectiveness but with less morbidity or costs.
- Long-term results, high quality EBM-based studies are lacking in most technologies to bring these new technologies up to an "established" level.
- Reproducibility of technology, application, knowledge transfer, transparent and not selective publication and reference is necessary.
- Energy control and highly precise energy application are more important than energy type of a technology.
- In oncology, tumor stages influence outcome more than technology. Do not compare data which are not tumor-related.
- Applicator's size or special form limits its use in the approach to a tumor.
- Borderline problems in long-term evaluation of results and development process with its problems are identical for all new techniques/technologies.

(VII) Participants Main Specialization

Participant	Technology	Kidney cancer	Prostate cancer	Prostate adenoma
Berges	TUMT			X
Blana	HIFU		X	
Braun	CRYO		X	
Brehmer	HIFU, RFA, CRYO	X	X	
Häcker	HIFU	X	X	
Muschter	LASER	X	X	X
Neubauer	LDR+HDR BRACHY		X	
Thüroff	HIFU, TUMT		X	X
Witzsch	HIFU, CRYO	X	X	

(VIII) Treatment Targets for Current Technologies

Technology	Kidney	Prostate	Seminal vesicles	Lymph nodes
HIFU	X	X	X	
CRYO	X	X	X	
RFA	X	X		
LASER	X	X		
MICROWAVE		X		
BRACHY	X	X		
RADIATION		X	X	X
SURGERY	X	X	X	X

Technical Principles of High Intensity Focused Ultrasound (HIFU)

A. Blana, A. Häcker

Introduction

Ultrasound is an acoustic mechanical wave that propagates within a medium. For diagnostic ultrasound scans low output powers are used. By focusing high energy ultrasound beams on a target area in the tissue, mechanical effects, e.g., cavitation, and thermal effects are obtained. This concept of tissue ablation was first proposed by Lynn et al. in 1942 [1] and clinically used by Fry et al. in 1955 [2]. Since that time the use of high intensity focused ultrasound (HIFU) has been extensively studied in different fields of urology.

Generation of HIFU

Ultrasound waves are generated by high frequency (0.5 to 10 MHz) vibration of a piezoelectric or piezoceramic transducer. They are focused by spherical arrangement, acoustic lens, or parabolic reflectors into a small, discrete region, the focal point. Ultrasound is coupled by degassed water between the source and patient's skin or rectal wall. Because of the comparable acoustic properties of water and tissue, the sound waves should penetrate the skin or rectum and further precursory tissue with only slight absorption and reflection. The power density of the converging ultrasound increases as it approaches the focal point.

The focal region is a cigar-shaped, 3-dimensional zone with its long axis perpendicular to the axis of wave propagation (Fig. 1). The dimensions of the focal zone depend on the frequency and the geometry of the source; they are generally in the order of 10 to 50 mm in length and 1 to 5 mm in diameter. A larger volume of tissue can be ablated by sequentially shifting the focal zone by incremental movements of the transducer combined with adjustment of the focal length. The extent of tissue ablation is approximately that of the physical focal zone, but it can be controlled within a limited range by power and duration of the ultrasound pulses [3]. By scanning the target using multiple pulses, larger areas of tissue can be ablated. The two major mechanisms of HIFU are mechanical and thermal effects.

Mechanical Effects of HIFU

Acoustic cavitation is complex and unpredictable, but the end result is cell necrosis induced through a combination of mechanical stress and thermal injury. Cavitation is caused by a process in which bubbles develop and acutely increase in size to the point at which resonance is achieved. The bubble formation is a consequence of the negative pressure of the ultrasound wave [4]. When the bubbles suddenly collapse, high pressures ranging from 20,000 to 30,000 bars develop and damage nearby cells.

Thermal Effects of HIFU

As an ultrasound wave propagates through a medium, it is progressively adsorbed, and the energy is converted to heat in any not-ideally

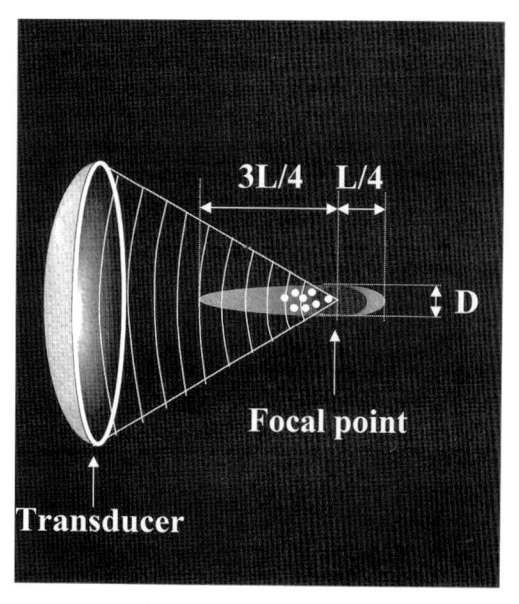

Fig. 1 Cigar-shaped HIFU lesion in the tissue growing from the focal point ¼ forward and ¾ backwards.

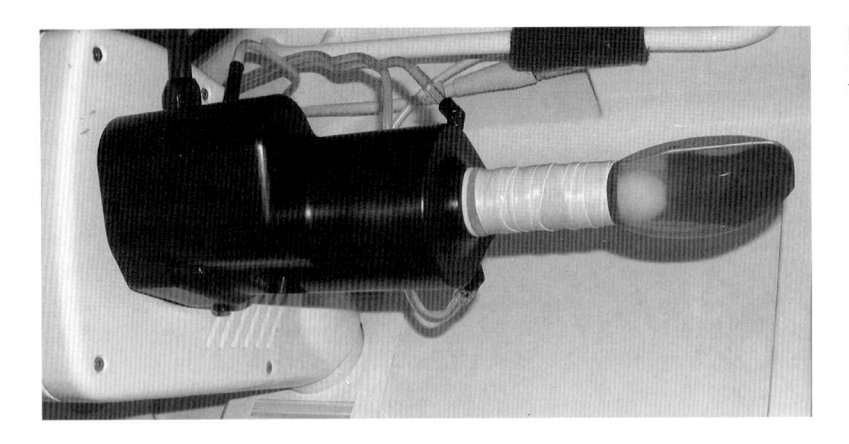

Fig. 2. Transrectal HIFU probe of the Ablatherm device.

viscoelastic medium, such as all biological tissues [5]. Tissue is rapidly heated to temperatures between 65 and 100 °C, causing irreversible cell damage and thermal coagulative necrosis. There is a steep temperature gradient between the focus and neighboring tissue, which is demonstrated by the sharp demarcation between the volume of necrotic (lesion) and normal surrounding cells on histology [6].

Current Technique of Transrectal HIFU for the Treatment of Prostate Cancer

The potential antitumor effect of transrectal HIFU has been shown by Chapelon et al. [7] who treated rats with two implanted sublines of Dunning tumor cells. The first clinical applications using HIFU were carried out simultaneously by Madersbacher et al. [8] in the treatment of benign prostatic hyperplasia (BPH) and by Gelet et al. [9] in the treatment of organ-confined prostate cancer.

Two HIFU devices for prostate cancer treatment are currently used. The *Sonablate-200* (Focus Surgery, Indianapolis, USA) offers a variety of rectal probes that have to be changed to use different focal lengths between 25 and 45 mm to create lesions according to the size of the prostate. The prostate is treated layer by layer (10 mm thick) from the apex to the base of the gland. This device has shown its efficacy so far only in studies with smaller patient groups [10].

A similar principle of adding lesions with a diameter of 17 mm and a length between 19 and 24 mm is used by the *Ablatherm* device (EDAP, Lyon, France). The HIFU probe is surrounded by a balloon with "degasified" coupling and liquid and consists of a motor driven unit with a treatment head (3 MHz) and a diagnostic 7.5 MHz ultrasound scanner (Kretz) (Fig. 2). The tablespoon-shaped therapeutic applicator fires with a power of up to 50 watts and incorporates a piezo element for rectum wall distance control. The Ablatherm was developed in a series of experiments and has shown its clinical efficacy in several studies [7, 9, 11–14].

References

[1] Lynn JG, Zweemer RL, Chick AJ, Miller AE. A new method for the generation and use of focused ultrasound in experimental biology. J Gen Physiol 1942; 26: 179–193
[2] Fry WJ, Barnard JW, Fry FJ, Kruminus RF, Brennan JF. Ultrasonic lesions in the mammalian central nervous system. Science 1955; 122: 517–518
[3] Häcker A, Köhrmann KU, Knoll T, Langbein S, Steidler A, Kraut O, Marlinghaus E, Alken P, Michel MS. High-intensity focused ultrasound for ex vivo kidney tissue ablation: influence of generator power and pulse duration. Endourol 2004; 18: 917–924
[4] Huber P, Debus J, Jenne J, Jöchle K, van Kaick G, Lorenz WJ, Wannemacher M. Therapeutic ultrasound in tumor therapy. Principles, applications and new developments. Radiologe 1996; 36: 64–71
[5] Barnett SB, Ter Haar GR, Ziskin MC, Nyborg WL, Maeda K, Bang J. Current status of research on biophysical effects of ultrasound. Ultrasound Med Biol 1994; 20: 211–219
[6] Chen L, Rivens I, ter Haar G, Riddler S, Hill CR, Bensted JP: Histological changes in rat liver tumours treated with high-intensity focused ultrasound. Ultrasound Med Biol 1993; 19: 67–74
[7] Chapelon JY, Margonari J, Vermier F, Gorry F, Ecochard R, Gelet A. In vivo effects of high-intensity ultrasound on prostatic adenocarcinoma Dunning R3327. Cancer Res 1992; 52: 6353–6357

8 Madersbacher S, Kratzik C, Susani M, Marberger M: Tissue ablation in benign prostatic hyperplasia with high intensity focused ultrasound. J Urol 1994; 152: 1956–1960

9 Gelet A, Chapelon JY, Bouvier R, Souchon R, Pangaud C, Abdebrahim AF, Cathignol D, Dubernard JM. Treatment of prostate cancer with transrectal focused ultrasound: Early clinical experience. Eur Urol 1996; 29: 174–183

10 Uchida T, Sanghvi NT, Gardner TA, Koch MO, Ishii, D, Minei S, Satoh T, Hyodo T, Irie A, Baba S. Transrectal high-intensity focused ultrasound for treatment of patients with stage T1b-2N0M0 localized prostate cancer: a preliminary report. Urology 2002; 59: 394–399

11 Gelet A, Chapelon JY, Bouvier R, Rouviere O, Lasne Y, Lyonnet D, Dubernard JM. Transrectal high-intensity focused ultrasound: minimally invasive therapy of localized prostate cancer. J Endourol 2000; 14: 519–528

12 Gelet A, Chapelon JY, Bouvier R, Rouviere O, Lyonnet D, Dubernard JM. Transrectal high intensity focused ultrasound for the treatment of localized prostate cancer: factors influencing the outcome. Eur Urol 2000; 40: 124–129

13 Thüroff S, Chaussy C, Vallancien G, Wieland W, Kiel HJ, Le Duc A, Desgrandschamps F, De La Rosette J, Gelet A. High-intensity focused ultrasound and localized prostate cancer: efficacy results from the European multicentric study. J Endourol 2003; 17: 673–677

14 Blana A, Walter B, Rogenhofer S et al. High intensity focused ultrasound for the treatment of localized prostate cancer: 5-year experience. Urology 2004; 63: 297–300

Status of High Intensity Focused Ultrasound (HIFU) in Urology in 2005

S. Thüroff, Ch. Chaussy

Introduction

The history of high intensive ultrasound goes back to 1927, where it first was used *non*-focused. In 1935 high intensive ultrasound was "bundled" with a concave lens and by this, the power in the focus increased: "HIFU" was born. Further developments brought up an "acoustic knife" in the 1950s. Different tests with the treatment of carcinomas in urology had been performed until, in the late 1980s and as first clinical therapy, transrectal ablation of prostate adenoma was started in larger series. The prostate was favorable for the HIFU treatment: "no movement, low blood flow, well reachable," so prostate adenoma and prostate cancer treatment was developed by Gelet et al. in cooperation with Chapelon (INSERM 556) and EDAP-TMS as the *Ablatherm*® which, in 1993, was introduced to clinical use. In the same period in USA the development of a similar technique started, which resulted in a device called *Sonablate*® (Focus Surgery). Within 10 years, HIFU for prostate cancer treatment had been performed in more than 6,500 patients treated by the Ablatherm® and some hundreds treated by the Sonablate® worldwide. Other indications for the HIFU technique have been studied and other devices have been constructed, such as the "Pyrotech®" as external HIFU device by EDAP (similar to a lithotripter, used by Vallencien, Paris) and studied on bladder cancer and a hand-held prototype device for renal HIFU application in recurrent renal cancer by Storz (used by Köhrmann/Alken, Mannheim). As prostate cancer treatment is the only HIFU treatment that has been in clinical practice for many years with representative treatment numbers and results, its application, indications, side effects, and results are shown in this chapter.

The technical equipment generally consists of an HIFU applicator, which is a motor-driven unit with a treatment head (3–4 MHz) and an integrated diagnostic ultrasound scanner (4–7.5 MHz) for localization and planning of the procedure. The treatment applicator has a longitudinal oval form. On its surface piezoelectric ceramics are placed which fire with a power up to 50 watt in a frequency of one shot per lesion every four to five seconds, in accord with the selected software/device. This application set-up was developed in different experiments, showing that the cell destruction is due to thermotherapeutic and cavitation effects. The applicator of Ablatherm®, in addition, recognizes and controls the rectal wall distance and avoids accidentally focusing on the rectum wall by autorepositioning or adequate alarms. The patient is positioned for the treatment on his right side or in the stone cut position under ITN or spinal anesthesia on a treatment table.

Preparation for treatment starts with cleaning and water-flushing of the rectum. After a sphincter ani dilatation, the condom-covered, special degassed transducer-liquid filled applicator is smoothly inserted into the rectum. The balloon, which covers the probe, is filled with about 150 mL of degassed transmitter liquid (e.g., ABLASONIC®) which circulates, driven by a roller pump, slowly through the rectum balloon into a cooling unit and back to the rectum at about 15 °C.

HIFU treatment planning starts at the apex of the prostate with a therapy planning on the computer screen, showing the transrectal ultrasound picture of the prostate in longitudinal and/or transverse position. According to the results of the TRUS-guided prostate biopsies, in regard to localization and volume of the prostate cancer, a complete treatment in *one* session is generally performed. In the case of the Ablatherm®, the prostate is divided into two or three "longitudinal blocks" and the entire gland is completely treated from apex to base. In the case of the Sonablate®, the gland is subdivided into two/three ventrodorsal layers which are treated one after the other. The treatment planning divides the prostate into transversal slices, starting at the apex of the prostate. 1.6-mm slices are subdivided into single lesions. The positions of slices and lesions are defined by the operator on the control screen, exposure is restricted within the capsule. Hundreds of single lesions, according to the size of the prostate are defined and coagulated.

HIFU therapy starts automatically at the apex after this planning procedure, going through all defined regions. For the precision of the thermal effect, an absolutely stable position without any movement of the patient is necessary. Treatment duration is about 2–3 hours with both devices. The postoperative course is painless, so analgesic medication is not necessary.

Antibiotic prophylaxis is mandatory until all catheters are removed postoperatively. Because of the risk of epididymitis, urethral burning, pain, and irritative or obstructive symptoms, at least Ablatherm® patients undergo in most cases TURP in the same anesthesia session.

Indications: More than 6,500 patients have been treated by the Ablatherm® up to now under different indications in different risk groups — all having in common that they were not suitable for radical prostatectomy, had no exclusion criteria and had signed patient informed consent. Because of the minimal invasive character of the treatment and the limited clinical consequences in case of negative lymph nodes, a pelvine lymph node dissection was *not* performed.

Contraindications are extremely rare: if the patient has no rectum, HIFU cannot be performed. If the rectal wall after radiation is thickened, HIFU should be avoided until the rectal wall is normalized. If the patient had brachy- or cryotherapy before, HIFU should be avoided because there is no experience about rectal injury with such pretreatment.

Follow up requires PSA every three months in the first years. TRUS-guided sextant biopsies are recommended between six and twelve months after HIFU to detect small, not PSA-relevant residual tumor volumes to be retreated by HIFU. If these biopsies are cancer free and PSA is low and stable (ASTRO), the patient is judged as a "complete remission" and will undergo only half-year PSA controls. Only in cases where PSA rises to pathological levels and a second local treatment would be a therapeutic consequence, repetitive biopsies are recommended and a second HIFU treatment or any other therapy may be performed. It is remarkable that a recurrent tumor after surgery or HIFU is not more aggressive as typically a recurrent tumor after hormonal ablation or radiation therapy have proved to be! Regarding indications, results, and side effects, there are significant differences between the two devices: the Sonablate® is recommended for the treatment of T1–2 localized Pca without TURP in limited prostate sizes and claims to have a very small number of therapy-induced side effects and a high potency preservation rate. Nevertheless only a small number of patients have been treated. The latest publications had a median follow-up time of 18 months in 61 patients.

With the Ablatherm® after more than 10 years of clinical use and prospective studies, experience for indications, results, and side effects in different indications and risk groups of prostate cancer patients is much larger. Generally efficacy (Table **1**) and side effects (Table **2**) of an oncological therapy have to be evaluated, balanced and related to initial tumor stage as well as with cancer- or therapy-induced morbidity in the case of no or alternative therapy. An analysis of Ablatherm® results and side effects is shown within 4 major different indication groups here based on the "München HIFU database" which registers prospectively all treated patients since 1996 (>1,100). Results of HIFU centers working with the same device and same application technique (>60 worldwide) proved to have identical results in comparative studies.

Indications

Primary therapy in localized not surgical treatable PCa, T1–2, G 1–3, Nx/0, M0, all PSA (Ablatherm® and Sonablate®)

Elderly men, who would be subject to radiation, hormonal ablation, or "wait and see," as patients whose condition does not allow the performance of radical surgery are included.

Low risk: PSA < 10 ng/mL, medium risk: PSA 10–20 ng/mL, high risk: PSA > 20 ng/mL. Side effects: risk profiles of primary therapy cases are identical or lower (hemostatic HIFU effect) compared to the risk profile of a classical TURP. Efficacy: see Table **1**.

Neoadjuvant local debulking in advanced cases, T 3–4, all G/PSA, N x/0, M0, (Ablatherm® only)

Patients with any not-localized Pca disease: in these cases local coagulation destroys all — even the non-hormone/radiation-sensitive cells, avoids local morbidity as there are bleeding, rectal infiltration, supra- and infravesical obstruction. Treatment goal is further to postpone hormonal

Table 1 München Harlaching prospective HIFU database

		Local low + middle risk PCa (surgery not indicated)	Local unilateral PCa (unilateral, potency protective)	Local high risk + advanced Pca	Salvage HIFU in recurrent PCa after surgery	Salvage HIFU in recurrent PCa after radiation	N+ M+
Grouping criteria	number of patients	412	44	557	35	34	59
	T	1–2b	1–2a	3–4	4	1–4	1–4
	N	0	0	0	0	0	1
	M	0	0	0	0	0	1
	Gleason score (1–5)	1–3	1–4	4–5	1–5	1–5	1–5
	number of + biopsies	1–3	1–3	> 3	1–x	1–x	1–x
	PSA i	< 20	< 20	> 20	all	all	all
	% of all patients	35.8	4.6	48.4	3.1	3.0	5.1
	age (median)	68	66	70	70	72	66
Staging results	targeted prostatic Vol.	> 80	< 80	> 80	> 90	> 90	> 80
	number of + biopsies	2	2	3.2	3	4	4 / 6
	Gleason % 1–3	100	80	29	33	20	17
	Prostate volume (mL)	35	21	25	4	14	32
	potent before therapy	68	80	45	4	18	32
	PSA initially	7	7	11/28	13	17	31 / 52
PSA [ng/mL]	nadir	0.0	0.5	0.0/0.1	0.2	0.7	0.15
	time to nadir (weeks)	10.3	x	9.2	x	x	7.4/2.7
	velocity (ng/year)	0.11	x	0.15/0.78	x	x	0.6/16.9
	stability (ASTRO)	80.7	83.3	73.2/23.1	x	x	x
	at last PSA test	0.4	2.1	0.7/2.7	0.3	2.6	3.3/10.4
%	negative biopsies	93.7	52	82	74	53	63
	if positive biopsies: reduced tumor volume	98	ipsi/contra: 38%/62%	85	35	60	70
	additional Pca therapy (not HIFU retreatment)	4.9	4.6	15/28	50	70	100
	severe complications	1.6	2	2.7	14	49	3.1
	EndoOR after HIFU	18	18	22	14	31	22
	retreatment rate	7.7	23	0	12/0		11
	follow-up (weeks)	114/332	90/203	133/305	25/257	52/150	102/132
	potent after HIFU	37	70	22	0	0	0

Table 2 Side effects Ablatherm®

	Side effect (%)	HIFU first	After RPE	After RAD	HIFU re X
1	No ejaculation	100	100	100	100
2	Infraves. obstruction	72.4	74.7	64.7	79.9
3	Erectile dysfunction	55	100	100	75
4	Urological Infection	9.5	13.6	8.7	31.7
5	Stress incontinence	1.7	2.9	2.9	2.2

ablation to a later moment and to postpone the moment of biochemical progression. Side effects: identical to primary HIFU. Efficacy: significant reduction of disease-induced morbidity. Survival – which should be longer – as well as quality of life are under evaluation (see Table 1).

Salvage HIFU in recurrent Pca, all rT/G/PSA, N x/o, M0 (Ablatherm® only)

Patients with local visible tumors after surgery, radiation, or progression under hormonal ablation are subjects for this group. Adapted treatment parameters/software in this group are necessary because radiated prostates absorb HIFU much better: modified in shot duration, delay time, power and application strategy, this avoids rectal morbidity and ensures high efficacy. **Side effects after long hormonal ablation/orchidectomy:** if there was no additional local pretreatment, identical to classical HIFU. HA-pretreated prostates shrink, are smaller, and less tissue has to be resected. **Side effects after surgery:** rPCa in these cases is in most cases a small volume tumor close to the sphincter externus. TURP is not necessary. Patients can leave hospital within 24 h. A urethral catheter for one week under antibiotics is sufficient. There is an elevated risk for stress incontinence. **Side effects after radiation:** radiation failures can occur after a few years – but even after 10 years. The longer ago the radiation was performed, the less are therapy-related problems. Rare, but problematic are cases radiated a few years ago and having an induced high rectal and/or vesical morbidity. If the patient still has rectal bleeding, if DRE is painful, or the rectal wall in TRUS is thicker than 3 mm the treatment should be postponed for one year. Rectal fistula with the special software in the CE marked Ablatherm® are extremely rare. But an elevated risk for stress incontinence and in the prototype version an elevated risk for fistula were registered. **Efficacy:** all treatments have to be considered as palliative treatments (see Table 1).

Partial therapy in unilateral, low-volume, low-Gleason cases. T1–2a, G 1–2, N x/0, Mo, PSAi < 20 ng/mL (Ablatherm® only)

Potent patients with an ultimative request for potency preservation can be included in this group, if they show up with low Gleason score, low tumor volume, and unilateral tumor. They have to be extensively informed that they have a high risk of local recurrence in the untreated prostatic lobe. They do not exclude any other definitive local treatment such as surgery, radiation, or complete HIFU, but they have to understand that they pay for potency preservation by strict controls being aware of Pca recurrence. Partial treatment postpones the moment of definitive local treatment for years. **Side effects:** as in normal, primary HIFU. **Efficacy:** Ipsilateral negative biopsy rate and recurrence rate are similar to local cases. But contralaterally, 1/3 showed cancer formation within the follow-up (see Table 1).

Summary: HIFU in Prostate Cancer

The classical therapeutic options for patients with prostate cancer are surgery, radiation, and hormonal ablation. Quite a few patients are not suitable for PVE because of their advanced tumor stage, their comorbidity, their fear of therapeutically induced complications such as impotence or incontinence. Palliative or "wait and see" strategies in many cases proved not to be sufficient in the long-term for a life without suffering from local or systemic progression of this widespread disease [3], because of their limited duration. Highly intensive ultrasound (HIFU) has tation. The incontinence rate after salvage cryosurgery is significantly lower than in patients undergoing salvage prostatectomy (7.5% vs. 45%), although patients have to be informed about this complication. Incontinence in these cases is caused by damage to the external sphincter. Lam et al. describe the placement of a temperature probe in the external sphincter area under direct cystoscopic vision and could reduce incontinence rate in their series down to less than 5% [10].

The overall results of salvage cryosurgery are inconsistent and depend on the used equipment. Although in this series a very good result in terms of cancer control could be achieved, the high number of adverse events (100%) led to a decreased use of cryosurgery. These problems can mostly be addressed to the equipment. For example, using the liquid nitrogen-based system, it was not easy to control the extent of the ice-ball exactly. Secondly, temperature probes were not available.

So looking at newer studies, in which the modern equipment was used, the overall results are comparable with the 5-year data of salvage surgery, although we have to admit that long-term results are still lacking [11–14] (Table 1).

In the form of salvage therapy (for secondary indications), cryotherapy represents a treatment alternative that is both of great value to patients and also, from an economic point of view, should be actively endorsed.

Therefore, for our clinic cryotherapy is not used as often as radiation therapy (external or interstitial), the secondary indication is actually the main indication. Even if the rate of postoperative morbidity seems to be somewhat higher, this should surely be regarded as acceptable in view of the good oncological outcomes.

Conclusion

Based on the results of clinical studies carried out by the U.S. Health Care Financing Administration (HCFA), cryotherapy has been approved for primary and secondary (radiation failure) therapy of adenocarcinoma of the prostate in the USA. For the same indications cryotherapy had received FDA approval. Hence, it can no longer be regarded as an experimental therapeutic procedure.

Apart from the fact that cryotherapy represents a valid curative therapy option for localized tumors, answering the justifiable desire of many patients for a minimally invasive form of treatment, cryotherapy also makes sense from an economic standpoint. When radiation therapy fails, often the only solution that has to be discussed is anti-androgen treatment with at best a palliative expectation.

In our view cryotherapy of the localized prostate carcinoma is as yet (still) not a substitute for an operation, which remains the standard therapy for this condition. Because of the long progression time for prostate cancer (up to 15 years), a balanced assessment can only be made following further studies. An important adjunct requirement for this therapy is that all cryotherapy patients be monitored in accordance with standardized parameters over long periods of time following treatment.

With regard to radiation, cryoablation can already today be considered a genuine alternative. This procedure is particularly interesting for clinics and medical centers that do not offer radiation therapy and have no license to handle radioactive substances, but still wish to offer their patients a promising semi-invasive therapeutic procedure.

Table 1 New studies of secondary (salvage) indications

Author	Number of Patients	PSA < 0.5 ng/mL	Negative Postoperative Biopsy
Ghafar [11]	38	74%	n. i.
Chin [12]	118	96%	94.1%
Izawa [13]	145		79%
de la Taille [14]	43	n. i.	66%

References

1 Mazur P, Miller RH. Survival of frozen-thawed human red cells as a function of the permeation of glycerol and sucrose. Cryobiology 1976; 13: 523–536
2 Gage AA, Guest K, Montes M, Caruana JA, Whalen DA Jr. Effect of varying freezing and thawing rates in experimental cryosurgery. Cryobiology 1985; 22: 175–182
3 Orpwood RD. Biophysical and engineering aspects of cryosurgery. Phys Med Biol 1981; 26: 555–575
4 Rabin Y, Steif PS, Taylor MJ, Julian TB, Wolmark N. An experimental study of the mechanical response of frozen biological tissues at cryogenic temperatures. Cryobiology 1996; 33: 472–482
5 Hoffmann NE, Bischof JC. The cryobiology of cryosurgical injury. Urology 2002; 60 (2 Suppl 1): 40–90
6 Homasson JP, Thiery JP, Angebault M, Ovtracht L, Maiwand O. The operation and efficacy of cryosurgical, nitrous oxide-driven cryoprobe. I. Cryoprobe physical characteristics: their effects on cell cryodestruction. Cryobiology 1994; 31: 290–304
7 Rabin Y, Julian TB, Wolmark N. A compact cryosurgical apparatus for minimally invasive procedures. Biomed Instrum Technol 1997; 31: 251–258
8 Leibovici D, Zisman A, Siegel YI, Lindner A. Cryosurgical ablation for prostate cancer: preliminary results of a new advanced technique. Isr Med Assoc J 2001; 3: 484–487
9 Touma NJ, Izawa JI, Chin JL. Current status of local salvage therapies following radiation failure for prostate cancer. J Urol 2005; 173: 373–379
10 Lam JS, Belldegrun AS. Salvage cryosurgery of the prostate after radiation failure. Rev Urol 2004; 6: 27–36
11 Ghafar MA, Johnson CW, de la Taille A, Benson MC, Bagiella E, Fatal M, Olsson CA, Katz AE. Salvage cryotherapy using an argon based system for locally recurrent prostate cancer after radiation therapy: the Columbia experience. J Urol 2001; 166: 1333–1337; discussion: 1337–1338
12 Chin JL, Pautler SE, Mouraviev V, Touma N, Moore K, Downey DB. Results of salvage cryoablation of the prostate after radiation: identifying predictors of treatment failure and complications. J Urol 2001; 165 (6 Pt 1): 1937–1941; discussion: 1941–1942
13 Izawa JI, Perrotte P, Greene GF, Scott S, Levy L, McGuire E, Madsen L, von Eschenbach AC, Pisters LL. Local tumor control with salvage cryotherapy for locally recurrent prostate cancer after external beam radiotherapy. J Urol 2001; 165: 867–870
14 de la Taille A, Hayek O, Benson MC, Bagiella E, Olsson CA, Fatal M, Katz AE. Salvage cryotherapy for recurrent prostate cancer after radiation therapy: the Columbia experience. Urology 2000; 55: 79–84

Prostate Brachytherapy

S. Neubauer, P. Derakhshani, G. Spira

Introduction

Brachytherapy is a form of radiation therapy in which a radiation source is placed either within or in close proximity to the tissue. In low-dose prostate brachytherapy, radionuclide sources are permanently implanted into the prostate gland, in high-dose rate brachytherapy the source is temporarily introduced into the prostate and removed after radiation treatment.

Developments in transrectal ultrasound, the use of a transperineal approach instead of retropubic implantation and the enormous advances in planning software have renewed the interest in prostate brachytherapy and led to an increasing use worldwide.

Physical advantages of brachytherapy result from the fact that radioactive sources are located within the target volume; thus, the distance radiation has to travel through tissue to reach its target is minimized. Prostate tumors can be treated without irradiating the skin or other dose-limiting organs. A second advantage is attributable to the "inverse square" law. The intensity of radiation decreases proportionally to the inverse of the square of the distance between source and target. Because of this exponential attenuation of radiation intensity, the dose decreases at a much greater rate near the radioactive source compared to external radiation techniques. With judicious source placement very high doses can be delivered to the tumor, and a minimum dose given to adjacent normal structures.

Several studies have shown the importance of physician experience for adequate dose delivery [1, 2].

At least 100 initial treatments and approximately 40–60 annual procedures will be necessary for every team to achieve high and reproducible implant quality.

Modern Prostate Brachytherapy Technique

In 1981, Holm in Denmark developed a transperineal implant method using transrectal ultrasound (TRUS) [3]. TRUS was used to guide percutaneous delivery of radioisotopes, achieving uniform seed distribution in the prostate and eliminating the guesswork previously used to guide the seeds in place. This formed the basis of the transperineal technique that is used today in brachytherapy, whether it is permanent or temporary, high-dose rate (HDR), or low-dose rate (LDR) brachytherapy.

The aim of permanent seed implants (PSI) is to deliver a tumoricidal dose to the entire prostate gland. The seeds employed may contain either the radio-isotope iodine 125(^{125}I) or palladium 103 (^{103}Pd). The seeds are introduced into the prostate gland by means of template-guided needles transperineally under transrectal ultrasound guidance. Dose planning software permits rapid planning of the seed position and dose profiles around the prostate capsule to ensure that an adequate dose is achieved around the periphery of the gland together with a suitable margin (Fig. 1). At the same time calculations are made to assure that adjacent organs receive as little dose as possible in order to limit side effects. Implant techniques vary from preloaded needles to afterloading the seeds once the needles are introduced into the gland. Stranded seeds (Fig. 2) are used preferably over loose seeds to prevent

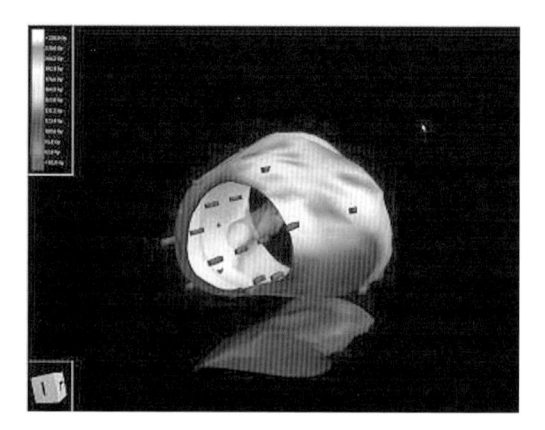

Fig. 1 Intraoperative planning in permanent seed implants: 3D-isodose calculation utilizing stranded iodine seeds.

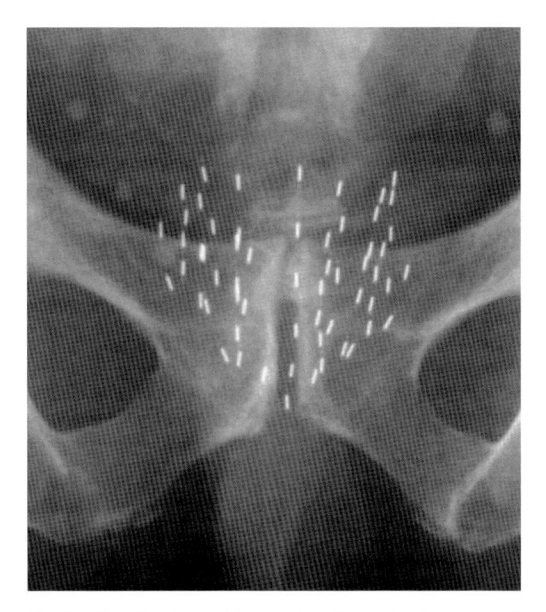

Fig. 2 Post-implant X-ray showing distribution of stranded iodine seeds.

seed migration and improve post implant dosimetry [4–7].
- At present most centers use an intraoperative technique, where planning and execution of the implant are done in a single session. A report from The American Brachytherapy Society in 2000 [8] recognized the following variations:
- *Preplanning:* Creation of a plan a few days or weeks before the implant procedure.
- *Intraoperative planning:* Treatment planning in the operating theatre; the patient and TRUS probe are not moved during the time between the volume study and seed insertion procedure.
- *Intraoperative preplanning:* Creation of a plan in the operating theatre just before the implant procedure, with immediate execution of the plan.
- *Interactive planning:* Stepwise refinement of the treatment plan using computed dose calculations derived from image-base needle position feedback.
- *Dynamic dose calculation:* Constant updating of calculations of dose distribution using continuous deposited seed position feedback.

After the seeds are implanted, a post-implant dosimetry is performed as a quality control measure to ensure that the dose delivered to the gland has been sufficient.

The influence on treatment efficacy of the technical modifications described above remains unclear at present.

In temporary prostate implants (TPI), afterloading needles are placed into the prostate under ultrasound guidance. A dose calculation based on ultrasound or CT images is performed. The radioactive sources are loaded into the needles according to the treatment plan only for the duration of the procedure. Optimized inverse planning provides greater flexibility for delivering individual dose distributions. A remote afterloading unit under robotic control is used to deliver treatments. This minimizes the radiation exposure to medical staff. A single radioactive source is moved along the afterloading needles. After the target dose is delivered, the source and the needles are removed. Recently intraoperative real-time planning has also been introduced to TPI [37]. The possibility of real-time modification in conjunction with ultrasound-based image acquisition in 1 mm slices enhances implant quality, possibly leading to improved clinical results in the future.

Patient Selection for Brachytherapy

Prostate brachytherapy is a multidisciplinary technique. Patient selection involves issues that relate to both urology and radiation oncology. The most commonly used risk stratification criteria appear in Table **1**. In accordance with the rec-

Table 1 Risk group stratification of localized prostate cancer patients

Risk group	Stage (AJCC 1992/2002)	Gleason score	PSA
Low	T1a–T2a	2–6	< 10 ng/mL
Intermediate, 1 factor	> T2b	> 7	> 10 ng/mL
High, 2 or more factors	> T2b	> 7	> 10 ng/mL

ommendations of the American Brachytherapy Society [9] and the EAU/ESTRO/EORTC [10], patients with low-risk prostate cancer may be treated with PSI alone. There are a number of studies that have shown good results with PSI alone or combined with external beam radiotherapy (EBRT) in patients with intermediate risk disease [11–13]. An RTOG study, now closed, randomized patients with intermediate risk disease to implant alone or implant combined with external beam radiotherapy and the results, although pending, should help to clarify the optimal treatment strategies for these patients.

For high-risk patients the role of brachytherapy is less certain. Patients with two or more adverse risk factors (PSA > 10 ng/mL, Gleason score > 6, or > T2a disease) are frequently treated with EBRT for 5 weeks before or after the implant. Despite these general guidelines, some experts believe that as long as an adequate margin is applied to the target volume there is no need for EBRT, whereas others routinely recommend the use of external beam in combination with brachytherapy [14–16].

Technical Considerations

For PSI the prostate size is optimal below 50 mL to avoid pubic arch interference. In experienced hands, larger prostates up to 70 mL volume can safely be treated if pubic arch interference is ruled out and IPSS is below 15 [17]. Volume reduction with an LHRH analogue may be indicated, if the pubic arch is narrow [18]; however, these patients have been shown to have a higher incidence of post-implant retention and irritative symptoms [19]. Patients must be able to flex their hips to 90°, have a pre-treatment IPSS of < 15, a maximum urinary flow rate above 10 mL/s, and should be clinically or urodynamically unobstructed [20, 21]. Prior transurethral resection of the prostate (TURP) is a relative contraindication to PSI, especially if there is a large or irregular resection defect or continence is marginal. Time interval between TURP and seed implant should be at least 6 months to avoid substantial urinary morbidity [22, 23]. With strict patient selection, PSI can be safely performed in patients after TURP.

As temporary implants do not cause prolonged radiation, urinary morbidity in general is lower in patients at risk (prior TURP, large prostate volume, high IPSS) [24]. Therefore, patients not suitable for permanent implants in terms of urinary tract status may be candidates for a temporary implant instead.

Clinical Results

Permanent seed implant monotherapy

Long-term results have been reported in the literature by many centers around the world. The first to publish 10-year results was the Seattle group in 1998 [25]. This series was comprised of the first cohort of patients ever treated with modern brachytherapy techniques. Risk stratification in patient selection was not well understood at the time. Of 152 patients in the series, 64% were treated with implant alone. Thirty-six percent, who were deemed at higher risk, were treated with a combination of implant (^{125}I or ^{103}Pd) and external beam radiotherapy. Biochemical disease-free survival (PSA < 0.5 ng/mL) at 10 years was 64%. The effect of the learning curve for the technique and the treatment in general could be appreciated when, in 2001, the same group published results for low-risk patients treated two years on [1]. There was a significant improvement in the results, 87% of patients treated had biochemical disease-free survival (PSA 0.2 ng/mL) at ten years follow-up.

Other centers, both in America and Europe, have produced similar long-term results as shown in Tables 2 and 3.

Table 2 PSA progression-free survival for patients with low risk prostate cancer treated with PSI as monotherapy

Series	No. of patients	PSA-failure definition	Follow-up (years)	PSA progression-free survival
Grimm 2001 [1]	125	ASTRO	10	87%
Beyer 2003 [26]	551	ASTRO	10	91%
Joseph 2004 [27]	421	ASTRO	8	84%
Potters 2004 [28]	733	ASTRO	7	84%

Table 3 PSA progression-free survival for patients with intermediate risk prostate cancer treated with PSI as monotherapy

Series	No. of patients	PSA-failure definition	Follow-up (years)	PSA progression-free survival
Beyer 2003 [26]	551	ASTRO	10	69%
Joseph 2004 [27]	245	ASTRO	8	74%
Battermann 2004 [29]	114	ASTRO	7	75%

Table 4 PSA progression-free survival for patients with intermediate/high-risk prostate cancer treated with PSI combined treatment

Series	No. of patients	PSA-failure definition	Follow-up (years)	PSA progression-free survival
Sylvester 2003 [11]	232	ASTRO	10	70%
Critz 2004 [12]	1,469	PSA < 0.2	10	80%/61%
Merrick 2004 [32]	46	ASTRO	7	85%
Stock 2004 [31]	132	ASTRO	5	86%

Currently a European multicenter database has been set up to follow the progress of 1,175 low and intermediate risk patients treated with PSI alone [30].

Combined permanent seed implant and EBRT

There are a number of publications on long-term follow-up of patients with intermediate and high-risk prostate cancer treated with PSI. Most authors advocate combined treatment with EBRT, although some authors reported similar results with PSI monotherapy [14–16, 31]. To date, it remains unclear whether high-risk tumors can be treated with PSI alone or need combined treatment. At present, it seems reasonable to treat patients with intermediate risk tumors with PSI monotherapy in selected cases (Table 4).

Stock el al. [31] treated 132 high-risk patients (Gleason score 8–10, PSA level > 20 ng/mL, stage T2c–T3 or positive seminal vesicle biopsy or two or more of the following: Gleason score 7, PSA level > 10–20 ng/mL, or stage T2b) with combined hormonal therapy (9 months), permanent radioactive seed brachytherapy, and external beam radiation. The actuarial overall freedom from PSA failure rate was 86% at 5 years. (97%/85%/76% for Gleason < 6/7/8–10).

Merrick et al. [32] reported on 46 consecutive T1c–T2b (1997 AJCC) patients with Gleason score 8 and 9 prostate cancer with a median follow-up of 58 months treated with ^{103}Pd and supplemental external beam radiation therapy (45 Gy). The utilization of hormonal therapy for 6 months or less resulted in a statistically not significant improvement in biochemical outcome (92.3% versus 81.8%, p = 0.393).

Critz et al. [12] treated 1,469 men (T1,T2, Nx,M0) with PSI followed by external irradiation with a median follow-up of 6 years. The overall 10-year disease-free survival rate (PSA < 0.2 ng/mL) was 83%. Median time to recurrence was 30 months (range 3 months to 8 years) and 24% of recurrences were after 5-year follow-up. 10-year DFS for low, intermediate, and high risk group was 93%, 80% and 61%, respectively (p < 0.0001). Pre-treatment PSA, Gleason score, and percent positive biopsies were significantly related to disease freedom in multivariate analysis, while stage and age were not. The authors concluded that outcome can be reasonably compared with radical prostatectomy performed in the PSA era.

Temporary prostate implants

Combined HDR-afterloading and EBRT

External beam radiation therapy (EBRT) with dose-escalating HDR brachytherapy (HDR-BT) boost produces excellent long-term outcomes in terms of biochemical control (BC), disease-free survival (DFS), and cause-specific survival (CSS) even in patients with high-risk prostate cancer even though there is no consensus about implant technique and protocol. Published studies report on 1 to 4 implants per patient, giving 1 to 4 fractions per implant. The target dose is 5.5–15 Gy per fraction leading to a total delivered HDR-boost dose of 18–30 Gy. This in conjunction with the applied external beam dose of 36–50 Gy (either before, during or after HDR-boosts) leads to a postulated total biological equivalent dose of 85–155 Gy. Therefore, any comparison of recent HDR-afterloading studies has to take into account the different treatment protocols.

Galalae et al. reported on 611 patients in three prospective series (Seattle, Kiel, William Beaumont) treated with EBRT and HDR-BT. The ASTRO definition for biochemical failure was used [33]. Five- and ten-year BC rates were 77%/73%, DFS 67%/49%, and CSS 96%/92%, respectively. Biochemical control for low-risk was 96%, 88% for intermediate, and 69% for high-risk patients at 5 years. These data represent excellent 5-year results for high-risk patients. CSS was 100%/99%/95%. The results were similar at all three institutions which showed the reproducibility of the results.

Kestin et al. [35] performed a matched-pair analysis to compare EBRT alone to EBRT + HDR. One hundred and sixty-one high-risk patients were prospectively and randomly matched with a group of EBRT-only patients according to PSA level, Gleason score, T stage, and duration of follow-up. After a median follow-up of 2.5 years EBRT + HDR patients demonstrated significantly lower PSA nadir levels (median, 0.4 ng/mL) compared to those receiving EBRT alone (median, 1.1 ng/mL) and 5-year BCR 67 vs. 44% (p < 0.001).

Martinez et al. [35] published results on 207 patients treated with EBRT+HDR-BT (5.5–11.5 Gy/fraction). They were divided into two groups. Group I: low-dose biologically effective dose < 93 Gy (58 patients); group II: high-dose biologically effective dose > 93 Gy (149 patients). Five-year BC for the low-dose group was 52%; the rate for the high-dose group was 87% (p < 0.001). Improvement also occurred in CSS of the high-dose brachytherapy group (p = 0.014). The authors concluded that with higher doses an incremental beneficial effect on biochemical control and cause-specific survival can be observed (Table 5). These results, coupled with the low risk of complications and the real-time interactive planning, defined a new treatment option for high-risk patients.

HDR-afterloading monotherapy

HDR-afterloading has recently gained interest as monotherapy in favorable prostate cancer (Fig. 3). Three pilot studies with a total of 160 patients have been published with a maximum follow-up of three years [24, 38, 39]. The technique involves a schedule of 38 Gy delivered in four fractions (2 treatment days). Initial results showed superior 3-year impotence rates as compared to palladium PSI (16% versus 45%) [24]. Urinary symptoms were less frequent but the rate of urethral stricture was 8% compared to 3% in PSI. Biochemical control was not significantly different in both treatment groups.

Whether HDR-afterloading as monotherapy can be regarded as a treatment option in se-

Table 5 Biochemical no-evidence-of-disease (bNED) for patients with intermediate/high prostate cancer treated with HDR-afterloading combined treatment

Series	No. of patients	PSA-failure definition	Follow-up (years)	bNED
Galalae 2004 [33]	611	ASTRO	10	73%
Kestin 2000 [34]	161	PSA < 0.2	5	67%
Martinez 2002 [35]	149	ASTRO	5	87%
Pellizon 2003 [36]	119	ASTRO	4	75%
Martin 2004 [37]	102	ASTRO	3	82%

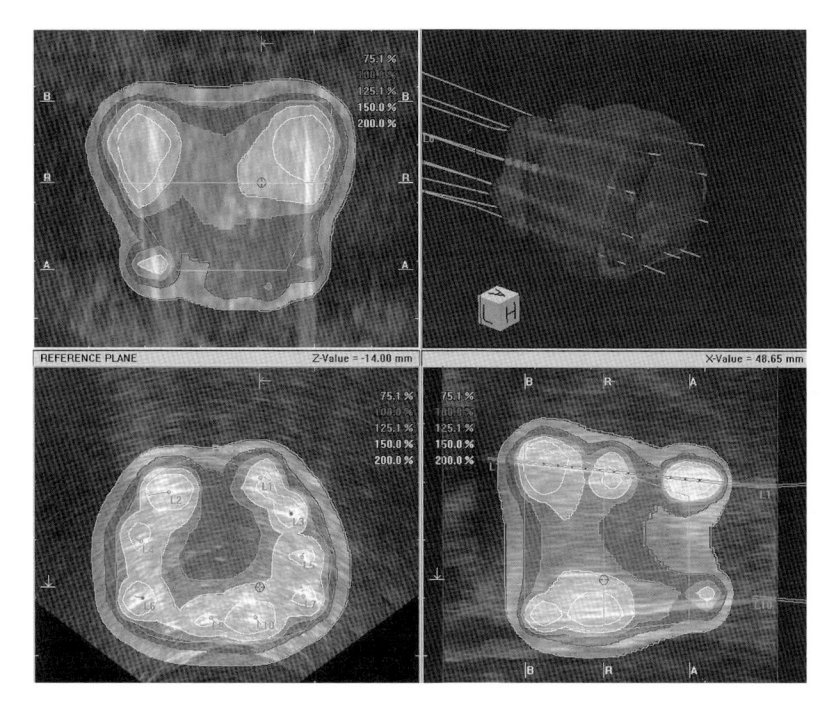

Fig. 3 Real-time ultrasound-based inverse-planning in HDR-afterloading temporary prostate implant.

lected low-risk patients needs further investigation.

LDR brachytherapy compared to other treatment options

There are no randomized controlled trials that compare brachytherapy with other treatment options and most of the data are retrospective. Non-comparable groups, incomplete follow-up, unclear definition, or insufficient information on prognostic factors and variation in outcome criteria make it difficult to evaluate the evidence.

Vicini et al. compared 6 treatment options in 7 institutions for 6,877 patients with localized prostate cancer and concluded that there was no difference in 5-year outcomes when pre-treatment stratification was consistent [40].

Kupelian et al. compared external beam radiotherapy, radical prostatectomy, and brachytherapy 5-year outcomes in 2,991 patients with T1–T2 localized prostate cancer. Biochemical failure rates were similar with all treatments with the exception of low-dose external beam radiotherapy (< 72 Gy) where outcomes were significantly worse [41].

Comparing seed implantation to radical prostatectomy Stoke reported no difference in 5-year PSA-free survival between patients with low- and intermediate-risk tumors [42]. Similar results were obtained by Sharkey comparing data from 1707 patients treated with RP or PSI [43]. Results showed similar bNED in the low-risk group (89% PSI vs. 94% RP). In the intermediate and high-risk group PSI +/– EBRT was superior to RP in terms of bNED (89%/88% PSI vs. 58%/43% RP).

Henderson reviewed the literature from 1988 to 2003 on quality of life changes following PSI and other treatments for early prostate cancer [44]. Results suggest that radical prostatectomy, external beam radiotherapy, and PSI offer good long-term health-related quality of life. However, differences exist in the toxicity of treatment in terms of erectile function, voiding difficulty, incontinence, and bowel function. These differences seem to persist for at least 3–5 years post-treatment. The authors conclude that PSI offers a high probability of maintaining continence, potency and normal rectal function though both storage and voiding urinary symptoms have been reported. Quality of life outcome following PSI compares favorably with other radical treatment options for the management of early prostate cancer [44].

In a systematic review of the clinical and cost effectiveness for prostate brachytherapy Norderhaug et al. concluded that the outcomes appear to be comparable for radical prostatectomy, external beam radiotherapy and brachytherapy in low-risk patients concerning the primary therapy [45].

The impact for every country should be taken into account when looking at costs. Brachytherapy may be a rapid and outpatient procedure with early recovery and return to normal activities compared to external beam radiation with daily therapies for 8–10 weeks. A German review of 200 patients younger than 56 years demonstrated a cost escalation due to a median loss of work-time of 104.4 days after radical prostatectomy [46]. Thus, treatment efficacy, side effects, and cost comparison will influence the choice of treatment for both physician and patient.

Complications and Management

Urinary morbidity

Incontinence is rare after low-dose brachytherapy but temporary irritative symptoms are common. The relationship between urethral dose and the severity of urinary symptoms had been the subject of many publications and has led to a modification of seed loading patterns with a view to limiting the dose to the urethra to a maximum of 150% of the minimal peripheral dose [47].

Henderson et al. conducted a prospective study of IPSS score and urinary toxicity in 216 patients in the UK who underwent prostate seed implant [20]. They reported that 95% of the patients experienced temporary deterioration in their urinary symptoms which persisted at clinically significant levels (IPSS increase > 3 points) for 9 months after the implant. The severity of the post-implant symptoms was closely related to the pre-implant IPSS score. Patients were routinely managed with α-blockers and returned to baseline values by nine months.

Merrick et al. reported similar findings in a group of 130 patients studied prospectively with IPSS and a dysuria severity score [48]. An α-blocker was either given two weeks prior to implant or withheld until the onset of post-implant urinary symptoms. Quality of life questionnaires were administered at baseline and then at 1, 3, 6, 12, 18, and 24 months. The maximum incidence of symptoms was 85% at 1 month after brachytherapy that resolved over time. Prophylactic α-blockers gave significantly lower maximum dysuria scores but did not affect the time to resolution of dysuria.

Stone et al. have reported on the long-term urinary morbidity in a prospective study that followed 248 patients for a median of 31 months after seed implantation [49]. They found that prostate brachytherapy is associated with minimal long-term urinary morbidity and that a cohort of patients with marked urinary symptoms prior to implantation improved after the procedure. This finding was also documented by Henderson et al.

Our own series of 516 patients treated with PSI between 2001 and 2004 showed similar results in terms of overall urinary morbidity. Interestingly, the group of patients with large prostate volumes above 40 mL with initial IPSS < 15 did not experience increased urinary toxicity as compared to smaller volumes [50].

Eapen et al. found a significant association between urinary toxicity and the number of periurethral needle manipulations (p = 0.025) [51].

Bucci et al. evaluated the incidence and duration of urinary retention requiring catheterization following prostate brachytherapy. Two hundred and eighty-two patients were treated with prostate brachytherapy alone [52]. Baseline IPSS was the most important predictive factor for post-implantation catheterization but the extent of post-implant edema was also predictive for the need and duration of catheterization. Urinary obstruction after prostate brachytherapy developed in 15% of patients with a median duration of catheter insertion of 21 days.

In our own series, prospective analysis of 742 patients treated with PSI, the routine use of NSAID in combination with alpha-blockers lowered our acute retention rate to 6%.

In TPI acute genitourinary (GU) EORTC grade 3 complications were reported in 4 to 8%, whereas GU EORTC grade 4 complications were 0%. Late GU complications grade 3 and 4 were reported in 2.1–5% and 0% of patients [35, 36].

Rectal morbidity

Proctitis is relatively uncommon and has been described in approximately 5% of cases [53–55]. Rectal toxicity increases when seed implants are combined with external beam radiotherapy. The relationship between rectal dose and rectal symptoms has been studied by Waterman et al. [56]. Rectal morbidity increases with increase in dose to the rectum and also with the percentage

Table 6 Potency rates following PSI

Study	No of patients	Mean age	Treatment	Potency rate and follow-up
Stock [58]	416	66	^{125}I/^{103}Pd	79% – 59%; 3 and 6 years after implant
Potters [59]	482	67	^{125}I/^{103}Pd	76%
Mabjeesh [60]	131	65	^{125}I	80% at 3 years, some with Sildenafil
Merrick [61]	181	65	^{125}I/^{103}Pd	52% at 6 years
Robinson [62], meta-analysis	172	67	^{125}I/^{103}Pd	76% at 1 year
Raina [63]	86	63	^{125}I	70% with Sildenafil

of the rectal surface that receives that dose. To limit the incidence of late morbidity to 1%, 3%, or 5% the maximum rectal dose should be limited to < 200, 250, 300 Gy, respectively.

In TPI as a boost to external radiotherapy acute lower gastrointestinal (GI) EORTC grade 3 complications were reported in 0 to 4.1%, whereas GI EORTC grade 4 complications were 0%. Late GI complications grade 3 and 4 were reported in 4.1–5% and 0–1% of patients [33, 35, 36].

Sexual function

Any treatment for prostate cancer can negatively affect sexual function (SF) and sexual bother (SB). Initial differences among different radiation treatment subgroups exist, but diminish with time. Speight et al. [57] reported on 992 men with newly diagnosed prostate cancer. SF changes associated with EBRT +/– BT were statistically significant and those for BT alone were not. Short-term androgen ablation appeared to confer only temporary and recoverable impairment of erectile function. Patient median age in all series is between 65 and 70 years at treatment and in radiotherapy worsening of SF appears over time. Therefore, definite causality of decreased SF remains unclear compared to radical prostatectomy (Table 6).

Conclusion

Prostate brachytherapy is increasingly being used in the treatment of localized prostate cancer. For patients with low- and intermediate-risk prostate tumors, results from the few comparative studies showed no difference in clinical effectiveness for prostate brachytherapy, radical prostatectomy, or external beam radiation therapy.

Team experience and further technical development will enhance outcome and reduce side effects if prognostic and selection criteria are respected. As recommended for challenging techniques, minimal yearly numbers of treatments per team should be mandatory. It is suggested for brachytherapy teams to perform a minimum number of implants annually in order to maintain adequate skill levels.

In patients with high-risk tumors the combination of HDR-BT and external beam therapy offers the advantages of further dose escalation with protection of organs at risk. Results presented so far showed excellent control for this tumor entity including low side effects.

For every patient presenting with newly diagnosed prostate cancer, all treatment options should be discussed including details of outcomes, toxicity, quality-of-life issues, salvage of treatment failure, and cost issues.

References

[1] Grimm PD, Blasko JC, Sylvester JE, Meier RM, Cavanagh W. 10-year biochemical (prostate-specific antigen) control of prostate cancer with (125)I brachytherapy. Int J Radiat Oncol Biol Phys 2001; 51: 31–40

[2] Neubauer S, Derakhshani P, Muskalla K, Metz J, Spira G. Iodine-125 prostate brachytherapy in localized prostate cancer: importance of team experience for dose delivery and toxicity. Radiother Oncol 2004; 71: S44

[3] Holm HH, Juul N, Pedersen JF et al. Transperineal 125-Iodine seed implantation in prostatic cancer guided by transrectal ultrasonography. J Urol 1983; 130: 283–286.

[4] Tapen EM, Blasko JC, Grimm PD, Ragde H, Luse R, Clifford S, Sylvester J, Griffin TW. Reduction of radioactive seed embolization to the lung following

prostate brachytherapy. Int J Radiat Oncol Biol Phys. 1998; 42: 1063–1067
5. Al-Qaisieh B, Carey B, Ash D, Bottomley D. The use of linked seeds eliminates lung embolization following permanent seed implantation for prostate cancer. Int J Radiat Oncol Biol Phys. 2004; 59: 397–399.
6. Fagundes HM, Keys RJ, Wojcik MF, Radden MA, Bertelsman CG, Cavanagh WA. Transperineal TRUS-guided prostate brachytherapy using loose seeds versus RAPIDStrand: a dosimetric analysis. Brachytherapy 2004; 3: 136–140
7. Lee WR, de Guzman AF, Tomlinson SK, McCullough DL. Radioactive sources embedded in suture are associated with improved postimplant dosimetry in men treated with prostate brachytherapy. Radiother Oncol 2002; 65: 123–127
8. Nag S, Ciezki JP, Cormack R, Doggett S, de Wyngaert K, Edmundson GK, Stock RG, Stone NN, Yu Y, Zelefsky MJ. Clinical Research Committee, American Intraoperative planning and evaluation of permanent prostate brachytherapy: report of the American Brachytherapy Society. Int J Radiat Oncol Biol Phys 2001; 51: 1422–1430
9. Nag S, Beyer D, Friedland J, Grimm P, Nath R. American Brachytherapy Society (ABS) recommendations for transperineal permanent brachytherapy of prostate cancer. Int J Radiat Oncol Biol Phys 1999; 44: 789–799
10. Ash D, Flynn A, Battermann J, de Reijke T, Lavagnini P, Blank L; ESTRA/EAU Urological Brachytherapy Group; EORTC Radiotherapy Group. ESTRO/EAU/EORTC recommendations on permanent seed implantation for localized prostate cancer. Radiother Oncol 2000; 57: 315–321
11. Sylvester JE, Blasko JC, Grimm PD, Meier R, Malmgren JA. Ten-year biochemical relapse-free survival after external beam radiation and brachytherapy for localized prostate cancer: the Seattle experience. Int J Radiat Oncol Biol Phys 2003; 57: 944–952
12. Critz FA, Levinson K. 10-year disease-free survival rates after simultaneous irradiation for prostate cancer with a focus on calculation methodology. J Urol 2004; 172: 2232–2238
13. Merrick GS, Butler WM, Wallner KE, Galbreath RW, Lief JH, Allen Z, Adamovich E. Impact of supplemental external beam radiotherapy and/or androgen deprivation therapy on biochemical outcome after permanent prostate brachytherapy. Int J Radiat Oncol Biol Phys 2005; 61: 32–43
14. Potters L, Cao Y, Calugaru E, et al. A comprehensive review of CT-based dosimetry parameters and biochemical control in patients treated with permanent prostate brachytherapy. Int J Radiat Oncol Biol Phys 2001; 50: 605–614
15. Critz FA, Tarlton RS, Holladay DA. Prostate specific antigen-monitored combination radiotherapy for patients with prostate cancer. I-125 implant followed by external beam radiation. Cancer 1995; 75: 2383–2391
16. Critz FA, Levinson AK, Williams WH et al. Simultaneous radiotherapy for prostate cancer: [125]I prostate implant followed by external-beam radiation. Cancer J Sci Am 1998; 4: 359–363
17. Merrick GS, Butler WM, Wallner KE, Allen Z, Galbreath RW, Lief JH. Brachytherapy-related dysuria. BJU Int 2005; 95: 597–602
18. Henderson A, Langley SE, Laing RW. Is bicalutamide equivalent to goserelin for prostate volume reduction before radiation therapy? A prospective, observational study. Clin Oncol (R Coll Radiol) 2003; 15: 318–321
19. Crook J, McLean M, Catton C, Yeung I, Tsihlias J, Pintilie M. Factors influencing risk of acute urinary retention after TRUS-guided permanent prostate seed implantation. Int J Radiat Oncol Biol Phys 2002; 52: 453–460
20. Henderson A, Ismail AK, Cunningham M, Aldridge S, Loverock L, Langley SE, Laing RW. Toxicity and early biochemical outcomes from 125iodine prostate brachytherapy in the UK. A prospective study. Clin Oncol (R Coll Radiol) 2004; 16: 95–104
21. Langley SE, Laing RW. Iodine seed prostate brachytherapy: an alternative first-line choice for early prostate cancer. Prostate Cancer Prostatic Dis 2004; 7: 201–207
22. Moran BJ, Stutz MA, Gurel MH. Prostate brachytherapy can be performed in selected patients after transurethral resection of the prostate. Int J Radiat Oncol Biol Phys 2004; 59: 392–396
23. Stone NN, Ratnow ER, Stock RG. Prior transurethral resection does not increase morbidity following real-time ultrasound-guided prostate seed implantation. Tech Urol 2000; 6: 123–127
24. Grills IS, Martinez AA, Hollander M, Huang R, Goldman K, Chen PY, Gustafson GS. High dose rate brachytherapy as prostate cancer monotherapy reduces toxicity compared to low dose rate palladium seeds. J Urol 2004; 171: 1098–1104
25. Ragde H, Elgamal AA, Snow PB, Brandt J, Bartolucci AA, Nadir BS, Korb LJ. Ten-year disease free survival after transperineal sonography-guided iodine-125 brachytherapy with or without 45-gray external beam irradiation in the treatment of patients with clinically localized, low to high Gleason grade prostate carcinoma. Cancer 1998; 83: 989–1001
26. Beyer DC, Thomas T, Hilbe J, Swenson V. Relative influence of Gleason score and pretreatment PSA in predicting survival following brachytherapy for prostate cancer. Brachytherapy 2003; 2: 77–84
27. Joseph J, Al-Qaisieh B, Ash D, Bottomley D, Carey B. Prostate-specific antigen relapse-free survival in patients with localized prostate cancer treated by brachytherapy. BJU Int 2004; 94: 1235–1238

28 Potters L, Klein EA, Kattan MW, Reddy CA, Ciezki JP, Reuther AM, Kupelian PA. Monotherapy for stage T1–T2 prostate cancer: radical prostatectomy, external beam radiotherapy, or permanent seed implantation. Radiother Oncol 2004; 71: 29–33

29 Battermann JJ, Boon TA, Moerland MA. Results of permanent prostate brachytherapy, 13 years of experience at a single institution. Radiother Oncol 2004; 71: 23–28

30 Langley S, Laing R, Henderson A, Aaltomaa S, Kataja V, Palmgren JE, Bladou F, Salem N, Serment G, Nava L, Losa A, Guazzoni G, Guedea F, Aguilo F. European collaborative group on prostate brachytherapy: preliminary report in 1175 patients. Eur Urol 2004; 46: 565–570

31 Stock RG, Cahlon O, Cesaretti JA, Kollmeier MA, Stone NN. Combined modality treatment in the management of high-risk prostate cancer. Int J Radiat Oncol Biol Phys 2004; 59: 1352–1359

32 Merrick GS, Butler WM, Wallner KE, Galbreath RW, Adamovich E. Permanent interstitial brachytherapy for clinically organ-confined high-grade prostate cancer with a pretreatment PSA < 20 ng/mL. Am J Clin Oncol 2004; 27: 611–615

33 Galalae RM, Martinez A, Mate T, Mitchell C, Edmundson G, Nuernberg N, Eulau S, Gustafson G, Gribble M, Kovacs G. Long-term outcome by risk factors using conformal high-dose-rate brachytherapy (HDR-BT) boost with or without neoadjuvant androgen suppression for localized prostate cancer. Int J Radiat Oncol Biol Phys 2004; 58: 1048–1055

34 Kestin LL, Martinez AA, Stromberg JS, Edmundson GK, Gustafson GS, Brabbins DS, Chen PY, Vicini FA. Matched-pair analysis of conformal high-dose-rate brachytherapy boost versus external-beam radiation therapy alone for locally advanced prostate cancer. J Clin Oncol 2000; 18: 2869–2880

35 Martinez AA, Gustafson G, Gonzalez J, Armour E, Mitchell C, Edmundson G, Spencer W, Stromberg J, Huang R, Vicini F. Dose escalation using conformal high-dose-rate brachytherapy improves outcome in unfavorable prostate cancer. Int J Radiat Oncol Biol Phys 2002; 53: 316–327

36 Pellizzon AC, Nadalin W, Salvajoli JV, Fogaroli RC, Novaes PE, Maia MA, Ferrigno R. Results of high dose rate afterloading brachytherapy boost to conventional external beam radiation therapy for initial and locally advanced prostate cancer. Radiother Oncol 2003; 66: 167–172

37 Martin T, Roddiger S, Kurek R, Dannenberg T, Eckart O, Kolotas C, Heyd R, Rogge B, Baltas D, Tunn U, Zamboglou N. 3D conformal HDR brachytherapy and external beam irradiation combined with temporary androgen deprivation in the treatment of localized prostate cancer. Radiother Oncol 2004; 71: 35–41

38 Martin T, Baltas D, Kurek R, Roddiger S, Kontova M, Anagnostopoulos G, Dannenberg T, Buhleier T, Skazikis G, Tunn U, Zamboglou N. 3-D conformal HDR brachytherapy as monotherapy for localized prostate cancer. A pilot study. Strahlenther Onkol 2004; 180: 225–232

39 Yoshioka Y, Nose T, Yoshida K, Oh RJ, Yamada Y, Tanaka E, Yamazaki H, Inoue T, Inoue T. High-dose-rate brachytherapy as monotherapy for localized prostate cancer: A retrospective analysis with special focus on tolerance and chronic toxicity. Int J Radiat Oncol Biol Phys 2003; 56: 213–220

40 Vicini FA, Martinez A, Hanks G, Hanlon A, Miles B, Kernan K, Beyers D, Ragde H, Forman J, Fontanesi J, Kestin L, Kovacs G, Denis L, Slawin K, Scardino P. An interinstitutional and interspecialty comparison of treatment outcome data for patients with prostate carcinoma based on predefined prognostic categories and minimum follow-up. Cancer 2002; 95: 2126–2135

41 Kupelian PA, Potters L, Khuntia D, Ciezki JP, Reddy CA, Reuther AM, Carlson TP, Klein EA. Radical prostatectomy, external beam radiotherapy <72 Gy, external beam radiotherapy > or =72 Gy, permanent seed implantation, or combined seeds/external beam radiotherapy for stage T1–T2 prostate cancer. Int J Radiat Oncol Biol Phys 2004; 58: 25–33

42 Stokes SH. Comparison of biochemical disease-free survival of patients with localized carcinoma of the prostate undergoing radical prostatectomy, transperineal ultrasound-guided radioactive seed implantation, or definitive external beam irradiation. Int J Radiat Oncol Biol Phys 2000; 47: 129–136

43 Sharkey J, Cantor A, Solc Z, Huff W, Chovnick SD, Behar RJ, Perez R, Otheguy J, Rabinowitz R. (103)Pd brachytherapy versus radical prostatectomy in patients with clinically localized prostate cancer: A 12-year experience from a single group practice. Brachytherapy 2005; 4: 34–44

44 Henderson A, Laing RW, Langley SE. Quality of life following treatment for early prostate cancer: Does low dose rate (LDR) brachytherapy offer a better outcome? A review. Eur Urol 2004; 45:134–141

45 Norderhaug I, Dahl O, Hoisaeter PA, Heikkila R, Klepp O, Olsen DR, Kristiansen IS, Waehre H, Bjerklund Johansen TE. Brachytherapy for prostate cancer: a systematic review of clinical and cost effectiveness. Eur Urol 2003; 44: 40–46

46 Herkommer K, Fuchs T, Hautmann R, Volkmer B. Radikale Prostatektomie bei Männern unter 56 Jahren: Eine Krankheitskostenanalyse. Der Urologe [A] 2004; Suppl 1: 77

47 Desai J, Stock RG, Stone NN, Iannuzzi C, DeWyngaert JK. Acute urinary morbidity following I-125 interstitial implantation of the prostate gland. Radiat Oncol Investig 1998; 6: 135–1341

48 Merrick GS, Butler WM, Wallner KE, Allen Z, Galbreath RW, Lief JH. Brachytherapy-related dysuria. BJU Int 2005; 95: 597–602
49 Stone NN, Stock RG. Prospective assessment of patient-reported long-term urinary morbidity and associated quality of life changes after 125I prostate brachytherapy. Brachytherapy 2003; 2: 32–39
50 Derakhshani P, Neubauer S, Muskalla K, Metz J, Spira G. Influence of intraoperative prostate volume on early urinary toxicity after permanent prostate brachytherapy. Radiother Oncol 2004; 71: S55
51 Eapen L, Kayser C, Deshaies Y, Perry GEC, Morash C, Cygler JE, Wilkins D, Dahrouge S. Correlating the degree of needle trauma during prostate brachytherapy and the development of acute urinary toxicity. Int J Radiat Oncol Biol Phys 2004; 59: 1392–1394
52 Bucci J, Morris WJ, Keyes M, Spadinger I, Sidhu S, Moravan V. Predictive factors of urinary retention following prostate brachytherapy. Int J Radiat Oncol Biol Phys 2002; 53: 91–98
53 Gelblum DY, Potters L. Rectal complications associated with transperineal interstitial brachytherapy for prostate cancer. Int J Radiat Oncol Biol Phys 2000; 48: 119–1124
54 Merrick GS, Butler WM, Wallner KE, Hines AL, Allen Z. Late rectal function after prostate brachytherapy. Int J Radiat Oncol Biol Phys 2003; 57: 42–48
55 Wust P, von Borczyskowski DW, Henkel T, Rosner C, Graf R, Tilly W, Budach V, Felix R, Kahmann F. Clinical and physical determinants for toxicity of 125-I seed prostate brachytherapy. Radiother Oncol 2004; 73: 39–48
56 Waterman FM, Dicker AP. Is it necessary to eliminate the posterior dose margin in prostate brachytherapy to achieve an acceptably low risk of late rectal morbidity? Int J Radiat Oncol Biol Phys 2003; 57: 293–299
57 Speight JL, Elkin EP, Pasta DJ, Silva S, Lubeck DP, Carroll PR, Litwin MS. Longitudinal assessment of changes in sexual function and bother in patients treated with external beam radiotherapy or brachytherapy, with and without neoadjuvant androgen ablation: data from CaPSURE. Int J Radiat Oncol Biol Phys 2004; 60: 1066–1075
58 Stock RG, Kao J, Stone NN. Penile erectile function after permanent radioactive seed implantation for treatment of prostate cancer. J Urol 2001; 165: 436–439
59 Potters L, Torre T, Fearn PA, Leibel SA, Kattan MW. Potency after permanent prostate brachytherapy for localized prostate cancer. Int J Radiat Oncol Biol Phys 2001; 50: 1235–1242
60 Mabjeesh N, Chen J, Beri A, Stenger A, Matzkin H. Sexual function after permanent (125)I-brachytherapy for prostate cancer. Int J Impot Res 2005; 17: 96–101
61 Merrick GS, Butler WM, Galbreath RW, Stipetich RL, Abel LJ, Lief JH. Erectile function after permanent prostate brachytherapy. Int J Radiat Oncol Biol Phys 2002; 52: 893–902
62 Robinson JW, Moritz S, Fung T. Meta-analysis of rates of erectile function after treatment of localized prostate carcinoma. Int J Radiat Oncol Biol Phys 2002; 54: 1063–1068
63 Raina R, Agarwal A, Goyal KK, Jackson C, Ulchaker J, Angermeier K, Klein E, Ciezki J, Zippe CD. Long-term potency after iodine-125 radiotherapy for prostate cancer and role of sildenafil citrate. Urology 2003; 62: 1103–1108

TUMT for Benign Prostatic Hyperplasia

R. Berges

Introduction

During the past 10 years, TUR-P treatment for benign prostatic hyperplasia has been increasingly challenged by minimally invasive procedures, among them transurethral microwave, radiofrequency, or laser sources.

In contrast to other procedures, microwave thermotherapy TUMT does not require general or regional anesthesia, thus it can be performed entirely as an outpatient procedure. Critics, however, state that TUMT has a relatively low impact on BPH relevant treatment parameters and a subsequent high retreatment rate, thus being far less effective than TUR-P. These objections prove to be wrong when a more detailed analysis differentiates between the various TUMT systems, because recent developments in TUMT technology have contributed to a boost in treatment effectiveness.

TUMT Techniques

The scope of thermal therapy increases with the advent of applicators delivering energy at levels between 42 to 70 °C. It is critical to understand that, in general, only TUMT systems that are able to deliver temperatures within the prostate above 55 °C are able to produce sufficient heat to cause tissue necrosis. These systems are referred to as high-energy (HE)-TUMT and are considered as ablative procedures. Systems delivering heat below this threshold are termed low-energy (LE)-TUMT and are regarded as non-ablative, thus treatment with these systems is symptomatic only.

In addition to these principal differences between TUMT systems, great efforts have been made to better understand heat transmission within the prostate. Although heat kills in a consistent and reproducible manner, microwave thermotherapy treatment outcome may vary to a great extent due to variations in the temperature applied with the same system in different patients, as tissue temperature in the prostate is mainly determined by three processes:

- application of heat through absorption of microwave energy,
- heat conduction in the tissue, and
- loss of heat through prostatic blood flow.

This relationship is reflected by the classic bioheat equation [1] (Fig. 1) which has been successful in modeling temperature distributions *in vivo*.

From this equation it is easy to understand that the major variable influencing heat absorption and thus treatment outcome in any individual prostate is "prostatic blood flow", as "heat conduction" is a tissue-specific constant and microwave power and treatment time are fixed values depending on the specific TUMT device. To compensate for a six-fold increase in blood flow it was calculated that the microwave power has to be increased three-fold to achieve the same biological treatment effect. This shows the tremendous significance of prostatic blood flow for TUMT [2].

Just recently, a third generation of high energy TUMT devices has been introduced that, for the first time, is able to continuously monitor actual temperature levels within the prostate during treatment at three different areas (prostatic base, middle, and apex). This "temperature feedback" enables the device to calculate blood flow within the prostate and then adjust both microwave power and treatment time in each individ-

$$\rho c \frac{dT}{dt} = \lambda \Delta T - \omega_b \rho_b c_b \rho (T - T_a) + Q_s + Q_m$$

temperature change — heat conduction — blood flow — microwave power

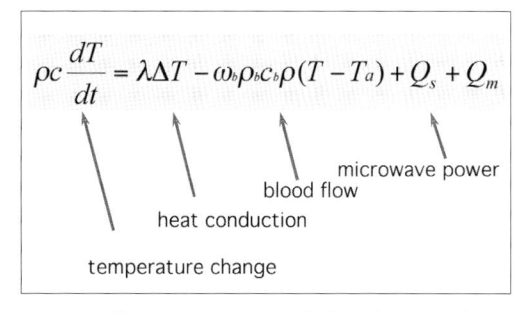

Fig. 1 Bioheat equation to calculate heat uptake in prostate tissue using microwave power (see text).

ual case resulting, again for the first time, in a predictable and reproducible amount of necrosis produced in each treatment [3].

Treatment Outcome

As stated above, microwave treatment outcome is largely dependent on the amount of energy delivered to the prostate. Currently more than 100,000 TUMT treatments/year are performed worldwide and there are more than 15 different TUMT systems available. Consistent and reliable clinical evidence, however, is available only for selected systems, namely the Prostatron®, Targis®, Urologix®, and Prostalund® devices, the latter of which is the only system enabling the aforementioned crucial intraprostatic temperature measurements.

Low energy TUMT

There have been 5 prospective clinical trials published since 1998 with a follow-up of 5 years, most of which have been conducted with the Prostatron® device [4–8]. In addition, there is evidence from one randomized study against TUR-P including 69 patients [9] (Table 1). Summarizing the results from these trials, there is no evidence of prostate volume reduction or significant reduction of prostatic obstruction and only a minor improvement in Q_{max} to the extent of 2–4 mL/s after LE-TUMT treatment. However, LE-TUMT leads to a significant reduction of LUTS in treated patients. Therefore, LE-TUMT is considered to be a symptomatic but not an ablative procedure.

High energy TUMT

Treatment outcome is largely dependent on the device used as there are substantial differences in treatment outcome when intraprostatic temperature measurements are applied, as with the Prostalund-feedback treatment PLFT®.

Evidence for non-PLFT high energy TUMT is available from several clinical trials that have been conducted either with the Urologix T3® [10], Prostatron® [11–14] or Tragis® [15] system. In addition, two meta-analysis [16, 17] have been published (not listed in Table 2) that, however, did not discriminate between PLFT and conventional HE-TUMT, and — to make matters worse — also included low-energy TUMT trials. Reported outcome from these meta-analyses are therefore questionable.

In summary, HE-TUMT has a comparable outcome regarding symptom improvement as LE-TUMT. In addition, HE-TUMT results in tissue necrosis, thus classifying this treatment modality as an ablative procedure. On average, HE-TUMT

Table 1 Studies and treatment outcome for low-energy TUMT

Author	Study design	n	Equipment used	Follow-up (years)	Symptom improvement	Q_{max} improvement (mL/s)	Re-treatment rate (%)
Keijzers et al. 1998	open prospective	231	Prostatron 2.0	5	4–5 pts. (Madson Iverson Score)	+2–3	41
Hallin et al. 1998	open prospective	187	Prostatron 2.0	4	–	–	66
Francisca et al. 1999	open prospective	1092	Prostatron 2.0	5	4–5 pts. (Madson Iverson Score)	+2–3	40
Daehlin et al. 2000	open prospective	91	Primus U+R	5	–37% (IPSS)	–	52
Tsai et al. 2001	open prospective	65	Prostcare	5	–31% at 6 months	+1 at 6 months	85
Dahlstrand et al. 1995/96	RCT	69	LE vs. TURP Prostatron 2.0	2	n. a.	n. a	n. a

Table 2 Studies and treatment outcome for high-energy TUMT (PLFT excluded)

Author	Study design	n	Equipment	Follow-up (years)	Symptom improvement	Q_{max} improvement (mL/s)	Re-treatment rate (%)
Ramsey et al. 1998	open prospective	155	Urologix T3	3	56% (AUA Score)	5.1	n. a.
d'Ancona et al. 1998	RCT	52	Prostatron 2.5. vs. TURP	2.4	13 pts. TUMT vs. 14 pts. TUR-P (IPSS)	4.3 TUMT vs. 9.2 TUR-P	12.5
Ahmed et al. 1997	RCT	60	Prostatron 2.5 vs. TURP	0.5	13 pts. TUMT vs.13 pts. TUR-P (IPSS)	1 TUMT vs. 5 TURP	n. a
Floratos et al. 2001; Delarosette et al. 2003	RCT	155	Prostatron 2.5 vs. TURP	3	40% TUMT vs. 85% TUR-P	3 TUMT vs. 17 TUR-P	22 TUMT vs. 13 TUR-P
Thalmann et al. 2002	open prospective	200	Targis	3.5	85%	8.5	22

results over time in a 35% reduction in prostate size and leads to an increase of Q_{max} by 70% (1 to –8.5 mL/s), which was always less than the flow improvement from TUR-P in direct comparison trials.

The pitfall for conventional TUMT treatment is the broad variance in treatment outcome, as common TUMT devices do not allow adjustments in heat intake during treatment. This results in an unfavorable retreatment rate of between 25 and 30% after only 3–4 years and it can be expected that retreatment rates will continue to increase with longer follow-up (Table 2).

ProstaLund feedback treatment (PLFT)

PLFT is the only currently available HE-TUMT device that attributes the different heat consumption within individual prostates, thus allowing for adjustment of microwave power and treatment time. In a randomized trial comparing 100 PLFT with 46 TUR-P cases with a published follow-up of 3 years no differences were observed in both treatment arms regarding symptom relief (–65%), improvement of symptom bother, or Q_{max} (8 mL/s, Fig. 2) [18]. Prostate volume reduction was less pronounced in TUMT, however, differences were not significant compared to TUR-P. 5-year follow-up data will be available soon proving continuous and comparable effectiveness with the TUR-P arm, making PLFT a possible candidate to really compete with the so-called gold standard TUR-P. (Data have been viewed by the author and are submitted for publication.) Similar results have been reported for PLFT treatment in a multicenter prospective trial with 102 patients with a current follow-up of 6 months treated in the USA [19].

In addition to the favorable treatment outcome of PLFT, further developments include the use of adrenalin injections administered through a modified transurethral catheter to reduce prostatic blood flow prior to treatment and so bringing treatment time uniformly below 35 min [20] regardless of prostate size, and a (prototype) stenting device abolishing the need for post-treatment catheterization (personal communication with S. Schelin) — a typical feature of all HE-TUMT treatments. These modifications have made this method in Sweden, the country of origin, already the number one choice in the therapy for obstructive BPH.

Adverse Events after TUMT Treatment

Apart from retreatment rates, both LE- and HE-TUMT are relatively safe procedures. However, especially for HE-TUMT a limited number of serious adverse events has been reported, emphasizing that this is not a harmless procedure if treatment indications and proposed device-specific operating procedures are neglected. Reported adverse events include rectum fistulas followed

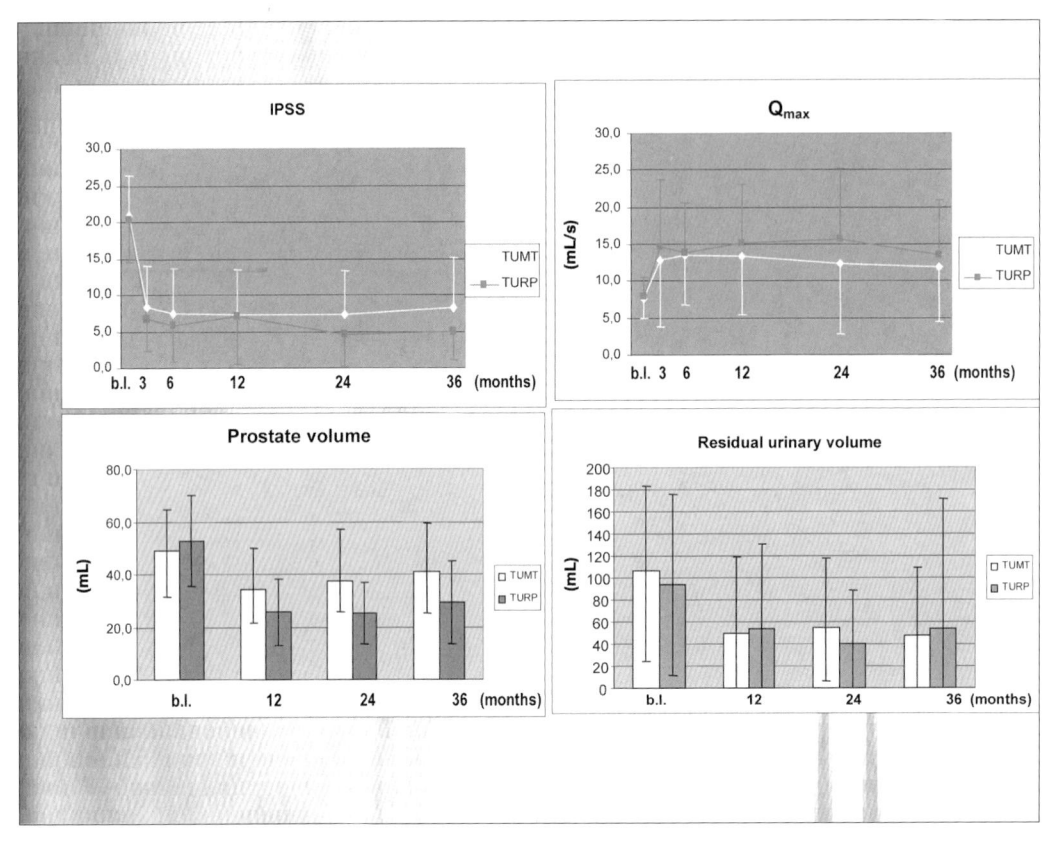

Fig. 2 3-year treatment outcome after PLFT vs. TURP (data from Urology 2002; 60: 292–299).

by colostomy, and penile burns up to complete necrosis followed by amputation [21].

References

1. Pennes HH. Analysis of tissue and arterial blood temperatures in the resting human forearm. J Appl Physiol 1948; 1: 93–122
2. Bolmsjö M, Sturesson C, Wagrell L, Andersson-Engels S, Mattiasson A. Optimizing transurethral microwave thermotherapy: a model for studying power, blood flow, temperature variations and tissue destruction. Br J Urol 1998; 81: 811–816
3. Wagrell L, Schelin S, Bolmsjo M, Brudin L. Intraprostatic temperature monitoring during transurethral microwave thermotherapy for the treatment of benign prostatic hyperplasia. J Urol 1998; 159: 1583–1587
4. Keijzers GB, Francisca EA, D'Ancona FC, Kiemeney LA, Debruyne FM, de la Rosette JJ. Long-term results of lower energy transurethral microwave thermotherapy. J Urol 1998; 159: 1966–1972
5. Hallin A, Berlin T. Transurethral microwave thermotherapy for benign prostatic hyperplasia: clinical outcome after 4 years. J Urol 1998; 159: 459–464
6. Francisca EA, Keijzers GB, d'Ancona FC, Debruyne FM, de la Rosette JJ. Lower-energy thermotherapy in the treatment of benign prostatic hyperplasia: long-term follow-up results of a multicenter international study. World J Urol 1999; 17: 279–284
7. Daehlin L, Frugard J. Transurethral microwave thermotherapy in the management of lower urinary tract symptoms from benign prostatic obstruction: follow-up after five years. Scand J Urol Nephrol 2000; 34: 304–308
8. Tsai YS, Lin JS, Tong YC, Tzai TS, Yang WH, Chang CC, Cheng HL, Lin YM, Jou YC. Transurethral microwave thermotherapy for symptomatic benign prostatic hyperplasia: long-term durability with Prostcare. Eur Urol 2001; 39: 688–692; discussion: 693–694
9. Dahlstrand C, Walden M, Geirsson G, Pettersson S. Transurethral microwave thermotherapy versus transurethral resection for symptomatic benign prostatic obstruction: a prospective randomized study with a 2-year follow-up. Br J Urol 1995; 76: 614–618

[10] Ramsey EW, Miller PD, Parsons K. Transurethral microwave thermotherapy in the treatment of benign prostatic hyperplasia: results obtained with the Urologix T3 device. World J Urol 1998; 16: 96–101

[11] d'Ancona FC, Francisca EA, Hendriks JC, Debruyne FM, de la Rosette JJ: The predictive value of baseline variables in the treatment of benign prostatic hyperplasia using high-energy transurethral microwave thermotherapy. Br J Urol 1998; 82: 808–813

[12] Ahmed M, Bell T, Lawrence WT, Ward JP, Watson GM. Transurethral microwave thermotherapy (Prostatron version 2.5) compared with transurethral resection of the prostate for the treatment of benign prostatic hyperplasia: a randomized, controlled, parallel study. Br J Urol 1997; 79: 181–185

[13] Floratos DL, Kiemeney LA, Rossi C, Kortmann BB, Debruyne FM, de la Rosette JJ. Long-term follow-up of randomized transurethral microwave thermotherapy versus transurethral prostatic resection study. J Urol 2001; 165: 1533–1538

[14] De la Rosette JJ, Floratos DL, Severens JL, Kiemeney LA, Debruyne FM, Pilar Laguna M. Transurethral resection vs. microwave thermotherapy of the prostate: a cost-consequences analysis. BJU Int 2003; 92: 713–718

[15] Thalmann GN, Mattei A, Treuthardt C, Burkhard FC, Studer UE. Transurethral microwave therapy in 200 patients with a minimum follow-up of 2 years: urodynamic and clinical results. J Urol 2002; 167: 2496–501

[16] Ramsey EW, Dahlstrand C. Durability of results obtained with transurethral microwave thermotherapy in the treatment of men with symptomatic benign prostatic hyperplasia. J Endourol 2000; 14: 671–675

[17] Hoffman RM, MacDonald R, Monga M, Wilt TJ. Transurethral microwave thermotherapy vs. transurethral resection for treating benign prostatic hyperplasia: a systematic review. BJU Int 2004; 94: 1031–1036

[18] Wagrell L, Schelin S, Nordling J, Richthoff J, Magnusson B, Schain M, Larson T, Boyle E, Duelund J, Kroyer K et al. Three-year follow-up of feedback microwave thermotherapy versus TURP for clinical BPH: a prospective randomized multicenter study. Urology 2004; 64: 698–702

[19] David RD, Grunberger I, Shore N, Swierzewski SJ 3rd. Multicenter initial U.S. experience with Core-Therm-monitored feedback transurethral microwave thermotherapy for individualized treatment of patients with symptomatic benign prostatic hyperplasia. J Endourol 2004; 18: 682–685

[20] Schelin S. Mediating transurethral microwave thermotherapy by intraprostatic and periprostatic injections of mepivacaine epinephrine: effects on treatment time, energy consumption, and patient comfort. J Endourol 2002; 16: 117–121

[21] FDA/Center for Devices and Radiologic Health. FDA Public Health Notification: Serious injuries from microwave thermotherapy for benign prostatic hyperplasia. US Food and Drug Administration, 2000 http://www.fda.ogv/cdrh/safety/bph.html. Accessed January 15, 2004

Radiofrequency (RF) Therapy of the Kidney: Indications, Technique, and Results

B. Brehmer, G. Jakse

Introduction

Renal cell carcinoma (RCC) is the most common primary malignancy of the kidney. Open surgery is the mainstay of treatment of localized disease, and may be the optimal treatment for patients with isolated solitary metastatic disease [1]. To decrease surgical morbidity, laparoscopic nephrectomy has been introduced as a minimally invasive surgical alternative. Laparoscopic radical nephrectomy is meanwhile established with considerable advantages; decreased postoperative morbidity, decreased analgesic requirements, improved cosmetic results, shorter hospital stay and convalescence [2]. The consistent effort to improve these advantages of the laparoscopic procedures as minimally invasive techniques is the introduction of RF therapy to the RCC treatment.

The first radiofrequency (RF) ablation was reported in 1976 by LeVeen and co-workers in 21 patients with different tumors [3]. This technique took a long time before in the 1990s it was accepted as a clinical treatment modality in oncology. Solbiati published in 1997 the treatment of 29 patients with 44 liver metastases treated with RF ablation [4], and Livraghi was the first to report the treatment of primary liver malignancy in 42 patients [5]. Zlotta reported in 1997 the first three patients treated with RF ablation for RCC [6]. Since these first publications more than 330 patients treated with RF ablation for RCC have been reported in the peer reviewed literature.

Basic Technical Aspects

RF delivers a high-frequency (460–500 kHz) alternating current into the tumor by an electrode, a thin needle, usually 21–14 gauge, that is electrically insulated along all but the distal 1 to 3 cm of the shaft. The application of RF current produces resistive friction in the tissue that is converted into heat and induces cellular destruction and protein denaturation at temperatures above 50 °C when applied for 4 to 6 minutes [7]. Temperatures above 105 °C result in gas formation, which reduces significantly creation of the RF current. Therefore, the goal of RF ablation is to induce temperatures of 50 to 100 °C [7].

Most RF systems used for the kidney are monopolar. Electrodes can be placed directly into tumors using ultrasound, computed tomography (CT), or magnetic resonance (MRI) guidance (Fig. 1). Efforts to increase RF-induced coagulation have led to modifications in the original design of the electrodes, including the development of various RF applicators such as multi-timed applicators [8, 9] or pulsed energy delivery [10]. Currently, there are three RF devices with FDA approval for soft tumor ablation (Radionics Inc., Burlington, MA; RadioTherapeutics Corp., Sunnyvale, CA; and RITA Medical Systems, Mountain View, CA). No study has yet demonstrated a clear advantage of any one device [7].

Indications/Contraindications

The gold standard of treatment in RCC remains surgical resection and should always be preferred if possible. At our institution, patient selection includes those with known contraindications to partial or complete nephrectomy as a result of comorbid conditions or patients with multiple bilateral RCCs. Also the combination of RF ablation and open surgery in multiple tumors in one or both kidneys is a successful concept.

Contraindications may include difficulty for successful treatment due to size (> 4 cm) or location of the tumor. Tumors in the hilum or central collecting system are unfavorable for RF ablation. In addition, if the tumor is located so that thermal injury may occur to the liver, colon, or other organs, RF ablation is not possible.

Clinical Studies

Gervais and co-workers have published the largest study; they examined RF ablation of 42 renal cell carcinomas in 34 patients [11]. Of the 42 tumors, 29 were exophytic, 2 were parenchymal, 4 were central, and 7 were mixed. All 29 exophytic

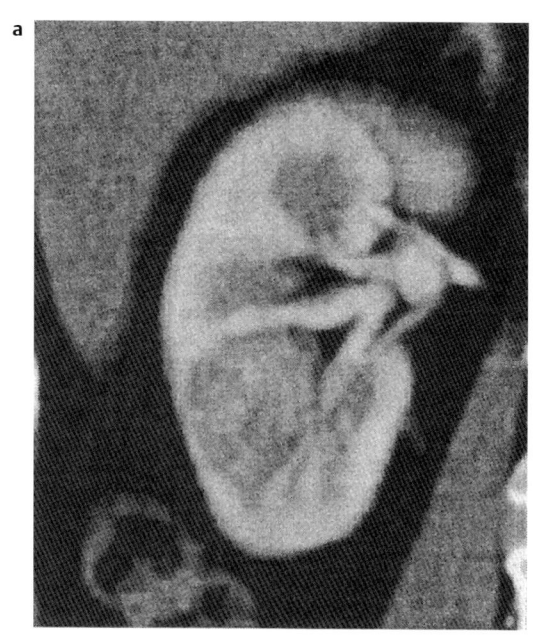

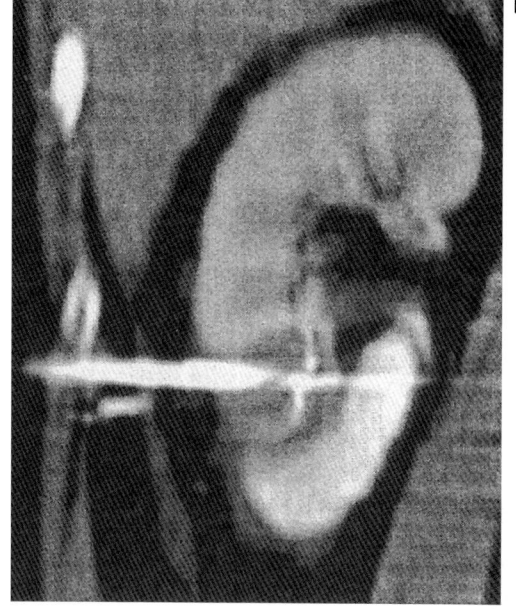

Fig. 1 RF ablation in RCC (cT1N0M0). CT before [a], during [b], and after [c] treatment.

tumors (mean size: 3.2 cm; size range: 1.1–5.0 cm) and 2 parenchymal tumors were ablated successfully. One of the central tumors (25%) and four of the mixed tumors (57%) were treated with technical success. The authors report that a significant negative predictor of technical success is a tumor larger than 3.0 cm with a component in the renal sinus, although 5 of 11 tumors of this type were treated successfully.

Su published the results of 29 patients with a total of 35 small renal tumors (mean size: 2.2 cm; range: 1.0–4.0 cm) [12]. The authors reported that 33 of 35 (94%) renal lesions required just a single RF ablation treatment during a

Table 1 Summary of published results

Study	Pat.	Mean tumor size (cm)	NED	Mean follow-up (months)
Gervais [16]	42	3.2	42	13.2
Mayo-Smith [13]	32	2.6	31	9.0
Su [12]	35	2.2	35	9.0
Farrell [17]	20	1.7	20	9.0
Aachen	16	3.4	16*	13.4

NED: no evidence of disease in CT scan.
* 1 Patient after partial resection of the kidney.

mean follow-up of 9 months, whereas the 2 remaining tumors were successfully retreated in a second session.

Mayo-Smith reported on the outcomes of 32 tumors in 32 patients (mean size: 2.6 cm; range: 1.0–5.0 cm) [13]. After either one or two sessions, 31 of the 32 tumors (97%) were treated successfully by CT. Six patients (19%) required a second session because of incomplete treatment during the first session.

At our institution 16 patients with 17 renal cell carcinomas were treated with RF ablation. Except in one tumor, all ablations were successful. In this case the residual tumor was resected 4 weeks after ablation and showed vital cancer on histology. No one of the 16 patients showed a recurrence at follow-up (mean: 17.1 months; range: 10–26 months) (Table 1).

Reported outcomes reveal a very low complication rate associated with RF ablation of renal masses. Only 3 experienced complications were described in 159 patients from the literature, including two ureteral strictures and a small liver burn. Of these, only the ureteral strictures required intervention [14]. Mayo-Smith reported a 5-mm skin metastasis at the electrode insertion site in one patient which was resected without recurrence [13]. It is important to note that the very low complication rate is reported in patients who were already deemed to be too high risk for surgical intervention because of advanced age or medical comorbidities.

In summary, RF ablation is a viable option for nonsurgical patients. It is safe with a low complication rate. Tumor size and location are the two most important factors for the successful treatment. Further clinical follow-up is required from ongoing clinical studies. Patients have to be evaluated jointly by a urologist and radiologist.

The extent of disease should be well established with sufficient imaging to verify the location and extent of local tumor. A biopsy before the procedure is not imperative. Long-term follow-up of thermal ablation with sonography has limited value. Contrast-enhanced CT or MRI is the mainstay of long-term imaging follow-up. Follow-up imaging is performed at 1 and 3 months, and every 3–4 months thereafter at our institution.

All reports in the literature are experimental laboratory examinations, single center experience or phase II studies with no follow-ups of more than 17 months [15]. Grade of evidence: 3a.

References

[1] Godley PA, Stinchcombe TE. Renal cell carcinoma. Curr Opin Oncol 1999; 11: 213–217

[2] Allan JD, Tolley DA, Kaouk JH, Novick AC, Gill IS. Laparoscopic radical nephrectomy. Eur Urol 2001; 40: 17–23

[3] LeVeen HH, Wapnick S, Piccone V, Falk G, Ahmed N. Tumor eradication by radiofrequency therapy. Responses in 21 patients. JAMA 1976; 235: 2198–2200

[4] Solbiati L, Goldberg SN, Ierace T, Livraghi T, Meloni F, Dellanoce M et al. Hepatic metastases: percutaneous radio-frequency ablation with cooled-tip electrodes. Radiology 1997; 205: 367–373

[5] Livraghi T, Goldberg SN, Lazzaroni S, Meloni F, Solbiati L, Gazelle GS. Small hepatocellular carcinoma: treatment with radio-frequency ablation versus ethanol injection. Radiology 1999; 210: 655–661

[6] Zlotta AR, Wildschutz T, Raviv G, Peny MO, van Gansbeke D, Noel JC et al. Radiofrequency interstitial tumor ablation (RITA) is a possible new modality for treatment of renal cancer: ex vivo and in vivo experience. J Endourol 1997; 11: 251–258

[7] Goldberg SN, Gazelle GS, Mueller PR. Thermal ablation therapy for focal malignancy: a unified ap-

proach to underlying principles, techniques, and diagnostic imaging guidance. AJR Am J Roentgenol 2000; 174: 323–331

[8] Curley SA, Izzo F, Ellis LM, Nicolas VJ, Vallone P. Radiofrequency ablation of hepatocellular cancer in 110 patients with cirrhosis. Ann Surg 2000; 232: 381–391

[9] Rossi S, Buscarini E, Garbagnati F, Di Stasi M, Quaretti P, Rago M et al. Percutaneous treatment of small hepatic tumors by an expandable RF needle electrode. AJR Am J Roentgenol 1998; 170: 1015–1022

[10] Goldberg SN, Stein MC, Gazelle GS, Sheiman RG, Kruskal JB, Clouse ME. Percutaneous radiofrequency tissue ablation: optimization of pulsed-radiofrequency technique to increase coagulation necrosis. J Vasc Interv Radiol 1999; 10: 907–916

[11] Gervais DA, McGovern FJ, Arellano RS, McDougal WS, Mueller PR. Renal cell carcinoma: clinical experience and technical success with radio-frequency ablation of 42 tumors. Radiology 2003; 226: 417–424

[12] Su LM, Jarrett TW, Chan DY, Kavoussi LR, Solomon SB. Percutaneous computed tomography-guided radiofrequency ablation of renal masses in high surgical risk patients: preliminary results. Urology 2003; 61: 26–33

[13] Mayo-Smith WW, Dupuy DE, Parikh PM, Pezzullo JA, Cronan JJ. Imaging-guided percutaneous radiofrequency ablation of solid renal masses: techniques and outcomes of 38 treatment sessions in 32 consecutive patients. AJR Am J Roentgenol 2003; 180: 1503–1508

[14] Hines-Peralta A, Goldberg SN. Review of radiofrequency ablation for renal cell carcinoma. Clin Cancer Res 2004; 10: 6328S–6334S

[15] Roy-Choudhury SH, Cast JE, Cooksey G, Puri S, Breen DJ. Early experience with percutaneous radiofrequency ablation of small solid renal masses. AJR Am J Roentgenol 2003; 180: 1055–1061

[16] Gervais DA, McGovern FJ, Wood BJ, Goldberg SN, McDougal WS, Mueller PR. Radiofrequency ablation of renal cell carcinoma: early clinical experience. Radiology 2000; 217: 665–672

[17] Farrell MA, Charboneau WJ, DiMarco DS, Chow GK, Zincke H, Callstrom MR et al. Imaging-guided radiofrequency ablation of solid renal tumors. AJR Am J Roentgenol 2003; 180: 1509–1513

Cryotherapy of Renal Cell Carcinomas

U. K. F. Witzsch

Introduction

Nephron-sparing surgery (NSS) for renal cell carcinoma (RCC) is an established procedure [1]. Due to a well-known impact on the quality of live [2] the question for less invasive procedures in the treatment of multimorbid patients was raised. Also there are sometimes contraindications for NSS or nephrectomy.

Cryoablation of RCC is a minimally invasive alternative to NSS. There is experimental and clinical evidence for its efficacy as shown below.

Principles of Cryotherapy

The outcome of cryotherapy of the kidney was experimentally investigated by Nakada et al. [3]. These experiments were done with a second generation cryotherapy device. First, the growth kinetics of implanted RCC in a canine model were defined.

Then 35 versus 35 versus 10 rabbits were sacrificed seven days after implantation. They were treated with cryotherapy at 15 min double freeze with 5 mm margin at –20 °C with nephrectomy, or with nothing. The cryotherapy group showed the same results as the nephrectomy group.

From a clinical point of view there are several reports on cryotherapy of renal masses. Lin et al. [4] described a case with bilateral RCC. In 1998 the patient underwent a left partial nephrectomy for RCC. In August 1999 he underwent a left laparoscopic cryotherapy for RCC. In January 2001 the patient underwent a right laparoscopic cryoablation for RCC. Six months afterwards a bilateral needle biopsy did not show histological signs of RCC. In August 2002 the patient underwent bilateral nephrectomy prior to transplantation due to renal insufficiency. There was no RCC found in the specimens.

Results of Cryotherapy

Steinberg et al. [5] treated 200 patients with NSS and 88 with cryotherapy for multiple tumors of the kidney, 4.5% of which were bilateral. All procedures were done laparoscopically.

The bilateral tumors were treated with partial nephrectomy of all tumors *(en bloc-lpn)* (n = 3), NSS of each single tumor *(lpn)* (n = 2), partial nephrectomy and cryotherapy *(lpn + cryo)* (n = 2), and cryotherapy only *(cryo)* (n = 6). Freezing time was 15 minutes (Table **1**).

There was no progression for one to 54 months. One *de novo* tumor was seen.

Nadler et al. [6] treated 15 patients with laparoscopic renal cryosurgery for renal masses. Freezing was done with a single, first generation (liquid nitrogen driven) probe. At least two freeze cycles interrupted by a passive thaw cycle were performed. The lesions were frozen with a 1 cm safety margin. Intraoperative biopsy showed RCC in 10 cases. Follow-up of seven out of ten patients was achieved. Five showed negative biopsies, one residual RCC (with a 3.2 cm tumor) and one multiple microfoci surrounding the tumor necrosis. Mean serum creatinine was elevated from 1.25 ng/mL preoperatively to 1.36 ng/mL postoperatively. Blood loss was 67 mL and thus less than in NSS, also no ischemia was necessary.

Table **1** Treatment of renal tumors

	Ischemia	Blood loss [mL]	Operation time [min]	Complications
en bloc-lpn	40 warm	117	230	1 pneumonia
2x lpn	40 cold	325	305	1 dvt
lpn + cryo	30 warm	175	262	1 sepsis
cryo		169	258	0

Table 2 Approaches to the kidney

	US quality	Min. equipment	Min. invasiveness	Control
Open	+++	++	–	++
Hand-assisted	+	+	+	+
Laparoscopic	++	–	++	+
Percutaneous	–	+++	+++	–

Third Generation Cryotherapy

Third generation cryotherapy is the latest technological evolution. This technology is described in the chapter on cryoablation of the prostate. The needle technology enables an easy percutaneous and laparoscopic approach which reduces the invasiveness of the procedure.

Regarding the approach to the kidney there are several modalities available for 3rd generation cryotherapy (Table 2).

The open approach gives the best control but also has most invasiveness. The laparoscopic approach has its advantage in minimally invasiveness and ultrasound quality. The percutaneous approach is the least invasive but offers less control of the procedure and inadequate US resolution.

Best guidance of the needles for homogeneous placement is ensured by use of a special cryotherapy template grid. The needle placement starts with positioning of a temperature sensor in the middle of the tumor. Then a circle of cryoneedles is placed around the temperature sensor to ensure complete freezing of the lesion. The dimensions of the ice ball are approximately 3 × 2 cm. This leads to a maximum diameter of treatable tumor of 4 cm approximately. The placement of the needles and the progress of freezing as well as the blood flow in and around the lesion are controlled by ultrasound. Two freeze thaw cycles are applied.

Discussion and Conclusion

The efficacy of cryotherapy for ablation of RCC is proven. Most authors have treated small peripheral masses. Depending on the technology used, a maximum size of three to four centimeters is recommended. Bigger lesions should be treated with NSS. Due to the fact that intrarenal masses are more difficult to reach, control seems only possible with high resolution ultrasound. On the other hand, ice formation is not directly visualized so this makes the control more difficult and indicates more or less NSS. Also damage of surrounding tissue due to damage of arteries while freezing bigger masses has been discussed. The mode of freezing was different due to different technologies used.

There is no consensus as to whether an intraoperative biopsy is mandatory or not. Regarding possible tumor cell spillage due to bleeding after the biopsy, only personal communications are available. Regarding side effects, blood loss is less than in NSS. All other side effects occur with almost the same probability as in NSS with the same approach.

Thus, cryotherapy of RCC is a minimally invasive alternative to NSS in selected cases in the hands of an urologist experienced in surgery of the kidney.

References

[1] Witzsch U, Humke U, Kollias A, Becht E. Organerhaltende Nierenchirurgie – Werkbankchirurgie und Autotransplantation. In: Plastisch-rekonstruktive Chirurgie in der Urologie, Schreiter F (ed), Thieme, Stuttgart, 1999

[2] Poulakis V, Witzsch U, de Vries R, Moeckel M, Becht E. Quality of life after surgery for localized renal cell carcinoma: comparison between radical nephrectomy and nephron sparing surgery. Urology 2003; 62: 814–820

[3] Nakada S, Jerde T, Warner T, Lee F. Comparison of cryotherapy and nephrectomy in treating implanted VX-2 carcinoma in rabbit kidneys. BJU Int 2004; 94, 632–636

[4] Lin C, Moinzadeh A, Ramani A, Gill I. Histopathological confirmation of complete cancer cell kill in excised specimens after renal cryotherapy. Urology 2004, 64: 590

[5] Steinberg A, Kilciler M, Abreu S, Ramani A et al. Laparoscopic nephron-sparing surgery for two or more ipsilateral renal tumors. Urology 2004; 64: 255–258

[6] Nadler R, Kim S, Rubenstein J, Yap R et. al. Laparoscopic renal cryosurgery: The Northwestern Experience. J Urol 2003; 170: 1121–1125

Extracorporeal Application of High Intensity Focused Ultrasound (HIFU) for Renal Tumor Thermoablation: Technical Principles and Clinical Application

A. Häcker, M. S. Michel, K. U. Köhrmann

Introduction

HIFU has the potential to be the least invasive of the currently available ablation methods for renal tumors, as the energy source needs not to be introduced directly into the tumor. Experimental trials on the kidneys started in 1992 by Vallancien [1, 2] revealed that, in principle, ablation of kidney tissue by means of focused ultrasound is possible. Thus far, clinical application of HIFU for the treatment of renal tumors has only been experimental in nature. To date (February 2005), treatment results of 14 patients have been published [3, 4] (evidence grade 4).

Technical Principles

The components of an HIFU system include a transducer to generate and focus ultrasound waves; an imaging device, usually a standard imaging ultrasound probe that can be placed in-line with the HIFU transducer to monitor the treatment under real-time conditions; a coupling device such as a water bath or water cushion to provide an interface for transmission of ultrasound energy from transducer to patient; a housing or gantry for the HIFU device; and a central computing unit from which the operator can control treatment parameters. These control parameters are power output, number of pulses, pulse duration, duration between the pulses, focal length, and treatment volume. Currently, two devices for clinical application have been used: The "UTT" (the prototype by Storz Medical, Switzerland; ultrasound probe is shown in Fig. 1) and the commercially available "Model JC Haifu Focused Ultrasound Tumor Therapeutic System" (Chongqing Haifu Technology, China).

Using the Storz device, ultrasound is coupled by degassed water in a water cushion between the ultrasound source and patient's skin (Fig. 2). Because of the comparable acoustic properties of water and tissue, the sound waves should penetrate the skin and further precursory tissue with only slight absorption and reflection. The power density of the converging ultrasound increases as it approaches the focal point. Tissue is rapidly heated to temperatures between 65 and 100 °C, causing irreversible cell damage and thermal coagulative necrosis. The focal region is a cigar-shaped 3-dimensional zone with its long axis perpendicular to the axis of wave propagation. The dimensions of the focal zone depend on the frequency and the geometry of the source; they are in the order of 10 to 50 mm in length and 1 to 5 mm in diameter. A larger volume of tissue can be ablated by sequentially shifting the focal zone by incremental movements of the transducer combined with adjustment of the focal length. By scanning the target using multiple pulses, larger areas of tissue can be ablated.

For clinical application, an important factor is the ability to monitor treatment accurately. This is achieved by using real-time ultrasound [5–7] or MRI [8]. HIFU treatments of kidney tissue can be monitored under real-time conditions by standard imaging ultrasound probes placed in-

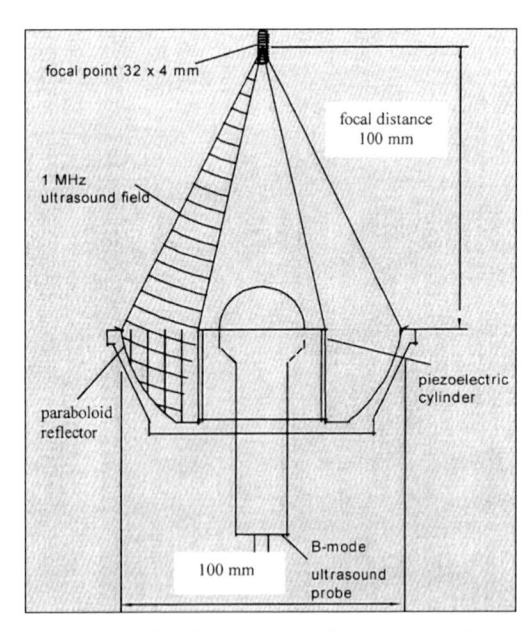

Fig. 1 Principle of extracorporeal HIFU device (Storz UTT).

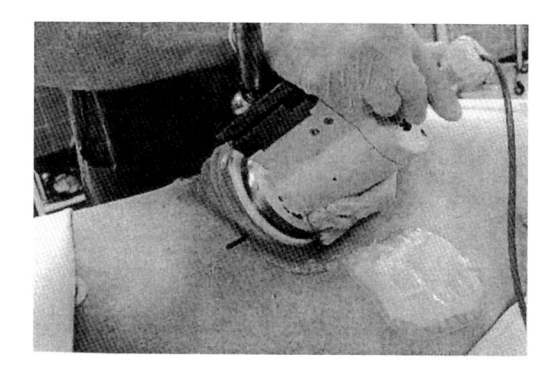

Fig. 2 Application of HIFU to the patient in flank position.

line with the therapeutic HIFU transducer. The position of the therapeutic focus can therefore be identified on the diagnostic image. The extent of the treatment can be monitored by recording post-treatment grey scale changes on the diagnostic images: However, the use of ultrasound for imaging lesions for precise targeting of tissue destruction is limited. Additional imaging modalities, such as duplex-Doppler, CT, and MRI, applied in an on-line thermometry system, are therefore necessary to target the tumor precisely and to monitor the ablation effect on-line. These new techniques are still under development and investigation. Today, no device exists for the treatment of renal tumors under MRI guidance. Because of movement of the kidney during breathing, tumor localization and targeting can be difficult. When using general anesthesia, ventilation can be stopped briefly, and movement of the kidney thus prevented, during application of ultrasound. General anesthesia is also required for managing pain when high energy levels are applied. However, HIFU treatments without general anesthesia have been described in the literature [4, 9].

Clinical Application

When treating healthy kidneys of eight patients with extracorporeally applied HIFU in a phase 1 study, Vallancien et al. [1] did not observe any significant changes in the usual laboratory parameters, except for a transient increase in creatine phosphokinase after a long pulse. Side effects included skin burns. Köhrmann et al. [10] applied HIFU to healthy kidney tissue of 24 patients immediately before nephrectomy. In 19 out of the 24 cases, hemorrhage or necrosis was detected macroscopically. Histologically, interstitial hemorrhages and fiber rupture, as well as collagen fiber shrinkage with eosinophilia, were detected in the focal area. In a phase 2 study, Vallancien et al. [1] treated four patients with T2-T3 renal tumors with HIFU 2, 6, 8, and 15 days before performance of nephrectomy. Histological examination of the treated kidneys revealed a coagulation necrosis in the targeted tumor area. In two cases a small edema formed in the perirenal fat tissue during surgery. No subcapsular or perirenal hematomas were noted. The muscle wall (lumbar incision) was normal in all cases, and there were no lesions of adjacent organs (colon, inferior vena cava, duodenum, ureter, and renal pelvis). During operations done on day 2 or 3, a clearly demarcated necrotic area was detected corresponding to the selected volume. No adverse systemic effects were observed. Two patients had localized first-degree and third-degree skin burns. Köhrmann and colleagues [3] reported on a patient with 3 renal tumors who underwent HIFU in three sessions under general or sedation anesthesia and who was followed by clinical examinations and MRI for 6 months. After HIFU treatment, MRI indicated necrosis in the two tumors of the lower pole of the kidney within 17 and 48 days. The necrotic area in these two tumors shrunk thereafter within 6 months (tumor 1: size 2.3 cm to 0.8 cm; tumor 2: size 1.4 cm to 1.1 cm). Unfortunately, one tumor in the upper pole (size 2.8 cm) was inadequately treated because of absorption of ultrasound energy by the interposed ribs. During one session a skin burn of grade 2 occurred. Wu et al. [4] reported on their preliminary experience using HIFU for the treatment of patients with advanced stage renal malignancy. HIFU treatment (median duration of therapy 5.4 h; range 1.5-9 h) was performed in 12 patients with advanced stage renal cell carcinoma and 1 patient with colon cancer metastasized to the kidney (median tumor size 8.7 cm; range 2-15). All patients received HIFU treatment safely, including 10 who had partial ablation and 3 who had complete tumor ablation. After HIFU, hematuria disappeared in 7 of 8 patients and flank pain of presumed malignant origin disappeared in 9 of 10 patients. Postoperative images showed a decrease in or absence of tumor blood supply in the treated region and significant shrinkage of the ablated tumor. Of the 13 patients, 7 died (median survival 14.1 months, range 2 to 27) and

6 were still alive with a median follow-up of 18.5 months (range 10 to 27). A minor skin burn was observed in the first patient, which had healed 2 weeks after HIFU.

HIFU is a noninvasive technique. It does not allow accurate pathological tissue diagnosis, staging and grading of the renal mass, which determine the prognosis of the patient. Therefore, a preablation biopsy of the renal mass is necessary [11, 12] for precise pathological diagnosis of the renal lesions (benign or malignant), which is critical for determining appropriate clinical and radiological follow-up. Radiographical follow-up using CT or MRI with contrast media application is necessary for tumor control.

HIFU is a promising but presently experimental procedure. It will achieve routine clinical application if technical problems concerning visualization of the target organ and lesion, precise control of lesion size, complete ablation of the tumor mass, and reduction in side effects (skin burns) can be resolved. The objectives of further developments are to optimize ultrasound coupling, creation of flexible lesion sizes, and to provide an on-line ablation imaging system to ensure complete tumor ablation. At this time, HIFU should be reserved for selected patients in well designed clinical studies.

References

[1] Vallancien G, Harouni M, Veilon B, Mombet A, Prapotnich D, Brisset JM, Bougaran J. Focused extracorporeal pyrotherapy: Feasibility study in man. J Endourol 1992; 6: 173–181

[2] Vallancien G, Chartier-Kastler E, Bataille N, Chopin D, Harouni M, Bourgaran J. Focused extracorporeal pyrotherapy. Eur Urol 1993; 23 (suppl 1): 48–52

[3] Köhrmann KU, Michel MS, Gaa J, Marlinghaus E, Alken P. High intensity focused ultrasound as noninvasive therapy for multilocal renal cell carcinoma: case study and review of the literature. J Urol 2002; 167: 2397–2403

[4] Wu F, Wang ZB, Chen WZ, Bai J, Zhu H, Qiao TY. Preliminary experience using high intensity focused ultrasound for the treatment of patients with advanced stage renal malignancy. J Urol 2003; 170: 2237–2240

[5] Wu F, Chen WZ, Bai J, Zou JZ, Wang ZL, Zhu H, Wang ZB. Pathological changes in human malignant carcinoma treated with high-intensity focused ultrasound. Ultrasound Med Biol 2001; 27: 1099–1106

[6] Madersbacher S, Schatzl G, Djavan B, Stulnig T, Marberger M. Long-term outcome of transrectal high-intensity focused ultrasound therapy for benign prostatic hyperplasia. Eur Urol 2000; 37: 687–694

[7] Chaussy C, Thüroff S. The status of high-intensity focused ultrasound in the treatment of localized prostate cancer and the impact of a combined resection. Curr Urol Rep 2003; 4: 248–252

[8] Hynynen K, McDannold N, Vykhodtseva N, Jolesz FA. Noninvasive MR imaging-guided focal opening of the blood-brain barrier in rabbits. Radiology 2001; 220: 640–646

[9] Visioli AG, Rivens IH, ter Haar GR, Horwich A, Huddart RA, Moskovic E, Padhani A, Glees J. Preliminary results of a phase I dose escalation clinical trial using focused ultrasound in the treatment of localised tumours. Eur J Ultrasound 1999; 9: 11–18

[10] Köhrmann K, Michel M, Back W. Non-invasive thermoablation in the kidney: first results of the clinical feasibility study. J Endourol 2000; 14 (suppl 1): A34

[11] Gill IS, Novick AC, Meraney AM, Chen RN, Hobart MG, Sung GT, Hale J, Schweizer DK, Remer EM. Laparoscopic renal cryoablation in 32 patients. Urology 2000; 56: 748–753

[12] Gervais DA, McGovern FJ, Arellano RS, McDougal WS, Mueller PR. Renal cell carcinoma: clinical experience and technical success with radio-frequency ablation of 42 tumors. Radiology 2003; 226: 417–424

Extracorporeal Shock Wave Therapy (ESWT) in Urology

Consensus

S. Lahme, G. Hatzichristodoulou, E. W. Hauck

After the first report of extracorporeal shock wave therapy (ESWT) in the field of urology by Bellorofonte in 1989, this technique has spread more and more, especially since the late 1990s. Among the different indications for ESWT, most data are available concerning Peyronie's disease (PD). As little is known about the pathophysiology of PD, ESWT is an empiric and symptomatic treatment modality. The mode of action still remains unclear. Hypothetically, shock waves lead to a disintegration of penile plaque formation or calcifications. There are hints that ESWT interferes with collagen structures resulting in a disorganization of the collagen formation. For the analgesic effect of ESWT hyperstimulation analgesia and alteration of pain receptors are discussed.

A wide variety of shock wave devices is available differing in mode of shock wave generation, focus size, focus geometry, intensity and positioning systems. It is recommended to use a shock wave device with a focus ranging from 3 mm to 20 mm. There is no evidence that a particular mode of shock wave generation is superior. According to the type of transducer, a positioning system, e.g., by ultrasound or a particular penile fixation device, may be beneficial. According to the literature so far no recommendation can be given for the technical parameters. It seems to be suitable to treat with 2000–3000 shock waves for several times.

Results of a meta-analysis and a placebo-controlled trial show that ESWT in PD resolves pain faster than during the natural course. No effect was detected concerning reduction of penile deviation, plaque size, and erectile dysfunction. Safety appears adequate since severe complications have not occurred so far.

The beneficial effect of ESWT on penile pain justifies further investigations of this treatment modality. Future studies should deal with the mode of action of ESWT, evaluation of further indications, such as prostatitis and indications in other fields of medicine (rheumatic diseases).

In summary, ESWT is an appropriate treatment modality to achieve pain reduction in Peyronie's disease within a short time. ESWT is not a therapeutic option to reduce penile deviation.

Etiology and Clinical Implications of Peyronie's Disease

G. Hatzichristodoulou, E. W. Hauck, S. Lahme

Definition and Epidemiology

Peyronie's disease (PD) was first mentioned by François de Lapeyronie in 1743. This disease leads to plaque formation on the penis, resulting in pain at erection and penile deviation [1]. Most of the plaques are localized on the dorsal side of the penis, less on the ventral or the lateral side.

About 1% of males suffer from PD and mainly white men are affected. This disease appears chiefly in the age group of 40 to 60 years, but has come up also in younger and older people. Investigations showed that the incidence rate is 26 per 100,000 men and the prevalence rate is 389 per 100,000 men [2].

Peyronie's disease is associated in many cases with the Dupuytren's contracture, a disease where the palmar aponeurosis shrinks [3]. The same causes for the two diseases have been discussed, but are not yet proven. Moreover patients, suffering from PD, have an increased prevalence of diabetes mellitus or arterial hypertension [4]. PD can also lead to an erectile dysfunction in about 50% [5, 6].

Pathophysiology

Although PD has been known for a long time, the pathophysiology largely still remains unclear. After an inflammatory infiltration of the soft tissue between the cavernous body and the tunica albuginea of the penis, a fibrosis of this tissue results. Various pathophysiological aspects and mechanisms are discussed.

Microtraumas have been mentioned as an etiologic factor for PD. These microtraumatizations occur during sexual intercourse and lead to a decreased compliance of the collagen structures of the penis, resulting in fibrosis [7]. Finally the elasticity of the cavernous body reduces. Due to this process, pain occurs during erection as well as a penile deviation. Today the opinion is supported that repetitive microtraumas only effect as a triggering factor for PD (Fig. 1).

β-blockers may also cause Peyronie's disease. There are investigations that show the significant role of metoprolol in the beginning of the disease. After stopping the metoprolol therapy, the symptoms of PD, such as pain and penile deviation, disappeared [8]. Nevertheless β-blockers

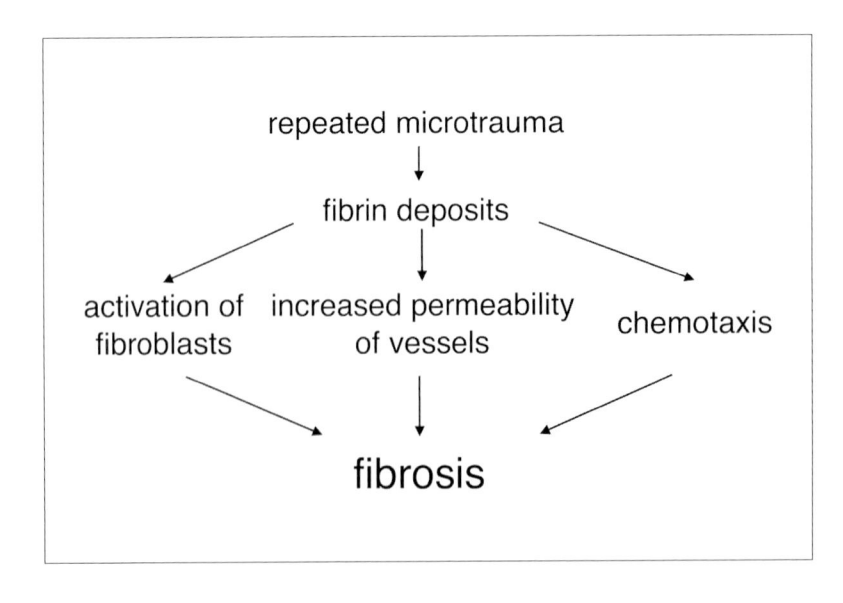

Fig. 1 Microtrauma as a cause of Peyronie's disease (Devine 1997).

repeated microtrauma
↓
fibrin deposits
↙ ↓ ↘
activation of fibroblasts · increased permeability of vessels · chemotaxis
↘ ↓ ↙
fibrosis

only have a secondary role in the generation of PD.

The high coincidence of Peyronie's disease and the Dupuytren's contracture of up to 78% [9] resulted in the hypothesis that both diseases belong to the circle of fibromatosis. Dupuytren's contracture as well as PD are mostly represented in men between 40 and 60 years [10, 11]. The incidence rate seems to be a little bit higher for Dupuytren's contracture than for PD, it is about 2.4% [12]. The clinical symptoms, such as an induration and a deviation, show the similarity of the two diseases. However, the differences in the pathophysiology and morphology dominate. In Dupuytren's contracture there is a proliferation of fibroblastic cells in the aponeurotic tissue, without an inflammation. In contrast to this, PD begins with an inflammation of the soft tissue between the cavernous body and the tunica albuginea, which leads to a fibrosis. Therefore, we have to assume that Dupuytren's contracture and PD belong to different groups of diseases [9].

Another interesting aspect for detecting the pathophysiology of PD, is the alteration of the collagen metabolism [13–15]. There does exist a significant reduction of the $\alpha 1$-proteinase inhibitor ($\alpha 1$-PI) in patients with PD compared with healthy men [16]. A deficiency of $\alpha 1$-PI may lead to changes of the collagen metabolism and to promotion of PD. This complex mechanism is currently a topic of research and may help in the basic understanding of the pathophysiology of PD (Fig. 2).

Symptomatology

Typically palpable plaques on the penis are found in patients affected with Peyronie's disease [6]. These indurations are mostly localized on the dorsal side of the penis. Only a few plaques are located on the ventral side or the lateral sides. Predominantly the plaque formation is found on the distal shaft of the penis [6]. The majority of the affected patients have one plaque on the penis, which measures usually about 1.5 to 3.0 cm. Bigger and smaller plaques are also mentioned, but in fewer cases [6]. In the course of the disease, existing plaques may calcify in 18% of the patients [17].

Patients complain about painful erection as well as pain in the flaccid penis [1, 18]. In about 70% pain at erection is reported [18]. In most cases pain regresses in the natural course of the disease [19].

Besides pain, there also exists a penile deviation. This deviation occurs at erection and is not apparent in the flaccid penis. Approximately 80% of all patients have a deviation to the dorsal side [6]. This corresponds with the localization of the majority of the plaques. A lateral deviation is also described in some cases [20]. After measurement, the deviation detected was up to 135°, with a mean deviation angle of 40° [6].

Due to the deviation and the pain at erection sexual intercourse can be difficult and problematic [21]. Some patients report about the impossibility of fulfilling coitus.

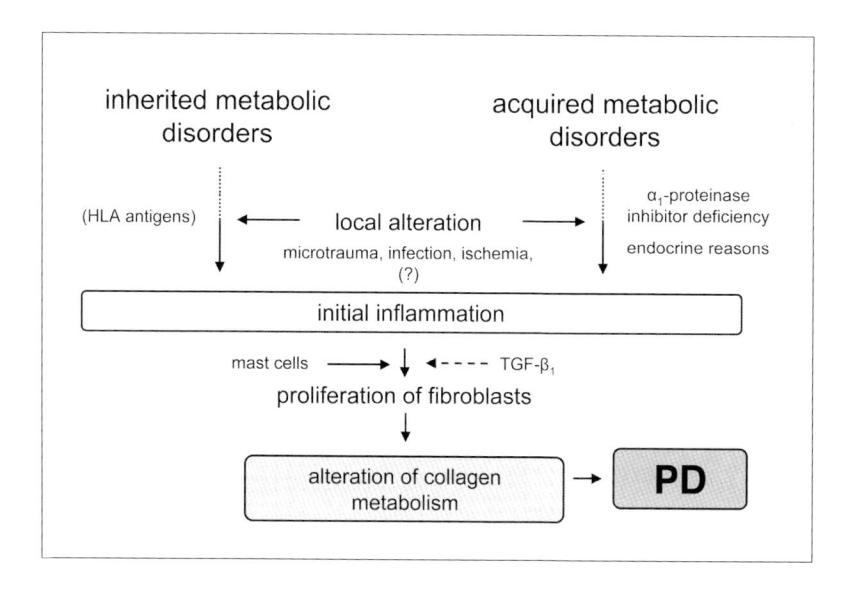

Fig. 2 Pathophysiology of Peyronie's disease (hypothesis).

During the natural course of Peyronie's disease, a spontaneous remission can be observed in about 40% [19]. Worth mentioning is the fact that pain ceases more often than the penile deviation. In cases in which the plaques are almost calcified, spontaneous remissions happen rarely. In none of the available studies a malignant degeneration was described.

Diagnostics

First of all, the patient has to be asked about the disease. Important points, such as existing pain or a penile deviation have to be found out. Moreover, the physician poses questions about penile indurations and erectile dysfunction. The patient will mention whether sexual intercourse is possible or more difficult, because of pain or deviation of the erect penis. The precise anamnesis also contains the duration of the disease, existence of Dupuytren's contracture, diabetes mellitus, or hypertension and if the patient is reminiscent of traumas in the genital region.

After anamnesis, the physician has to examine the flaccid penis in order to determine the number and the dimensions of the plaques as well as other pathological changes. An examination of the hands should also be done for detecting a possible Dupuytren's contracture.

The next step of diagnostics is ultrasound examination. The extent of the plaques can be defined sufficiently by using high-frequency transducers with at least 7.5 MHz. Extensive scars appear in the penile sonography with a dorsal signal quenching [22]. Around 70% of all plaques are visible on sonography [23, 24].

The decisive hint for the physician results from the autophotographies, made by the patient in two planes, from the side and from above [25]. These photographs allow an exact estimation of the penile deviation.

An alternative for detecting the grade of deviation is the intracavernous injection test with prostaglandin E_1. This may be the more sensitive method because it is taken by the physician and therefore has fewer sources of errors.

Further diagnostic steps comprise magnetic resonance imaging (MRI), which is very suitable for detecting acute inflammatory changes of the cavernous body. The comparison of MRI and sonography is continuing to be analyzed in recent investigations [17] (Fig. 3).

Therapy

Because of the lack of pathophysiological knowledge, to date there is no causal therapy of Peyronie's disease. All therapeutic attempts can only improve the symptoms of the disease, such as pain on erection or the penile deviation.

Two drugs seem to be helpful in the conservative treatment of PD. Potassium *para*-aminobenzoate (Potaba®) is one of them. Some studies have verified a significant reduction of the symptoms of the disease [26, 27]. Vitamin E is believed to be anti-inflammatory and so reduces the pain and the penile deviation [28]. However, the therapeutic effect of the above-mentioned

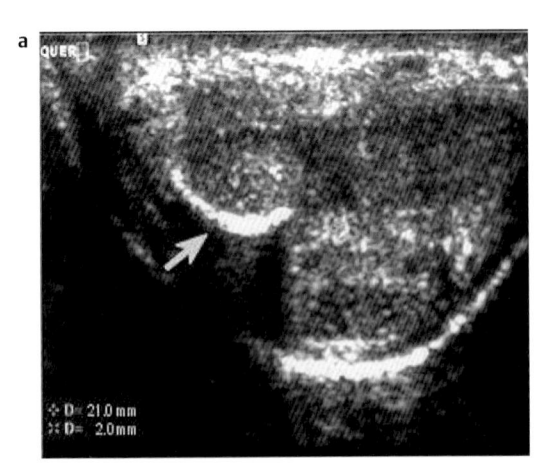

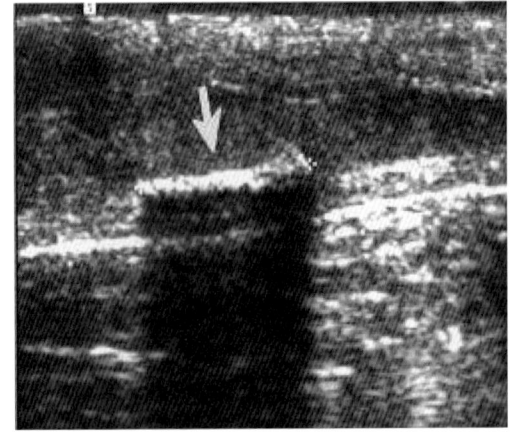

Fig. 3a, b Penile plaques and calcifications in Peyronie's disease detected by ultrasound examination. **a** Transversal examination, **b** longitudinal examination.

- different types of plaque treatment
  - intervention without plaque removal
  - laser ablation of plaques
  - plaque incision
  - partial plaque excision
  - complete plaque excision
- procedures with or without plication sutures
- different types of defect coverage of the tunica albuginea after plaque incision/excision
  - dorsal penile vein
  - saphenous vein
  - collagen fleece
  - small intestine submucosa
  - dacron
  - goretex

Fig. 4 Different types of surgical treatment in Peyronie's disease.

substances is still a topic of controversial discussion. In addition, tamoxifen and colchicine are also being used as a therapeutic trial [29–33]. In all, the therapeutic success of oral pharmacotherapy is unsatisfactory.

Extracorporeal shock wave therapy (ESWT) for patients suffering from Peyronie's disease was first described by Bellorofonte in 1989 [34]. ESWT is a therapeutic modality for pain reduction, with a low rate of side effects. It has no effect on reduction of the penile deviation [35–38]. Therefore, ESWT cannot replace the operative therapy of penile deviation due to PD. The expectancy of patients with regard to an improvement of penile deviation is enormous, but ESWT mainly can be recommended for patients with predominant pain at erection. The patient has to be informed about that, before starting this therapy. It remains to be seen to what extent ESWT will be used in the clinical daily routine in the future.

When conservative trials and ESWT are not successful, there remains only operative therapy. But surgical treatment only can be used for correction of the penile deviation, without having any chance of healing or influencing the disease. Several surgical procedures are used, e. g., plication procedures and incision or excision procedures [39–41]. Undesirable side effects after surgery may be a shortening of the penis or the possibility of relapses. An erectile dysfunction may also occur. Therefore the indication for the surgical correction of penile deviation in patients with PD has to be strictly made (Fig. 4).

As there is a severe lack of any causal therapies for PD the aim of any treatment modality must be to decrease the clinical symptoms like pain and penile deviation with minimal morbidity. ESWT provides minimal morbidity and is therefore one of the most important treatment modalities discussed for PD.

References

[1] Byström J, Rubio C. Induration penis plastica. Peyronie's disease. Clinical features and etiology. Scand J Urol 1975; 10: 12–20

[2] Lindsay MB, Schain DM, Grambsch P et al. The incidence of Peyronie's disease in Rochester, Minnesota, 1950 through 1984. J Urol 1991; 146: 1007–1009

[3] Rompel R, Mueller-Eckhardt G, Schroeder-Prinzen I et al. HLA antigens in Peyronie's disease. Urol Int 1994; 52: 34–37

[4] Muralidhar S, Kumar B, Sharma SK et al. Etiologic factors in Peyronie's disease. Int J Dermat 1997; 36: 579–581

[5] Lopez JA, Jarow JP. Duplex ultrasound findings in men with Peyronie's disease. Urol Radiol 1991; 12: 199–202

[6] Weidner W, Schroeder-Prinzen I, Weiske WH. Sexual dysfunction in Peyronie's disease: an analysis of 222 patients without previous local plaque therapy. J Urol 1997; 157: 325–328

[7] Devine CJ, Somers KD, Jordan GH, Schlossberg SM. Proposal: Trauma as the cause of Peyronie's Lesion. J Urol 1997; 157: 285–290

[8] Yudkin JS. Peyronie's disease in association with metoprolol. The Lancet 1977; 1355

9 Mohr W. Sind Peyronie-Krankheit und Dupuytren-Kontraktur gleichartige Leiden? Akt Urol 2001; 32 (Suppl. 1): 18–24
10 Mohr W. Gelenkpathologie, historische Grundlagen, Ursachen und Entwicklungen von Gelenkleiden und ihre Pathomorphologie. Springer, Berlin-Heidelberg, 2000
11 Heite HJ, Siebrecht HH. Beitrag zur Pathogenese der Induration penis plastica. Dermatol Wochenschr 1950; 121: 1–10 and 25–34
12 Brenner P, Mailaender P, Berger A. Epidemiology of Dupuytren's disease. In: Dupuytren's disease, Pathobiochemistry and clinical management. Berger A, Delbrueck A, Brenner P, Hinzmann R (eds), Springer, Berlin-Heidelberg, 1994; pp 244–254
13 Bichler KH, Lahme S, Feil G, Goetz T, Koempf J, Tomiuk J. Investigations on the metabolism of collagen tissue in patients suffering from Peyronie's disease. J Urol 1999; 161, 204
14 Bichler KH, Lahme S, Mattauch W, Petri E. Untersuchungen zum Kollagenstoffwechsel bei Induratio penis plastica (IPP). Urologe A 1998; 37: 306–311
15 Somers KD, Sismour EN, Wright Jr GL, Devine Jr CJ, Gilbert DA, Horton CE. Isolation and characterization of collagen in Peyronie's disease. J Urol 1989; 141: 629–631
16 Lahme S, Feil G, Bichler KH. Untersuchungen zum Kollagenstoffwechsel bei Patienten mit Induratio penis plastica. Akt Urol 2001; 32 (Suppl. 1): 37–40
17 Vosshenrich R, Schroeder-Prinzen I, Weidner W et al. Value of magnetic resonance imaging in patients with penile induration (Peyronie's disease). J Urol 1995; 153: 1122–1125
18 Levine L, Coogan CL. Penile vascular assessment using color duplex sonography in men with Peyronie's disease. J Urol 1996; 155: 1270–1273
19 Gelbard MK, Dorey F, James K. The natural history of Peyronie's disease. J Urol 1999; 144: 1376–1379
20 Porst H. Congenital and acquired penile deviations and penile fractures. In: Penile Disorders, Porst H (ed), Springer, Berlin-Heidelberg, 1997, pp 37–56
21 Hauck EW, Heitz M, Schreiter F et al. Übersicht Induratio penis plastica (Peyronie's disease). Akt Urol 1999; 30: 386–404
22 Wilbert DM. Induratio penis plastica – eine Übersicht. Akt Urol 2001; 32 (Suppl. 1): 7–9
23 Andersen R, Wegner HEH, Miller K, Banzer D. Imaging modalities in Peyronie's disease. Eur Urol 1998; 34: 128–135
24 Balconi G, Angeli E, Nessi R, de Flavis L. Ultrasonographic evaluation of Peyronie's disease. Urol Radiol 1988; 10: 85–88
25 Kelami A. Autophotography in evaluation of functional penile disorders. Urology 1983; 21: 628–629
26 Weidner W, Schroeder-Prinzen I, Rudnick J, Krause W, Weiske WH, Drawz B, Rebmann U, Pastermadjeff L, Kallerhoff M, Lenk S, Sperling H, Kliesch S, Schnittker J, Aulitzky W. Randomized prospective placebo-controlled therapy of Peyronie's disease (IPP) with Potaba® (aminobenzoate potassium). J Urol 1999; 161 (Suppl): 205, Abstract 785
27 Carson CC. Potassium para-aminobenzoate for the treatment of Peyronie's disease. Is it effective? Tech Urol 1997; 3: 135–139
28 Pryor JP, Farell CR. Controlled clinical trial of vitamin E in Peyronie's disease. Prog Reprod Biol Med 1983; 9, 41–45
29 Ralph DJ, Brooks MD, Bottazo GF, Pryor JP. The treatment of Peyronie's disease with tamoxifen. Br J Urol 1992; 70, 648–651
30 Apaydin E, Semerci B, Kefi A, Cikili N, Guersan A, Muelazimoglu N. The use of tamoxifen in the treatment of Peyronie's disease. Int J Impt Res 1998; 10 (Suppl. 3): 57, Abstract 421
31 Teloken C, Rhoden EL, Meyer Grazziotin T, Da Ros CT, Sogari PR, Vargas Souto CA. Tamoxifen versus placebo in the treatment of Peyronie's disease. J Urol 1999; 162: 2003–2005
32 Akkus E, Carrier S, Rehmann J, Breza J, Kardioglou A, Lue TF. Is colchicine effective in Peyronie's disease? A pilot study. Urology 1995; 44: 291–295
33 Kardioglou A, Tefekli A, Koeksal T, Usta M, Erol H. Treatment of Peyronie's disease with oral colchicine: long-term results and predictive parameters of successful outcome. Int J Impot Res 2000; 12: 169–175
34 Bellorofonte C, Ruoppolo M, Tura M, Zaatar C, Tombolini P, Menchini Fabris GF. Possibilita di impigeigo del litotritore piezoelettrico nel trattamento delle fibrsi caverbosi gravi. Arch It Urol 1989; LXI: 417–422
35 Butz M. Treatment of Peyronie's disease by extracorporeal shock wave (ESW). J Endourol 1995; 5 (Suppl): 165
36 Hauck EW, Altinkilic BM, Ludwig M, Luedecke G, Schroeder-Prinzen I, Arens C, Weidner W. Extracorporeal shock wave therapy in treatment of Peyronie's disease. Eur Urol 2000; 38: 663–670
37 Husain J, Lynn NNK, Jones DK, Collins GN, O'Reilly PH. Extracorporeal shock wave therapy in the management of Peyronie's disease: initial experience. Br J Urol Int 2000; 86, 466–468
38 Michel MS, Ptaschyk T, Musial A, Martinez-Portillio F, Koehrmann KU, Alken P. 18-month follow-up after extracorporeal shock wave treatment for Peyronie's disease. J Urol 2001; 165 (Suppl): 202
39 Bichler KH, Lahme S, Goetz T. Kollagenvlies zur Deckung nach Plaque-Exzision bei Patienten mit Induratio penis plastica. Akt Urol 2001; 32 (Suppl 1): 77–80
40 Essed E, Schroeder FH. New surgical treatment of Peyronie's disease. Urology 1985; 25: 580–582
41 Ralph DJ, Al-Akraa M, Pryor JP. The Nesbit operation for Peyronie's disease: 16-year experience. J Urol 1995; 154: 1362–1363

ESWT in Peyronie's Disease

E. W. Hauck, G. Hatzichristodoulou, S. Lahme

Introduction

During the last years the use of extracorporeal shock wave therapy (ESWT) for the treatment of Peyronie's disease as a semi-invasive therapeutic approach has been widely spread. Due to the lack of efficacy of most conservative therapeutic approaches, patients and their physicians seek for alternatives. However, despite the clinical spread of this method many aspects concerning this alternative treatment remain unclear.

Mode of Action

The rationale for the use of ESWT in Peyronie's disease has still not been clarified. Basic research on animal models and histological clinical investigations that can definitely explain the effect of ESWT in Peyronie's disease are not available. Until today only one study has been performed that investigated the effect of ESWT on the penis of the rat [1]. This controlled approach in an animal model resulted in no different effects concerning hemodynamic and histopathology parameters comparing the group treated by ESWT with the control group. Only one study investigated histological effects on specimens of penile punch biopsy in patients who received ESWT [2]. A reduction in packing and clumping of the collagen fibers has been observed by histological examination of the plaques after ESWT [2]. Such findings were not observed in patients after clinically unsuccessful treatment.

ESWT was introduced for the treatment of Peyronie's disease because this disorder resembles various calcified and non-calcified orthopedic diseases [3, 4] that are treated by shock waves. Peyronie's disease is also an inflammatory disease at the initial stage with fibrosis of the tunica albuginea or calcified plaques during its course. In orthopedics, mainly tendinosis calcarea of the shoulder also called "periarthritis humeroscapularis," the tennis or golfer elbow, epicondylopathia humeri radialis, calcaneal spur, and pseudarthrosis are treated [3]. However, a definite mode of action has not been described even in these orthopedic approaches yet. An improvement of vascularization with consecutive resorption of calcification or dissolution has been discussed as one possible mechanism of ESWT [3, 4]. Concerning the non-calcified diseases, a change in the milieu of the free radicals or a direct disturbance of pain receptors could be the reason for the pain-relieving effect [4]. Another possible effect could be analgesia after hyperstimulation of the pain receptors by shock waves [3]. In summary, these are the current hypotheses for the possible mode of action in orthopedic administrations of ESWT. Perhaps similar processes are responsible for the effects in Peyronie's disease. But basic research demonstrating the mode of action in Peyronie's disease is not available.

Clinical Studies

Twenty-one original papers [2, 5–25], one meta-analysis [26] and two review articles [27, 28] have been published. On the major international and many local meeting levels, an incredible flood of abstracts of very different kind of scientific value has been presented during the last years. For further evaluation only the results from the studies that have been published as original articles have been considered. Twenty-one papers have been published from 15 groups of authors. From five study groups with increasing series, only the most recent papers are included [2, 9, 14, 18, 21].

Only five of the 21 studies represent prospective controlled approaches according to their own definitions [2, 14, 15, 18, 25]. A case-controlled design was only performed by one study group [13]. No single-blinded approach – real vs. simulated ESWT – as described in orthopedic studies has been performed yet [31].

Thus, the evidence level is low. The experience with ESWT relies on the reports of clinical series. However, as described in the methodology of our explorative meta-analysis, there are several aspects why a direct comparison of these studies is very difficult and should be carefully assessed

[26]. The study groups differ considerably in the medical history of the subjects and severity of symptoms (Table 1). While in some studies only pretreated patients have been considered — including also patients who underwent surgery previously — in other series ESWT was performed as first-line therapy. The measurement of outcomes is not standardized. Effect size categorization is poorly documented and inconsistent. What constitutes a clear success, a modest success, or no success at all, varies from study to study. Treatment protocols vary widely, and some of them may be more effective than others. In the 15 studies, ESWT was performed by 7 different types of lithotripters (Table 2). The most common type was the lithotripter Storz Minilith SL1 that has been used in 9 studies. Moreover, shock waves were applied by the lithotripters Wolf Piezolith 2300, Wolf Piezolith 2500, EDAP LT-02, Siemens Lithostar, Siemens Multiline, and ReflecTron. The technical parameters of the settings covered a wide range from 1–5 settings between 2 and 90 days. Only in the series using the Storz Minilith SL1 did the energy applied seem to be of an energy low density of 0.11–0.17 mJ/mm^2 per shock wave.

Safety

Only penile pain during administration of ESWT, and frequently skin hematoma, and rarely hematuria relating to urethral bleeding were observed after the intervention. No severe complications were reported. Thus, the current evidence on the safety of ESWT seems to be adequate.

Results

Success rates vary widely for all outcomes. Reduction of plaque size from 0 to 68% of the patients, reduction of penile curvature from 21 to 74%, reduction of penile pain from 56 to 100%, and improvement of sexual function from 12 to 80% (Table 3 modified after [26, 32]).

Despite changes of the symptoms by varying percentages in the different studies, the quantity of improvement of each symptom should be regarded. Only the two most recent studies published in high-ranked journals [14, 25] provide exact data on the change of plaque size. In these two studies no significant changes of plaque size were observed on comparing the total number of patients before and after the intervention [14,

Table 1 Patient characteristics of the 15 studies on ESWT in Peyronie's disease (modified after [26, 32])

Study Group	Number of patients (n)#	Age (years, mean, range)	History (months, mean, range)	Penile curvature (°, mean, range)	Treatment before ESWT
Abdel-Salam [7]	24	55 (36–67)	26 (6–240)	?	?
Baumann [9]	74	54 (29–70)	19 (12–72)	?	+
Bellorofonte [5]	9	41 (32–65)	?	?	?
Butz [10]	72	55 (26–74)	17 (3–96)	?	?
Colombo [11]	82	54 (44–74)	23 (3–120)	?	?
Hamm [12]	28	57 (34–72)	>12	?	?
Hauck [14]	96	53 (24–69)	27 (3–52)	48 (15–90)	+
Husain [15]	34	56 (24–69)	19 (4–60)	51 (20–90)	?
Kiyota [16]	4	52 (35–65)	?	20 – 40	+
Lebret [17]	54	56 (29–76)	16 (3–60)	48 (20–110)	-
Manikandan [18]	42	55 (32–72)	17 (3–60)	20–75	+
Michel [20]	35	58	34	50	?
Mirone [2]	380	47 (32–71)	>6	?	+
Oeynhausen [24]	30	55 (28–72)	25 (4–96)	>30–>60	+
Strebel [25]	52	55 (29–77)	19 (4–168)	40 (0–80)	?

The number of patients included in the follow-up is provided.

Table 2 Technical parameters (modified after [26, 32])

Study Group	ESWT technique	Shock waves per setting (n)	Energy per shock wave	Number of settings (n)	Time between settings (days)
Abdel-Salam [7]	Siemens Lithostar	4000	15–21 kV	5 (4–10)	?
Baumann [9]	Wolf Piezolith 2500	2500	3	6	14–28
Bellorofonte [5]	Wolf Piezolith 2300	800	40–100 Mpa	6	7
Butz [10]	Storz Minilith SL1	3000	?; 0.09–0.14 mJ/mm^2	3–5	1–7
Colombo [11]	Storz Minilith SL1	3000	4; 0.11 mJ/mm^2	4	2
Hamm [12]	Storz Minilith SL1	3000	2–5; 0.04–0.17 mJ/mm^2	3.9 (3.5)	?
Hauck [14]	Storz Minilith SL1	4000	4–5; 0.11–0.17 mJ/mm^2	1–4	= 90
Husain [15]	Storz Minilith SL1	3000	4–5; 0.11–0.17 mJ/mm^2	3	?
Kiyota [16]	EDAP LT-02	?	450–960 bar	3–5	?
Lebret [18]	Siemens Multiline	3000	0.3 mmJ/mm^2	1.6 (1–3)	90
Manikandan [19]	Storz Minilith SL1	3000	4–5; 0.11–0.17 mJ/mm^2	3–6	2 groups: 1 versus 30
Michel [21]	Storz Minilith SL1	1000	3–5; 0.07–0.17 mJ/mm^2	5	7
Mirone [2]	Storz Minilith SL1	?	?	3	2
Oeynhausen [24]	ReflecTron	2000–4000	0.13–0.15 mJ/mm^2	4.5 (3–6)	30
Strebel [25]	Storz Minilith SL1	3000	4–5; 0.11–0.17 mJ/mm^2	5	7

25]. This tendency was confirmed by another well-designed study that reported on no significant differences concerning plaque size before and after ESWT [21].

Concerning the changes of penile curvature, the situation is similar. An early study described a significant (p < 0.001) decrease of mean curvature by 12.8° [15]. This tendency of statistical significant improvements of curvature could not be confirmed by 3 further studies that provide information concerning the quantity of changes for the total population of patients [14, 21, 25]. The more subjective symptoms of penile pain and the changes in sexual function are more difficult to quantify as no standardized instruments have been used in most studies. Thus, most results defining a positive response after ESWT rely on the more or less subjective assessment of the patient and/or the clinician.

Only one early study was performed in a case-controlled approach [13] comparing the effect of ESWT with untreated patients representing the natural course of the disease. In this series only a borderline significant effect on the decrease of penile curvature was observed. There were no significant differences concerning changes of plaque size, penile pain, or the subjective assessment of sexual function compared with the controls [13].

Explorative meta-analysis

Due to the lack of controls in the majority of studies, an exploratory meta-analysis of the studies published as peer-reviewed papers or abstracts at the annual meetings of the American Urological Association or the European Association of Urology has been performed [26]. As mentioned above, an exploratory meta-analysis was carried out because a methodologically sound meta-analysis *lege artis* did not appear appropriate since the treated groups differed con-

Table 3 Results of treatment by ESWT (modified after [26, 32])

Study Group	Follow-up (months, mean, range)	Reduction of plaque size (n, %)	Reduction of penile curvature (n, %)	Reduction of pain during erection (n, %)	Improvement of sexual function (n, %)
Abdel-Salam [7]	3–9	14/24 (58%)	14/24 (58%)	17/24 (72%)	14/24 (58%)
Baumann [9]	24 (4–69)	?	37/74 (50%)	42/47 (89%)	41/74 (55%)
Bellorofonte [5]	12	?	3/9 (33%)	?	5/9 (55%)
Butz [10]	12	?	36%	66%	50%
Colombo [11]	< 1	34/82 (41%)	24/78 (31%)	31/44 (70%)	?
Hamm [12]	?	?	18/28 (64%)	13/16 (81%)	20/28 (71%)
Hauck [14]	9 (3–53)	41/96 (43%)	28/96 (29%)	26/37 (76%)	25/96 (26%)
Husain [15]	8 (5–11)	?	15/32 (47%)	12/20 (60%)	?
Kiyota [16]	< 1	1/4 (25%)	0/4 (0%)	4/4 (100%)	?
Lebret [18]	13 (3–?)	23/54 (43%)	29/51 (54%)	31/34 (91%)	6/24 (25%)
Manikandan [19]	6 (2–18)	?	22/38 (58%)	21/25 (84%)	5/42 (12%)
Michel [21]	18	0	5/24 (21%)	16/17 (94%)	9/35 (26%)
Mirone [2]	?	260/380 (68%)	?	312/340 (92%)	303/380 (80%)
Oeynhausen [24]	4	20/30 (67%)	17/29 (58%)	13/16 (81%)	17/30 (56%)
Strebel [25]	11 (4–17)	?	16/52 (31%)	28/30 (93%)	11/40 (28%)

siderably concerning their structure, the selection of outcome measures was inconsistent, and the measurements were not standardized. Four control groups taken from the literature were included, two from reports on the natural history [29, 30] and two comparison groups from series on ESWT [2, 13], respectively.

The results of this exploratory meta-analysis have been summarized [26] as follows. ESWT seems to have an effect on penile pain during erection and on the improvement of sexual function. It seems that pain resolves faster after ESWT treatment than during the course of the natural history. The effect on plaque size and penile curvature is less impressive. Deducing from the data of this exploratory meta-analysis, the effect on plaque size and curvature remains questionable. ESWT is not an evidence-based therapy at the present time.

Results of a placebo-controlled, prospective, randomized, single-blind study

From October 2002 until July 2004, 102 patients suffering from Peyronie's disease (PD) were included in this monocenter study performed by the Department of Urology, University of Tübingen. It is the first placebo-controlled, randomized, and single-blind study, up to now, for detecting the efficacy of extracorporeal shock wave therapy (ESWT) in PD. Each group consisted of 51 patients. All patients were treated six times at weekly intervals, comprising 2000 shock waves each session. The Piezoson 100 (Richard Wolf Company, Knittlingen, Germany) was used. ESWT was performed in the flaccid penis without any anesthesia. The energy was 0.29 mJ/mm^2 and 180 shock waves were applied per minute. Six weeks after the last ESWT session, a follow-up examination took place and the status was compared with that before therapy.

There was a significant reduction of pain at erection in the main group detected, in contrast to the placebo group (Fisher exact test, p = 0.0023). Mean pain score on a visual analogue scale (VAS) dropped from 4 to 1.5. The effect on reduction of the penile deviation was without significance (Wilcoxon test, p = 0.652). Complications worthy of mention were not observed, merely petechial bleeding in 80.7% and small hematomas in 4.9% occurred in the main group. Nothing was observed in the placebo group.

From the above-mentioned results, it can be concluded that ESWT is not effective for the reduction of penile deviation. It can be recommended for analgesia. Patients with predominant penile deviation, requiring a straightening of the penis, should be managed by a surgical intervention.

Discussion

ESWT seems to have a good effect on penile pain during erection. Evidently pain seems to resolve faster after ESWT treatment than during the natural course of the disease. However, the question remains if it is really of value to treat the symptom pain that usually resolves spontaneously with time.

It is very difficult to assess the ability of performing sexual intercourse. In most studies no standardized or validated instrument for the assessment of sexual function has been used. Hypothetically, it is the relief of pain that improves the performance of sexual intercourse. It is more than questionable if the rather limited success rates concerning the decrease of penile curvature are really the reason for improvements of sexual function.

It seems remarkably that in the latest well designed studies [14, 21, 25] no statistically significant effect on the decrease of penile curvature was evident regarding the total populations. The question still remains if a described statistically significant decrease of penile curvature in certain subgroups or in some studies is really of clinical value for the patient.

Exact data on changes of plaque size have been only reported in the two most recent studies [14, 21]. In these studies no change of mean plaque size was evident in contrast to other studies reporting a decrease of plaque size in a certain percentage of the patients. The question arises if a softening or decrease of plaque size as described in some studies is of real clinical value for the patient.

Several studies concluded that a controlled, single-blinded multi-center study, with a careful, detailed documentation of the disease symptoms before the intervention and of the outcomes is required to investigate the real effect of ESWT. However, deducing from the data of the available clinical studies and the exploratory meta-analysis doubts arise if such a design could reveal statistically and clinically significant effects of ESWT.

Conclusion

Until today ESWT is no evidence-based therapy for Peyronie's disease. If the uncontrolled studies are analyzed carefully, the efficacy concerning the objective symptoms penile curvature and plaque size remains more than questionable. It seems that pain relief is faster after ESWT than during the natural course. However, the question remains if a symptom that usually disappears with the natural course is worthy of treatment by an expensive, time-consuming method like ESWT.

Considering this vague situation concerning the efficacy of ESWT, the official statement of the German Urological Society (DGU) was that ESWT should not be recommended as first line or standard therapy for Peyronie's disease [33]. This statement is also supported by the National Institute of Clinical Excellence in the United Kingdom. The guidelines recommend, in the scope of the evidence on efficacy, that ESWT does not appear adequate for use of this procedure without special arrangements for consent and for audit or research The National Institute of Clinical Excellence is not undertaking further investigations at present [34].

Summarizing, ESWT seems to be a safe procedure without severe side effects. However, the data published do not provide evidence to take ESWT into account as a standard procedure for the treatment of Peyronie's disease.

References

[1] Kadioglu A, Tefekli A, Erol B, Nurten A, Kilicaslan I, Armagan A, Kara I, Tellaloglu S. Hemodynamic and histopathologic effects of extra-corporeal shock waves (esw) on rat penis: preliminary results. Int J Impotence Res 2001; 13 (suppl 1): S59 abstract M80

[2] Mirone V, Imbimbo C, Palmieri A, Longo N, Fusco F, Tajana G. A new biopsy technique to investigate Peyronie's disease associated histologic alterations: results with two different forms of therapy. Eur Urol 2002; 42: 239–244

[3] Wild C, Khene M, Wanke S. Extracorporeal shock wave therapy in orthopedics. Assessment of an emerging health technology. Int J Technol Assess Health Care 2000; 16: 199–209

[4] Haupt G. Use of extracorporeal shock waves in the treatment of the pseudarthrosis, tendinopathy and other orthopedic diseases. J Urol 1997; 158: 4–22

[5] Bellorofonte C, Ruoppolo M, Tura M, Zaatar C, Tombolini P, Menchini Fabris GF. Possibility of using the

piezoelectric lithotripter in the treatment of severe cavernous fibrosis [in Italian]. Arch Ital Urol Nefrol 1989; 61: 417–422

[6] Butz M, Teichert HM. Treatment of Peyronie's disease (PD) by extracorporeal shock waves (ESW). J Urol 1998; 159 (suppl 5): 118 abstract 457

[7] Abdel-Salam Y, Budair Z, Renner C, Frede T, Rassweiler J, El-Annany F, El-Magraby H, El-Akkad M. Treatment of Peyronie's disease by extracorporeal shock wave therapy: evaluation of our preliminary results. J Endourol 1999; 13: 549–552

[8] Baumann M, Tauber R. Peyronie's disease: Extracorporeal shock wave therapy (EPT) as a new treatment [in German]. Akt Urol 1998; 29: 1–5

[9] Baumann M, Böhme H, Tauber R. Extracorporeal shock wave therapy (ESWT) in combination with local verapamil injections in the treatment of IPP (induratio penis plastica) [in German]. Akt Urol 2001; 32 (suppl 1): 61–64

[10] Butz M. Extracorporeal shock wave therapy (ESWT) in Induratio penis plastica – Development and topical ranking [in German]. Akt Urol 2001; 32 (suppl 1): 55–57

[11] Colombo F, Massimiliano N. Shock waves in the treatment of La Peyronie's disease. Outcomes evaluation by ultrasonography. La Peyronie's disease [in Italian]. Arch Ital Urol Androl 2000; 72; 388–391

[12] Hamm R, Mclarty E, Ashdown J, Natale S, Dickinson A. Peyronie's disease – the Plymouth experience of extracorporeal shock wave treatment. BJU Int 2001; 87: 849–852

[13] Hauck EW, Altinkilic BM, Ludwig M, Lüdecke G, Schroeder-Printzen I, Arens C, Weidner W. Extracorporeal shockwave therapy (ESWT) in the treatment of Peyronie's disease – first results of a case-controlled approach. Eur Urol 2000; 38: 663–670

[14] Hauck EW, Hauptmann A, Bschleipfer T, Schmelz HU, Altinkilic BM, Weidner W. Questionable efficacy of extracorporeal shock wave therapy in Peyronie's disease: results of a prospective approach. J Urol 2004; 171: 269–299

[15] Husain J, Lynn NNK, Jones DK, Collins GN, O'Reilly PH. Extracorporeal shock wave therapy in the management of Peyronie's disease: initial experience. BJU Int 2000; 86: 466–468

[16] Kiyota H, Ohishi Y, Asano K, Hasegawa N, Madarame J, Miki K, Kato N, Kimura T, Ishiyama T, Maeda S, Shimomura T, Shiono Y, Miki J. Extracorporeal shock wave treatment for Peyronie's disease using EDAP LT-02: preliminary results. Int J Urol 2002; 9: 110–113

[17] Lebret T, Herve JM, Lugane PM, Barre P, Orsini JL, Butreau M, Botto H. Extracorporeal shock wave lithotirpsy (ESWL) in the treatment of La Peyronie's disease. Use of a standardized lithotripter (Siemens multilinie) on "young" plaques (less than 6 months) [in French]. Prog Urol 2000; 10: 65–70

[18] Lebret T, Loison G, Hervé JM, Mc Eleny KR, Lugagne PM, Yonneau L, Orsoni JL, Saporta F, Butreau M, Botto H. Extracorporeal shock wave therapy in the treatment of Peyronie's disease: experience with standard lithotripter (Siemens-multiline). Urology 2002; 59: 657–661

[19] Manikandan R, Islam W, Srinivasan V, Evans CM. Evaluation pf extracorporareal shock wave therapy in Peyronie's disease. Urology 2002; 60: 795–800

[20] Michel MS, Ptaschynk T, Musial A, Martinez Portillo FJ, Köhrmann KU, Alken P. Shock wave therapy of Peyronie's disease: 18 months follow-up of a prospective study for standardised and objective evaluation of symptom changes under artificial erection [in German]. Akt Urol 2001; 32 (suppl 1): 68–71

[21] Michel MS, Ptaschnyk T, Musial A, Braun P, Köhrmann KU, Lenz ST, Alken P. Objective and subjective changes in patients with Peyronie's disease after management with shock wave therapy. J Endourol 2003; 17: 41–44

[22] Mirone V, Imbimbo C, Palmieri A, Fusco F. Our experience on the association of a new physical and medical therapy in patients suffering from induratio penis plastica. Eur Urol 1999; 36: 327–330

[23] Mirone V, Palmieri A, Granata AM, Piscopo A, Verze P, Ranavolo R. Ultrasound guided extra shock wave treatment of La Peyronie's disease [in Italian]. Arch Ital Urol Androl 2000; 72: 384–387

[24] Oeynhausen D, Oelbracht K, Zumbé J. Extracorporeal shock wave therapy (ESWT) in the treatment of Peyronie's disease [in German]. Akt Urol 2001; 32 (suppl 1): 58–60

[25] Strebel RT, Suter S, Sautter T, Hauri D. Extracorporeal shock wave therapy for Peyronie's disease does not correct penile deformity. Int J Impotence Res 2004; 16: 448–451

[26] Hauck EW, Mueller UO, Bschleipfer T, Schmelz HU, Diemer T, Weidner W. Extracorporeal shock wave therapy for Peyronie's disease: exploratory meta-analysis of clinical trials. J Urol 2004; 171: 740–745

[27] Michel MS, Köhrmann KU, Alken P. Treatment of Peyronie's disease by shock waves: a critical review [in German]. Akt Urol 2001; 32 (suppl 1): 65–67

[28] Groth T, Monga M. Extracorporeal shock wave therapy for Peyronie's disease. Arch Androl 2003; 49: 205–213

[29] Kadioglu A, Tefekli A, Erol B, Oktar T, Tunc M, Tellaloglu S. A retrospective review of 307 men with Peyronie's disease. J Urol 2002; 168: 1075–1079

[30] Gelbard MK, Dorey F, James K. The natural history of Peyronie's disease. J Urol 1990; 144: 1376–1379

[31] Rompe JD, Hopf C, Nafe B, Burger R. Low-energy extracorporeal shock wave therapy for painful heel: a prospective controlled single-blind study. Arch Orthop Trauma Surg 1996; 115: 75–79

[32] Hauck EW, Weidner W. Extracorporeal shock wave therapy (ESWT) in Peyronie's disease. In: Levine LA

(ed), Peyronie's disease: A guide to clinical management. Humana Press, Totowa (in press)

[33] Weidner W, Hauck EW. Significance of extracorporeal shock-wave therapy (ESWT) in plastic penile induration. Statement of the DGU [in German]. Urologe A 2004; 43: 597–598

[34] Dillon A. Extracorporeal shock wave therapy for Peyronie's disease. National Institute of Clinical Excellence, 2003, www.nice.org.uk/IP182overview

ESWT in Orthopedics

Physical-Technical Principles of ESWT

M. Maier, T. Tischer, L. Gerdesmeyer

Introduction

Since the first successful application of extracorporeal shock waves for lithotripsy of renal stones in 1980 [2], the use of shock wave therapy has rapidly expanded in medicine. For the first time in 1985, extracorporeal shock waves were used for the fragmentation of gallstones [13]. Today, besides treating renal stones and gall stones, also salivary stones, pancreatic stones, nonunion of long bones, epicondylitis humeri radialis, plantar fasciitis, and calcific tendinitis of the shoulder are being treated with varying success rates [10, 17, 24, 26, 34, 36–38].

In the beginning, an exact characterization of the working mechanisms of extracorporeal shock waves was not necessary for fragmentation of renal stones. Side effects like hemorrhages and skin injuries were accepted. In contrast, due to the changed requirements in orthopedic shock wave application, where different clinical goals were set for various indications, further information about shock waves, shock wave generators, and treatment modalities became necessary in order to maximize treatment success and concurrently minimize side effects. Today, the working mechanisms of shock waves for renal lithotripsy are well-known. In contrast, cellular and molecular working mechanisms for efficiency of ESWT in the treatment of disorders of the skeletal system are only partly understood, especially the pain-mediating effect of ESWT [9, 16, 21, 22, 31]. For clinical use, a detailed knowledge of the physical parameters of shock waves is necessary in order to maximize treatment success and better understand the working mechanisms of shock waves.

This article gives the reader an overview about shock wave parameters and characteristic properties of shock waves. They are partly derived form the international "standard recommendation" IEC 61846 (International Electrotechnical Commission, Geneva, Switzerland) of the "consensus group shock wave therapy," that gave a recommendation on what physical parameters should be defined for the shock waves and their generators [45].

Physical Characteristics of Extracorporeal Shock Waves

Definition of an extracorporeal shock wave

Shock waves are defined as transient pressure changes which propagate rapidly in three-dimensional space. Typically, these pressure pulses are characterized by reaching a very high maximum pressure in a very short time. In most shock wave generators used for medical application, the pressure maximum is reached in a few nanoseconds (ns) only. In addition to the very fast pressure rise and the emerging pressure maximum, shock waves are further characterized by a first positive pressure phase, followed a negative pressure phase (also called the "tensile phase") [14]. The physical shock wave parameters are described in Fig. 1 [16, 35, 45].

- *Positive maximum pressure (P_+):* P_+ is defined as the difference between the maximum positive pressure of the shock wave and the ambient pressure. P_+ reaches values between 5 Megapascal (MPa) und 120 MPa.
- *Negative maximum pressure (P_-):* P_- is defined as the maximum negative pressure during the second phase of the shock wave. P_- reaches values between 10% and 20% of P_+.
- *Rise time (T_r):* T_r is defined as the interval in which the pressure climbs from 10% of P_+ to 90% of P_+. T_r typically is between 1 and 500 ns.
- *Pulse amplitude (T_w):* T_w is defined as the time interval when the pressure first reaches 50% of P_+ and then falls under 50% of P_+ again (during the exponential pressure decline during the first phase of the shock wave). The duration of T_w is between 200 and 500 ns. Synonymous to T_w is also the term "full-width-half-maximum" (FWHM). The duration of T_w directly influences the energy flow density (EFD; see following sections for description) of shock waves.

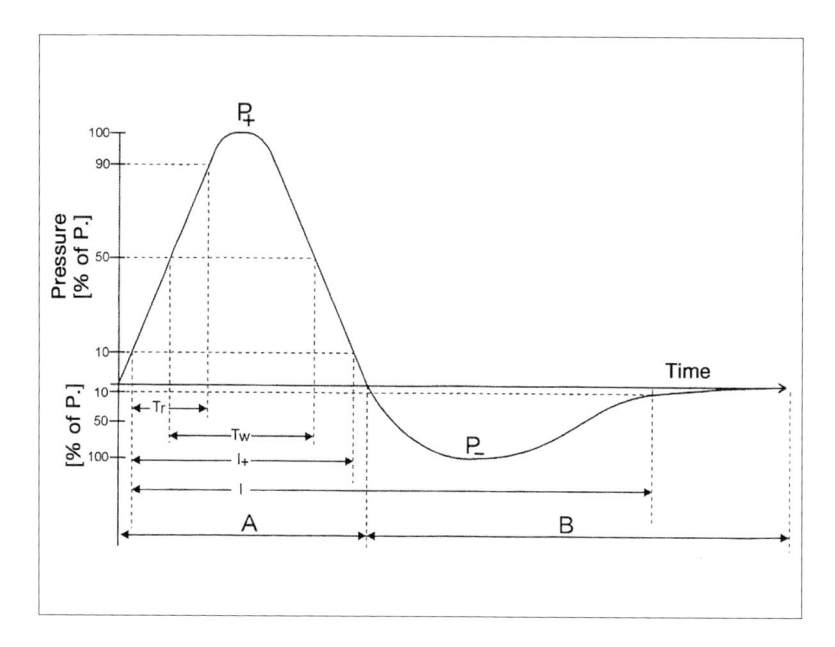

Fig. 1 Graphical representation of a standard shock wave, displaying shock wave pressure as a function of time. A: first shock wave part with positive pressure; B: second part with negative pressure. P_+ = maximum positive pressure; P_- = maximum negative pressure. T_r = rise time; T_w = pulse width; I_+ = standard time interval for calculation of the so-called "positive energy" of the shock wave; I = standard time interval for calculation of the so-called total energy of the shock wave.

The values of P_+, P_-, T_r, and T_w of the shock wave depend on the used shock wave generator and the generator settings [25, 27]. The phase of the shock wave during which the pressure is negative can also be called tensile phase. This tensile phase of the shock wave is noticeably longer than the first phase of the shock wave (positive pressure). In contrast, the amount of P_- is always smaller than P_+. Furthermore due to physical principles, the amplitude of P_- is, in contrast to P_+, more limited. During the "tensile phase," when negative pressure acts on the tissue, the cohesion force on the surrounding medium can be transgressed, leading to the formation of gas-filled "negative pressure bubbles" — so-called cavitation bubbles [25]. A complete shock wave has a duration of a few microseconds (μs) only; the frequency spectrum includes a range between 16 Hz up to 20 MHz.

Shock wave focus

By focusing extracorporeal shock waves, a three-dimensional shock wave field arises, that possesses a complex spatial and temporal distribution of positive and negative pressures. Therefore, the characterization of the shock wave field demands the registration of pressure-time distributions. An important parameter of this shock wave field is the so-called shock wave focus, which can be defined in different ways:

– (1) First, the shock wave focus can be defined as the area in which the pressure reaches at least 50% of P_+ (so called "–6 dB focus," $f_{-6\,dB}$). The outer boundary (that is all points, where exactly 50% of P_+ is reached) is formed by the so called "–6 dB isobar." In currently used shock wave generators the –6 dB focus has the form of an elliptical cigar, that is defined by its three axes f_x, f_y, and f_z (Fig. 2). These three axes

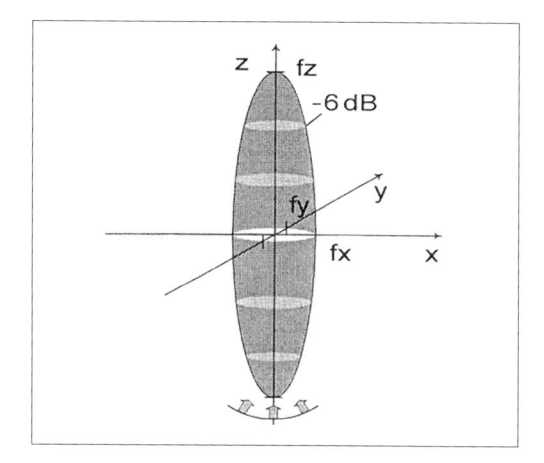

Fig. 2 Three-dimensional shape of the –6 dB shock wave focus, as defined by its three axes f_x, f_y, and f_z. According to the definition, the shock wave pressure, in the shaded area, is over 50% of the maximum pressure (P_+).

spark-plug of a car. The spark discharges lead to the generation of plasma bubbles in the surrounding medium. The plasma bubbles by themselves compress the tissue and, in that way, pressure waves (shock waves) are generated. The spherically propagating pressure waves are focused by an elliptical mirror and concentrated in the focal point (f_2). The main disadvantage of this process is the consumption of the sparking plug, which has to be changed after a defined number of discharges. Furthermore, the generated shock waves vary somewhat in regard to their energy and form [1]. But most likely these variations have no impact on clinical application.

- *Electromagnetic principle* (Figure **4B**): During this process eddy currents are induced with a pancake coil on a thin cooper foil. Due to the effect of the Lorentz force, explosion-like excursions of the foil are generated. Consequently, the adjacent water column will be deflected proportional to the voltage and thereby the pressure pulse is carried forward to the following medium. The generated shock wave will be focused by an acoustic lens in the target tissue (f_2).
- *Piezoelectric principle* (Figure **4C**): During this process multiple small pressure pulses will be generated by many tiny piezo crystals that are positioned in the center of a spherical bowl. Since the single crystals are positioned in a half shell, the shock waves can be easily focused (f) [43].
- *Ballistic principle* (Figure **5**): In this process a projectile will be accelerated in a barrel by compressed air in an extremely short amount of time. Comparable to a projectile fired by a gun, the projectile hits an applicator, over which the energy is then transferred to the target tissue. The tip of the applicator is the focus from which the shock wave propagates in a radial direction. During this kind of shock wave generation no focusing process, comparable to the sources mentioned above, takes place. However, using a special adapter, the radial shock waves can be focused. Due to the radial propagation, the pressure and energy of the shock wave field declines with of the depth of penetration in the tissue. Superficially located targets, e. g., many types of tendon and muscle disorders are well suited for the application of ballistic shock waves. Also the classic indication calcific tendinitis of the shoulder is an established indication for radial shock waves. Treating painful trigger points is an important indication to use this method. Currently, a number of studies report promising clinical results with ballistic shock wave generation.

At present it is believed that the basic biomedical effects of shock waves generated by different physical-technical principles do not differ (see also [20]). More importantly, differences in form, size, and energy flux density of the shock wave focus generated by different devices have to be taken into account. Detailed information about the physical parameters of commonly used shock wave generators are listed on the home page of the German and International society for extracorporeal shock wave therapy (http://www.ismst.org/fach/index.html).

Techniques in Pressure Measurements of Extracorporeal Shock Waves

The acoustic pressure of extracorporeal shock waves is measured using so-called hydrophones. They are capable of recording transient pressure changes (absolute values) in water. These hydrophones may be calibrated and then convert the pressure impulse proportional to the intensity to an electrical signal. In particular, measurements of the rise time (T_r) and of the maximum negative pressure (P_-) of the shock wave – but not the maximum positive pressure (P_+) – depend on the used hydrophone and ambient conditions [4]. Moreover, reliable, reproductive measurements are only possible with degassed, deionized water.

In general, there are four different methods available for measuring the pressure of extracorporeal shock waves.

- *Piezoelectric crystal hydrophones:* These devices were the first pressure transducers that were available for this kind of measurements. They consist of piezoelectric crystals of varying size. Unfortunately, these sensors allowed no reproducible measurements in the circumscribed focus fields. This is due to the fact that the diameter of the pressure transducer is bigger than the shock wave focus. This leads to inaccuracies that rely on reflections and interferences of the incoming shock waves with the pressure transducer. Today, piezoelectric crystal hydrophones are in use for measuring the overall constancy of the shock wave pressure of the shock wave generators, but they are no

longer used for measurements of selected physical parameters like P_+ or P_-.
- *Piezoelectric polymembranes from polyvinylidine fluoride (PVDF):* Unlike piezoelectric crystal hydrophones, these devices are composed of very small pressure transducers [8, 18, 40]. This allows point-like measurements within the acoustic field. Their use is restricted by the short half-life of the polymembranes and high costs.
- *PVDF pressure transducer:* Compared to PVDF polymembranes these devices have an improved durability and are much cheaper. The tip of these devices consists of a sharp metal needle that is covered with a thin film of PVDF. Today, they are widely used [13, 14]. The only disadvantage is that — due to complex interactions between the metal tip and the shock waves — the maximum negative pressure can only be approximated. But with P_- contributing only 10 to 20% to the total energy flux density, measurements are still quite accurate [44].
- *Fiberoptic hydrophones (laser fiber hydrophones):* These devices use a different measuring technology [7]. Laser fiber hydrophones consist of a light source, which is coupled to a glass fiber. The tip of the glass fiber is inserted in the acoustic field. The shock wave then changes the density of the surrounding medium, leading to changes in the intensity of the reflected light, which is recorded with a photodiode. In contrast to PVDF devices, these devices have a long lifetime.

It has to be remarked that, up to now, there are no systematic studies in the literature that investigate and compare pressure measurements of the different devices.

In principle, besides these electrical techniques there exist some nontechnical techniques for measuring the pressure of extracorporeal shock waves, but until now these methods have no practical use. One of these techniques, which is mainly used in urology, is based on the destruction of a defined amount of standard stones by the shock waves [5, 39]. The number of shock wave impulses necessary for the destruction of defined specimens — defined by the situation when all particles are reduced under a defined size — is recorded. According to the international standardization recommendation IEC 61846 (International Electrotechnical Commission, Geneva, Switzerland) of the consensus group "shock wave therapy," these techniques are not suitable for the quantitative characterization of extracorporeal shock waves.

Propagation of Extracorporeal Shock Waves in Tissue

Usually, shock waves are generated in water to facilitate the transmission in tissue with similar acoustic properties. The pressure pulses propagate in wave-like form in tissues like water, gas, or solid bodies.

The typical shape of a shock wave, with its steep and short rise of pressure until the P_+ is reached, is caused by asymmetric absorbability. This steepening phenomenon is caused through the different absorptions of individual frequencies and the dependence of the sound conduction velocity upon temperature and pressure. The sound conduction velocity is proportional to the density of the medium, through which the shock wave travels. This leads to the phenomenon that later shock wave impulses, which travel through already condensed medium (from earlier shock waves), travel faster and catch up with the earlier shock wave [35]. This pressure- and temperature-dependent phenomenon as well as the locally different absorption of shock wave parts — which also rely on the local phase velocity — lead to an increasing asymmetrical transformation and steepening of the pressure pulse, finally becoming the typical shock wave [35]. In the acoustic focus the shock wave has its typical asymmetric, wave-like configuration characterized by a steep pressure rise followed by a slower pressure decline. After passing the focus point, the shock waves loose their typical asymmetric form and return to normal pressure pulses (defocusing).

Influence of the acoustic impedance

The acoustic impedance (AI) — in short impedance — describes the resistance of the media to the passing shock waves. This resistance is dependent on the density of the traversed tissue and is important for the effect of the shock waves. In the ideal case, when no absorption takes place in the traversed tissue, the following Equation (2) is valid:

$$W_0 = p \times v^{-1} \qquad (2)$$

where P stands for the density of the medium, v for the velocity. The unit is [Ns/m^3]. Because of

Table 1 Speed of sound and acoustic impedance of various materials and tissues as reported in the literature [27]

Material/tissue	Speed of sound [m/s]	Acoustic impedance [×10³ Ns/m³]
Air	343	429
Fat	1450	1380
Water	1483	1480
Steel	5790	45700
Lung	650–1160	260–460
CNS	1560	1600
Kidney	1570	1630
Muscle	1545–1630	1650–1740
Bone	2700–4100	3200–7400
Renal stone	4000–6000	5600–14400

the similarity to Ohm's law (in electronics), this law is also called Ohm's law for the velocity of sound. When the shock wave hits the interface between two media, like water and air, or muscle and bone, it is partly absorbed and reflected depending on the size of the difference in impedance. Therefore it is necessary to minimize these differences when coupling shock waves to human tissue. That is the reason why shock waves are generated in water, since the acoustic impedance of water is similar to that of human skin. The acoustic impedance values are listed in Table 1.

Depending on the angle of arrival at the interface, the passing shock wave will be partly reflected, and only the nonreflected part of the shock wave will travel on in the following tissues [16]. This leads to the transformation of acoustic energy into mechanical energy, causing the destruction, for example, of calcific stones [26, 29]. The part of the acoustic energy which is transformed to mechanical energy depends on the amount of the impedance difference between two media and on the angle of arrival. When the shock wave traverses water (acoustic impedance of about 1.49 [Ns/m³]) and hits on a medium with higher acoustic impedance (e.g., a renal stone, impedance greater than 15 [Ns/m³]), most of the acoustic energy is transmitted to the stone [44]. On the back side of the stone, the contrary happens: when transmitting from tissue with high acoustic impedance to tissue with low acoustic impedance, most of the acoustic energy is reflected within the stone and mechanical energy is released. This explains why most effects of shock waves can be seen at the back side of the stones.

Effect of Extracorporeal Shock Waves in Biological Tissues

High pressure pulses are effective independent of the generator device and exert direct and indirect actions [9, 23, 45]. Furthermore, there are three different ways how shock waves can act directly or indirectly. Besides thermal and chemical effects, which are thought to play only a minor role, shock waves act mechanically. Basic principle is the transformation of acoustic energy to mechanical, thermal, or chemical energy. This is only possible when the shock wave hits tissues with different acoustic impedances (see Table 1). The resulting direct mechanical action is proportional to the difference in impedance and is clinically used for the destruction of renal stones or the disintegration of calcific depots [23, 28, 42]. Thermal actions, which are produced by the high pressure amplitudes and rapid changes between compression and decompression, play only a minor role. Under strong local compression the temperature rises measurably, but without clinical impact, since the time of the temperature rise is only extremely short.

An important indirect working mechanism is the induction of cavitation [1, 12]. Cavitation describes a phenomenon where gas-filled bubbles are generated in fluids under the influence of negative pressure. Pressures of only a few negative MPas, like those in the tensile phase of the shock wave, are necessary for the generation of these bubbles. If the cohesion forces of the transmitted medium are below the negative pressure of the shock wave, vacuum spaces are generated. The negative pressure leads to the evaporation of fluids next to the cavitation bubble, making it possible that the bubble can still grow in size. In water, cavitation bubble of about some millimeters in size can be generated. After the pressure wave has passed, the pressure ratio is normalized and the bubble collapses. Since this collapse is seldom symmetrical, during the asymmetrical collapse, local high speed currents (up to 800 m/s; jet-stream) are generated [46]. In this context, the application rate of the shock wave is of importance. If the frequency is very high, it may be possible that the just created cavitation bubble has not been collapsed when the following shock wave already arrives [9]. Under these circumstances the cavitation bubble is forced to asymmetrical collapse in best time, literally speaking they are shot dead. These bubbles, generated by forced asymmetrical collapse, are much more dominant and have higher local destructive properties [19, 25]. Another indirect effect of shock waves is the generation of free radicals. Similar to the clinically nonrelevant increase in temperature, it is believed that through high temperature, big pressure gradients, and released mechanical energy, free radicals will be generated, which also should have only negligible clinical effects.

As a basic principle, during laboratory situations, some working mechanisms have been demonstrated. Which effect these exert on biological tissue is not fully known. Recently, the release of some mediators like substance P [30] or the activation of cellular cascades has been reported [3]. The release of substance P was worldwide the first molecular working mechanism for the analgesic effect mediated by ESWT. Undisputed are the mechanical destructive properties, although they may differ between individuals in the clinical setting [11, 41]. What influence the single anatomic structures have on the effectiveness of shock waves can only be estimated. It is sure that the parameters estimated under laboratory settings cannot be transferred unchanged to *in vivo* situations. There are some hints, for example, that the shock wave focus can vary substantially concerning geometrical size and energy [6].

Practical Conclusion

Technical achievements in the generation of shock waves and new methods for the measurement of shock waves have vastly expanded our knowledge about the acoustic mechanical properties of shock waves. According to the general consensus agreement, the manufacturer of shock wave devices for use in medicine has to point out these technical parameters, which also should be mentioned in any scientific publication. This should lead to a high degree of transparence for the user and should simplify the interpretation of clinical and laboratory data. The exact molecular and biological working mechanisms of shock waves in the human body are still only partly understood. The mechanical destructive properties of shock waves are well-known, but whether or not there are deeper cellular effects is still not fully answered. Today, the measurement of the physical parameters of shock waves is relatively accurate, but still these parameters have not been compared to possible clinical effects and side effects. Until this is achieved, the discussion about physical parameters is of scientific interest only, but useless for clinical application.

References

[1] Bailey MR, Blackstock DT, Cleveland RO, Crum LA. Comparison of electrohydraulic lithotripters with rigid and pressure-release ellipsoidal reflectors. II. Cavitation fields. J Acoust Soc Am 1999; 106: 1149–1160

[2] Chaussy C, Brendel W, Schmiedt E. Extracorporeally induced destruction of kidney stones by shock waves. Lancet 1980; 2: 1265–1268

[3] Chen YJ, Kuo YR, Yang KD, Wang CJ, Sheen Chen SM, Huang HC, Yang YJ, Yi-Chih S, Wang FS. Activation of extracellular signal-regulated kinase (ERK) and p38 kinase in shock wave-promoted bone formation of segmental defect in rats. Bone 2004; 34: 466–477

[4] Chow GK, Streem SB. Extracorporeal lithotripsy. Update on technology. Urol Clin North Am 2000; 27: 315–322

[5] Chuong CJ, Zhong P, Preminger GM. A comparison of stone damage caused by different modes of shock wave generation. J Urol 1992; 148: 200–205

[6] Cleveland RO, Lifshitz DA, Connors BA, Evan AP, Willis LR, Crum LA. In vivo pressure measurements of lithotripsy shock waves in pigs. Ultrasound Med Biol 1998; 24: 293–306

[7] Coleman AJ, Draguioti E, Tiptaf R, Shotri N, Saunders JE. Acoustic performance and clinical use of a fibreoptic hydrophone. Ultrasound Med Biol 1998; 24:143–151

[8] Coleman AJ, Saunders JE. A survey of the acoustic output of commercial extracorporeal shock wave lithotripters. Ultrasound Med Biol 1989; 15: 213–227

[9] Delacretaz G, Rink K, Pittomvils G, Lafaut JP, Vandeursen H, Boving R. Importance of the implosion of ESWL-induced cavitation bubbles. Ultrasound Med Biol 1995; 21: 97–103

[10] Delius M. Twenty years of shock wave research at the Institute for Surgical Research. Eur Surg Res 2002; 34: 30–36

[11] Delius M, Enders G, Heine G, Stark J, Remberger K, Brendel W. Biological effects of shock waves: lung hemorrhage by shock waves in dogs – pressure dependence. Ultrasound Med Biol 1987; 13: 61–67

[12] Delius M, Ueberle F, Eisenmenger W. Extracorporeal shock waves act by shock wave-gas bubble interaction. Ultrasound Med Biol 1998; 24: 1055–1059

[13] Delius M, Ueberle F, Gambihler S. Destruction of gallstones and model stones by extracorporeal shock waves. Ultrasound Med Biol 1994; 20: 251–258

[14] Folberth W, Kohler G, Rohwedder A, Matura E. Pressure distribution and energy flow in the focal region of two different electromagnetic shock wave sources. J Stone Dis 1992; 4: 1–7

[15] Gerdesmeyer L. Extrakorporale Stoßwellentherapie – Schwerpunkt radiale Technologie, Grundlagen, klinische Ergebnisse. Norderstedt: Books on demand, 2004; 340

[16] Gerdesmeyer L, Maier M, Haake M, Schmitz C. Physical-technical principles of extracorporeal shock wave therapy (ESWT). Orthopaede 2002; 31: 610–617

[17] Gerdesmeyer L, Wagenpfeil S, Haake M, Maier M, Loew M, Wortler K, Lampe R, Seil R, Handle G, Gassel S, Rompe JD. Extracorporeal shock wave therapy for the treatment of chronic calcifying tendonitis of the rotator cuff: a randomized controlled trial. JAMA 2003; 290: 2573–2580

[18] Granz B, Holzapfel R, Koehler G. Measurement of shock waves in the focus of a lithotripter. IEEE Ultrasonic Symposium, 1989; 991–994

[19] Greenstein A, Matzkin H. Does the rate of extracorporeal shock wave delivery affect stone fragmentation? Urology 1999; 54: 430–432

[20] Haake M, Boddeker IR, Decker T, Buch M, Vogel M, Labek G, Maier M, Loew M, Maier-Boerries O, Fischer J, Betthauser A, Rehack HC, Kanovsky W, Muller I, Gerdesmeyer L, Rompe JD. Side-effects of extracorporeal shock wave therapy (ESWT) in the treatment of tennis elbow. Arch Orthop Trauma Surg 2002; 122: 222–228

[21] Haake M, Thon A, Bette M. Absence of spinal response to extracorporeal shock waves on the endogenous opioid systems in the rat. Ultrasound Med Biol 2001; 27: 279–284

[22] Hausdorf J, Schmitz C, Averbeck B, Maier M. Molecular basis for pain mediating properties of extracorporeal shock waves. Schmerz 2004; 18: 492–497

[23] Howard D, Sturtevant B. In vitro study of the mechanical effects of shock-wave lithotripsy. Ultrasound Med Biol 1997; 23: 1107–1122

[24] Howell DA. Pancreatic stones: treat or ignore? Can J Gastroenterol 1999; 13: 461–465.

[25] Huber P, Jochle K, Debus J. Influence of shock wave pressure amplitude and pulse repetition frequency on the lifespan, size and number of transient cavities in the field of an electromagnetic lithotripter. Phys Med Biol 1998; 43: 3113–3128

[26] Iro H, Zenk J, Waldfahrer F, Benzel W, Schneider T, Ell C. Extracorporeal shock wave lithotripsy of parotid stones. Results of a prospective clinical trial. Ann Otol Rhinol Laryngol 1998; 107: 860–864

[27] Krause H. Physik und Technik medizinischer Stoßwellensysteme. In: Extrakorporale Stoßwellentherapie, Rompe JD (ed), Chapman and Hall, Weinheim, 1997, pp 15–34

[28] Loew M, Jurgowski W, Mau HC, Thomsen M. Treatment of calcifying tendinitis of rotator cuff by extracorporeal shock waves: a preliminary report. J Shoulder Elbow Surg 1995; 4: 101–106

[29] Lokhandwalla M, Sturtevant B. Fracture mechanics model of stone comminution in ESWL and implications for tissue damage. Phys Med Biol 2000; 45: 1923–1940

[30] Maier M, Averbeck B, Milz S, Refior HJ, Schmitz C. Substance P and prostaglandin E2 release after shock wave application to the rabbit femur. Clin Orthop 2003; 406: 237–245

[31] Maier M, Milz S, Wirtz DC, Rompe JD, Schmitz C. Basic research of applying extracorporeal shockwaves on the musculoskeletal system. An assessment of current status. Orthopaede 2002; 31: 667–677

[32] Maier M, Staupendahl D, Duerr HR, Refior HJ. Castor oil decreases pain during extracorporeal shock wave application. Arch Orthop Trauma Surg 1999; 119: 423–427

[33] Maier M, Ueberle F, Rupprecht G. Physical parameters of extracorporeal shock waves. Biomed Tech (Berl) 1998; 43: 269–274

[34] Mulagha E, Fromm H. Extracorporeal shock wave lithotripsy of gallstones revisited: current status and future promises. J Gastroenterol Hepatol 2000; 15: 239–243

[35] Ogden JA, Toth-Kischkat A, Schultheiss R. Principles of shock wave therapy. Clin Orthop 2001; 387: 8–17

[36] Rompe JD, Decking J, Schoellner C, Nafe B. Shock wave application for chronic plantar fasciitis in running athletes. A prospective, randomized, placebo-controlled trial. Am J Sports Med 2003; 31: 268–275

[37] Rompe JD, Decking J, Schoellner C, Theis C. Repetitive low-energy shock wave treatment for chronic lateral epicondylitis in tennis players. Am J Sports Med 2004; 32: 734–743

[38] Rompe JD, Rosendahl T, Schollner C, Theis C. High-energy extracorporeal shock wave treatment of nonunions. Clin Orthop 2001; 387; 102–111

[39] Sass W, Steffen K, Matura E, Folberth W, Dreyer H, Seifert J. Experiences with lithotripters: measurements of standardized fragmentation. J Stone Dis 1992; 4: 129–140

[40] Schafer ME. Cost-effective shock wave hydrophones. J Stone Dis 1993; 5: 73–76

[41] Seidl M, Steinbach P, Hofstadter F. Shock wave induced endothelial damage – in situ analysis by confocal laser scanning microscopy. Ultrasound Med Biol 1994; 20: 571–578

[42] Steinbach P, Hofstaedter F, Nicolai H, Roessler W, Wieland W. Determination of the energy-dependent extent of vascular damage caused by high-energy shock waves in an umbilical cord model. Urol Res 1993; 21: 279–282

[43] Tavakkoli J, Birer A, Arefiev A, Prat F, Chapelon JY, Cathignol D. A piezocomposite shock wave generator with electronic focusing capability: application for producing cavitation-induced lesions in rabbit liver. Ultrasound Med Biol 1997; 23: 107–115

[44] Ueberle F. Shock wave technology. In: Extracorporeal shock waves in orthopaedics, W. Siebert W, Buch M (eds), Springer Berlin, 1997, pp 59–87

[45] Wess O, Ueberle F, Duehrssen R et al. Working Group Technical Developments – Consensus Report. In: High Energy Shock Waves in Medicine, Chaussy C, Eisenberger F, Jocham D, Wilbert D (eds), Thieme, Stuttgart, 1997, pp 59–71

[46] Zhong P, Cioanta I, Cocks FH, Preminger GM. Inertial cavitation and associated acoustic emission produced during electrohydraulic shock wave lithotripsy. J Acoust Soc Am 1997; 101: 2940–2950

Basic Research in Orthopedic Extracorporeal Shock Wave Application — An Update

T. Tischer, L. Gerdesmeyer, M. Maier

Introduction

Twenty years ago, when the treatment of renal stones was revolutionized by the introduction of extracorporeal shock wave lithotripsy (ESWL) [5], no one thought of application of these shock waves for the treatment of disorders of the musculoskeletal system. After the evaluation of possible side effects of shock waves on bone tissue (e. g., on the iliac bone, which can be in the focus area of the shock waves during treatment of renal stones) reproducible effects of shock waves on bone tissue were noted: in particular, primary osteocyte damage was seen, which converted after 72 hours to osteoblastic stimulation [19]. To further evaluate these effects, some interdisciplinary working groups between urologists and orthopedic surgeons began to work specifically on the effects of shock waves for the stimulation of bone healing. Subsequently in some animal models a decrease in the time necessary for fracture healing was found [22, 27, 71]. In contrast, some working groups noticed a delay of new bone formation and fracture healing [1, 16, 45]. These opposed, unsatisfying results did not prevent the introduction of extracorporeal shock wave application (ESWA) for the clinical treatment of delayed fracture healing and nonunion of long bones [58, 67, 70]. Moreover, ESWA was further introduced for the treatment of chronic tendinopathies of the heel, the elbow, the shoulder, and, recently, for experimental treatment of femoral head necrosis (see [55]), without further evaluation of the working mechanisms of shock waves in basic scientific investigations.

This fact questions the use and necessity of basic extracorporeal shock wave research on the musculoskeletal system. In this chapter, therefore, the outstanding benefit of basic research will be outlined. For a full understanding of the biological and molecular working mechanisms, a good knowledge about the physical principles of shock waves is necessary [3, 17, 50]. Especially during the first years of ESWA the lack of knowledge about physical definitions like energy flux density (EFD), acoustic fields, different focus zones, and different shock wave generator technologies contributed to the seemingly different results. Today, the most important parameter for the characterization of shock wave effects is the energy flux density ([mJ/mm^2]), which can be estimated relatively exactly. Just recently, the generator voltage necessary for the production of shock waves was used as a parameter, but these values differ vastly between different devices and it has been shown that there is no correlation between the generator voltage and the biological effects of shock waves from the different devices [42]. Also, the number of impulses and the size of the focus (e. g., it varies with different EFD) are important [12, 65].

The reader will be presented with the most important cell culture and animal studies on the effects of extracorporeal shock waves on the musculoskeletal system, ending with a short forecast of future basic research possibilities.

Clinical Application of Extracorporeal Shock Waves on the Musculoskeletal System

The current clinical use of shock waves in the treatment of tendinosis calcarea, epicondylitis humeri radialis, plantar fasciitis, delayed bone healing, and nonunion of long bones is described elsewhere in this book [2, 18, 49, 56]. A new, still experimental indication is the treatment of aseptic femur head necrosis [23, 31]. Here, the treatment is thought to induce added angiogenesis and to break up the sclerotic zone by microfracturing.

Currently, clinical ESWA is based on a sound scientific fundament [2, 18, 49, 56]. Numerous clinical studies have shown the effectiveness of this therapeutic method in comparison to other, conservative treatment modalities. It is of particular importance that there are already more scientific studies about the application of shock waves than most other treatment modalities. Even so, the scientific investigations about shock wave application are still not finished, either with regard to clinical studies or basic science research. Some authors still question the effec-

tiveness of shock waves in single studies [11, 21]. Unfortunately, there are no universally accepted treatment protocols with standardized energy flux densities, number of shock wave pulses, and frequency of treatment. In particular, the following questions should be addressed.
- The molecular working mechanisms of ESWA on the musculoskeletal system are still not fully understood. Positive effects in different diseases like tendinosis calcarea of the shoulder, the plantar fasciitis, aseptic pseudarthrosis, and aseptic femoral head necrosis heighten the suspicion that there is not merely one working mechanism, but many [36].
- In contrast, the assumption of many working mechanisms can lead to unwanted side effects with the application of shock waves. The induction of new bone formation, which is wanted during fracture repair or in the treatment of nonunions of long bones, may lead to difficulties in the treatment of tendinopathies like epicondylitis humeri radialis or plantar fasciitis, where healthy bone is also in the shock wave focus. Reciprocally, healthy tendons or muscle tissue may be damaged during the treatment of aseptic pseudarthrosis, where they are also in the shock wave focus. Especially, the treatment of aseptic pseudarthroses with ultra-high shock waves — as currently suggested (in one study up to 4 mJ/mm^2, [26]) — may damage these healthy tissues. For shock waves of this energy, various authors have shown that they negatively act on the integrity of tendons in the focus [35, 37, 41].
- Moreover, regardless which of these pathological processes were treated with ESWA, a 100% success rate was not achieved. This indicates that there must be unknown differences regarding shock wave interaction with the pathological process. In three disease patterns (tendinosis calcarea, epicondylitis humeri radialis, plantar fasciitis) first signs for individual differences have been demonstrated [38–40]. For example, the presence of a bone marrow edema of the calcaneus in MRI is a positive predictive value for therapeutic success during the treatment of plantar fasciitis [39]. Experiments have shown that variations in renal stones influence the outcome after treatment with shock waves [15, 59]. It was further shown that, with increasing mineral content, the stones were more susceptible for ESWL.
- Finally, the clinical studies differ regarding to the application modalities of extracorporeal shock waves. Especially, the magnitude of the used energy flux density, as well as used number of impulses, duration of treatment, and treatment at different time points vary strongly. In most of the studies, no reason was given why the used application modalities were chosen or why they were changed. This stands in sharp contrast with the results from basic science investigations where it is shown that ESWA effects depend on the used energy flux density and the number of applied shock wave impulses [35, 57, 75].

The clarification of the above-mentioned questions will considerably add to the successful clinical application of extracorporeal shock waves in orthopedic surgery and help to establish this form of treatment as a scientifically based therapy, not merely to be used as the method of last choice (after all other known treatment methods have been tried), but to be chosen earlier, maybe in some indications even as the therapy of first choice. A fast treatment success by ESWA, based on specific predictive factors and scientific knowledge, would also be desirable for economical aspects.

In the following sections it will be shown that some studies that begin to answer these questions are already available. Based on the encouraging results, coordinated efforts in the intensification of research in basic science and clinical application will be helpful.

Cell Culture and Animal Models in the Application of Extracorporeal Shock Waves on the Musculoskeletal System

It seems neither possible nor wise to present all published cell culture and animal studies on the application of shock waves to the musculoskeletal system. Instead, some general aspects will be pointed out and only selected studies introduced. For an overview, especially on older basic science studies, one might look at the superb works from Maier et al. and Rompe et al. [36, 55].

Table **1** lists the results of a PubMed query (http://www.pubmed.com) on March 1, 2005, on commonly used animal studies on the musculoskeletal system. Many different animal models are used, with rabbits and dogs being the most common. This is partly due to the fact that shock waves can be easily applied to rabbits and dogs, combined with the relatively moderate costs for animal care.

Table 1 Results of a PubMed query on March 3, in 2005, regarding which experimental animal model (animal model, rabbit, dog, ...) was used for the application of extracorporeal shock waves (shock wave or shockwave) on the musculoskeletal system (bone or tendon or cartilage)

First key word	Second key word	Third key word	1 + 2	1 + 2 + 3
Shock wave or **Shockwave**			4440	
-"-	Bone		139	
-"-	Tendon		52	
-"-	Cartilage		5	
-"-	Animal model	Bone or **tendon** or **cartilage**	26	6
-"-	Rodent	-"-	109	15
-"-	Rat	-"-	74	13
-"-	Mouse	-"-	32	1
-"-	Canine	-"-	32	6
-"-	Dog	-"-	78	10
-"-	Rabbit	-"-	79	21
-"-	Pig	-"-	78	5
-"-	Swine	-"-	75	5
-"-	Cow	-"-	16	1

Table **2** lists the basic scientific studies about the effects of shock waves on the musculoskeletal system; reviews are not included. The difference in the total number of studies in Tables **1** and **2** is related to works that were found twice (e. g., "canine" and "dog"). The results are summarized in the following paragraphs.

Application of Extracorporeal Shock Waves on Pathologically Altered Tissue

No basic science studies in an animal model of aseptic femoral head necrosis, plantar fasciitis, or epicondylitis radialis humeri have been accomplished.

Aseptic pseudarthrosis

There is only one basic scientific study available [27]. Starting point of this study were former reports about an increase in fracture healing after the application of extracorporeal shock waves [19, 22], whereas in other works a delay in bone healing was noted [1, 16]. Johannes et al. [27] used a model of nonunion of the radius (no callus formation or bridging of the fracture gap after 12 weeks) in dogs. After 12 weeks, half of the dogs (n = 5) were treated with extracorporeal shock waves with an energy flux density of 0.54 mJ/mm^2 (4 × 1000 impulses; time interval between treatment sessions not specified). After 12 more weeks, all treated dogs showed bony bridging on X-rays of the fracture gap, whereas only one of the five control animals showed this. These findings were confirmed by histological investigations. Unfortunately, no biomechanical analyses were performed to answer the question of how stable the bony bridge was. No data were presented about postoperative treatment, whether immobilization was carried out or not.

Fracture healing

Most of the basic science studies deal with the effect of shock waves on fracture healing (see Table **2**). In recent works, the influence of shock waves on the healing of bone defects was investigated, with shock waves being applied in the early phase of healing [1, 7, 8, 10, 16, 22, 66, 71, 75, 80]. The results of many of these studies have only limited significance for clinical application of ESWs, firstly since osteotomies or segmental bone defects without immobilization of the respective extremity are not used on patients and, secondly, the currently used energy flux densities are sometimes higher than the EFD

Table 2 Results of a PubMed query on March 3, 2005, regarding experimental animal studies on the application of extracorporeal shock wave on the musculoskeletal system. The studies marked with * are *in vitro* investigations

Study	Author	Year	Animal model	ESWA application
[81]	Yeaman	1989	Rat	Epiphysis
[68]	Van Arsdalen	1991	Rabbit	Epiphysis
[22]	Haupt	1992	Rat	Fracture model in the humerus
[28]	Kaulesar Sukul	1993	Rabbit*	Intact femur, intact tibia
[16]	Forriol	1994	Sheep	Fracture model of the tibia
[27]	Johannes	1994	Dog	Pseudarthrosis of the radius
[1]	Augat	1995	Sheep	Fracture model of the tibia
[14]	Delius	1995	Rabbit	Intact Femur
[45]	McCormack	1996	Rabbit	Osteotomy of the radius
[57]	Rompe	1998	Rabbit	Intact Achilles tendon
[66]	Uslu	1999	Rabbit	Bone defect in the radius
[26]	Ikeda	1999	Dog	Intact femur
[69]	Vaterlein	2000	Rabbit	Intact cartilage of the femur
[30]	Kusnierczak	2000	Cell culture	Human osteoblasts
[71]	Wang	2001	Dog	Fracture of the tibia
[77]	Wang	2001	Cell culture	Human bone marrow cells
[78]	Wang	2002	Rat	Bone marrow cells
[79]	Wang	2002	Rat	Bone marrow cells
[35]	Maier	2002	Rabbit	Intact femur
[64]	Tischer	2002	Rabbit	Intact femur
[41]	Maier	2002	Rabbit	Intact quadriceps tendon
[72]	Wang	2002	Dog	Bone-tendon junction
[32]	Maier	2003	Rabbit	Intact femur
[80]	Wang	2003	Rat	Segmental bone defect
[73]	Wang	2003	Rabbit	Bone-tendon junction
[33]	Maier	2003	Rabbit	Intact femur
[44]	Martini	2003	Cell culture	Human osteoblast-like cells
[43]	Martini	2003	Cell culture	Human osteoblasts
[48]	Narasaki	2003	Rabbit	Tibial bone lengthening
[7]	Chen	2003	Rat	Segmental bone defect in the femur
[76]	Wang	2004	Cell culture	Human osteoblasts
[13]	Da Costa Gomez	2004	Horse *	Cortical bone
[75]	Wang	2004	Rat	Fracture model of the femur
[52]	Pauwels	2004	Horse *	Cortical bone
[25]	Hsu	2004	Rabbit	Collagenase induced patellar tendinopathy
[10]	Chen	2004	Rat	Segmental bone defect
[8]	Chen	2004	Rat	Segmental bone defect
[9]	Chen	2004	Rat	Collagenase induced tendonitis of Achilles tendon
[34]	Maier	2004	Rabbit	Intact femur

used in a few studies for treatment in animals. In particular, the group around Wang et al. has revealed first molecular working mechanisms for the effects of shock waves during fracture healing. The application of ESWA on bone defects in the femur of rats leads to an increased expression of "bone morphogenetic proteins" (BMP 1, 2, and 4) [80]. In following studies it was shown that the effects of BMP and TGF-β1 release are most likely triggered by a Gi-protein triggered osteoblastic cascade [7]. Recently, in an early step, the activation of different mitogen-activated protein kinases (MAPK) by ESWA was shown. The "extracellular signal-regulated kinase" (ERK) and "p38 kinase" play an important role in the growth and differentiation of osteoblasts which initiate ESWA-mediated new bone formation [8]. After histologically and radiologically proven new bone formation, Wang et al. also showed superior mineral content and superior biomechanical strength of the bone tissue in a fracture model in rats [75]. Recently the role of TGF-β 1 in new bone formation was confirmed and also the increased production of the angiogenetic growth factor "vascular endothelial growth factor" (VEGF-A) in the treated area was shown, which leads to increased angiogenesis and therefore improved healing [10].

With these studies, molecular cascades — up to their origin — activated by the application of extracorporeal shock waves have been shown to induce new bone formation in fracture models.

Tendinitis/tendinosis calcarea

The destruction of "bonn stones" implanted in the rotator cuff of pigs was simulated *in vitro* [53]. For fragmentation of these stones at least 2000 shock wave impulses with an energy flux density of 0.42 mJ/mm^2 were necessary. The clinical significance of this work is low, since the implantation of artificial stones does not simulate the complex pathological alterations as seen in tendinosis calcarea. Moreover, the results are dependent on the physical and chemical composition of the artificial stones, which do not match with the composition of calcific depots in tendinosis calcarea. The interindividual variation of the chemical composition of calcific depots between patients could not be investigated.

The influence of shock waves in an experimental model of tendinitis (induced by injection of collagenase), either of the Achilles tendon or the patellar tendon, was also investigated [9, 25]. Briefly, low energy shock waves effectively promoted healing in the rat Achilles tendon, whereas higher energy shock waves elicited inhibitory effects [9]. Shock wave application can also increase collagen synthesis and cross-linking in the rabbit patellar tendinopathy [25].

Application of Extracorporeal Shock Waves in Cell Culture Models

With all restrictions coming from investigations on cell cultures, it has been shown that the use of high energy shock waves led to cell destruction, but when using lower energy shock waves, osteoblasts could be stimulated (rise in alkaline phosphatase, increased production of osteocalcin) [30, 43, 44]. In cell cultures treated with ESW an increased production of TGF-β1 could be demonstrated [79]. Moreover, the treatment with ESW leads to hyperpolarization of the membranes from osteoblasts, which leads to the activation of the *ras*-cascade, which then induces the activation of the osteogenic transcription factor cbfa-1, which finally causes osteoblastic differentiation [77]. In this experiment, for the first time, the influence of biophysical parameters (shock waves) on biochemical parameters (osteoblastic differentiation) could be shown.

Application of Extracorporeal Shock Waves on Intact Tissue

Most published studies about basic research on ESWA on the musculoskeletal system investigate the effects on various intact tissues like bone [14, 26, 32, 35, 64], tendon [41, 57], bone-tendon-junction [72–74], cartilage [69], nerve [54], dermis [51, 63], etc.

Bone

After application of extracorporeal shock waves, new bone formation can be seen in the intact femur, especially in the focus zone of the shock waves [14, 64]. The following etiological factors have been discussed: the creation of microfractures [26], an increase in regional blood flow, [35] and the release of the neurotransmitters prostaglandin E_2 and substance P [32]. Substance P mediates complex central pre- and postsynaptic effects and can induce peripherally a neurogenic inflammation as well as stimulation of the proliferation of different cells (e. g., osteoblasts) [32, 36]. In terms of the hyperstimulation hypothesis of Melzack, long-lasting pain relief follows an initial hyperstimulation algesia [36].

In the animal model, the high energy ESW-induced new bone formation is not only limited to the focus zone, but can extend over long distances. This should be taken into account for clinical applications of high energy shock waves [64].

To investigate the effects on growing tissue, immature kidneys and femur bones were treated with shock waves. Six months later, no signs of growth retardation were found during histological and radiological examinations on either the kidneys or the femur bone [68]. In contrast to these results, the Yeaman's group noticed a clear growth retardation in the growth plate of rats after high energy ESW [81]. Therefore, until proven otherwise, no ESWA should be performed on the growing skeleton. An actual study of Haupt [82] investigated the effects of radial shock waves in bony tissue in a rabbit model. Using pressures of 3.0 and 4.0 bar, two days after ESWT a reactive hyperemia of the focus zone was described. At this time point the beginning of new bone formation within the focus zone was detected. 60 days after application a significant new bone formation within the focus zone was found. These results allow the conclusion that radial shock waves have comparable effects in bone as known from focused shock waves. However, the number and intensity of side effects are less in radial ESWT. According to his results, Haupt [82] recommends the potential application of radial shock waves in the therapy of nonunions and for the induction of new bone formation (e. g., in parodontitis).

Tendon

Maier et al. and Rompe et al. showed dose-dependent tendon damage after treatment with high energy shock waves (EFD up to 1.2 mJ/mm^2) [41, 57]. Low-dose shock waves did not exert any negative effect on tendon morphology.

The tendon-bone interface was also a subject of study [72–74]. Shock wave therapy induces the ingrowth of neovascularization associated with the early release of angiogenesis-related markers at the Achilles tendon-bone junction in rabbits. This neovascularization may play a role to improve blood supply and tissue regeneration at the tendon-bone junction [73]. Also, shock wave treatment significantly improves the healing rate of the tendon-bone interface in a bone tunnel in rabbits [74].

Cartilage

Only one study has been done to investigate the effects of ESWA on mature cartilage. Healthy rabbits (n = 24) were treated with high energy shock waves (EFD = 1.2 mJ/mm^2), and up to 24 weeks later no pathological changes could be observed macroscopically, radiologically, or histologically [69].

Impact of Basic Research on Clinical Application of Shock Waves

It has to be remarked that, in some studies, shock waves were applied on intact, non-damaged tissue, and not like in clinical practice on pathological changed tissue. Nonetheless, these studies are of considerable significance for clinical practice, either for the investigation of possible side effects during ESWA, since often also healthy tissue is in the focus zone, and for the investigation of molecular working mechanisms of shock waves on the musculoskeletal system. This will be demonstrated in the following examples.

– Repeatedly it was shown, that high energy shock waves — as used in clinical practice for the treatment of aseptic pseudarthroses — can lead to significant morphological damage on intact tendon tissue [41, 57]. This should be considered, when the use of ultra-high energy shock waves for the treatment of aseptic pseudarthroses — as currently suggested in one study (up to 4 mJ/mm^2, [26]) — is considered. Moreover, even if shock waves are used and lead to no morphological alterations in tissues, they still can weaken the biomechanical stability of these tissues. This was recently shown in an animal model of calcifying tendon of the medial gastrocenemius muscle of turkeys [37].
– When investigating the molecular working mechanisms of the analgesic effects of shock waves, neural tissue comes to the fore. This is based on the detection of a shock wave-induced action potential in ischiadic nerve of frogs *in vitro* [60] and on the hypothesis that the analgesic effect may be archived by the so-called hyperstimulation theory of Melzack [24, 32, 46].
– The model of the intact bone is well suited for the investigation of dose-effect relations between shock wave energy and biological effects. This would be of uttermost importance for clinical application.

Conclusion and Outlook

All so far conducted studies on the effects of extracorporeal shock waves on the musculoskeletal system have provided valuable insights about working mechanisms and especially on possible side effects. Moreover, first results about molecular working mechanisms are now available, which allow insights into the complex interaction of shock waves with molecular mechanisms. Through coordinated intensification of basic animal research it seems possible, to put clinical shock wave application on top of a sound scientific knowledge in the near future:

- It is likely, that the most valuable hints for the optimization of extracorporeal shock wave therapy will come from animal experiments on established models of clinical diseases. The availability of established animal models of aseptic pseudarthrosis [4], epicondylitis radialis humeri [20], degenerative tendon damage in the rotator cuff (without calcifications), [62]) and aseptic femoral head necrosis [47] will serve as starting point for further investigations.
- The combination of these animal models with other controlled-experimental conditions like the application of nicotine [61] or nonsteroidal anti-inflammatory drugs [29] will allow us to answer other clinically relevant questions, like the influence of smoking and NSAI on the effect of ESWA, especially during the treatment of aseptic pseudarthrosis.
- Above all, transgenic or knock-out animals may help in the investigation of molecular pathways of extracorporeal shock waves on the musculoskeletal system. For example, the influence of endogenous opioids on the analgesic effect can be investigated in so-called "mu-opioid receptor knock-out" mice [6], which lack the mu-opioid receptor. For a detailed analysis of the influence of substance P on ESWA-mediated analgesia, the "PPT-A knock-out" mouse (pre-protachykinin A) or the "NK1-receptor knock-out" mouse (neurokinin 1) is available. In these animals, either the gene coding for substance P (PPT-A knock-out) or for the receptor of substance P (NK1-receptor knock-out) is missing.

Practical Conclusions

At the present time, the clinical use of extracorporeal shock waves is already based on a sound scientific knowledge. During numerous clinical studies the influence of ESW was investigated, and demonstrates the relevance of this therapy as an alternative procedure to other conservative therapies in the treatment of the described diseases. It is remarkable that already more scientific data exist for ESWA than for many of more often used conservative treatments. Recent experimental works have provided insights into the molecular working mechanisms of extracorporeal shock waves on the musculoskeletal system. In the long run, it seems possible that ESWA will be used as an accepted therapy for the treatment of aseptic pseudarthrosis, tendinosis calcarea of the shoulder, epicondylitis radialis of the humerus, plantar fasciitis, and aseptic femoral head necrosis, not only in the last instance, but increasingly in earlier stages of therapy. In future studies most value should be give to suitable application parameters of shock waves, like the number of pulses and the energy flux density or pressure. Standardized values of these parameters are of great value for clinical applications.

References

[1] Augat P, Claes L, Suger G. In vivo effect of shock waves on the healing of fractured bone. Clin Biomech (Bristol, Avon) 1995; 10: 374–378

[2] Biedermann R, Martin A, Handle G, Auckenthaler T, Bach C, Krismer M. Extracorporeal shock waves in the treatment of nonunions. J Trauma 2003; 54: 936–942

[3] Brendel W. Shock waves: a new physical principle in medicine. Eur Surg Res 1986; 18: 177–180

[4] Brownlow HC, Simpson AH. Metabolic activity of a new atrophic nonunion model in rabbits. J Orthop Res 2000; 18: 438–442

[5] Chaussy C, Brendel W, Schmiedt E. Extracorporeally induced destruction of kidney stones by shock waves. Lancet 1980; 2: 1265–1268

[6] Chen H, Seybold VS, Loh HH. An autoradiographic study in mu-opioid receptor knockout mice. Brain Res Mol Brain Res 2000;76: 170–172

[7] Chen YJ, Kuo YR, Yang KD, Wang CJ, Huang HC, Wang FS. Shock wave application enhances pertussis toxin protein-sensitive bone formation of segmental femoral defect in rats. J Bone Miner Res 2003; 18: 2169–2179

[8] Chen YJ, Kuo YR, Yang KD, Wang CJ, Sheen Chen SM, Huang HC, Yang YJ, Yi-Chih S, Wang FS. Activa-

tion of extracellular signal-regulated kinase (ERK) and p38 kinase in shock wave-promoted bone formation of segmental defect in rats. Bone 2004; 34: 466–477
9 Chen YJ, Wang CJ, Yang KD, Kuo YR, Huang HC, Huang YT, Sun YC, Wang FS. Extracorporeal shock waves promote healing of collagenase-induced Achilles tendinitis and increase TGF-beta1 and IGF-I expression. J Orthop Res 2004; 22: 854–861
10 Chen YJ, Wurtz T, Wang CJ, Kuo YR, Yang KD, Huang HC, Wang FS. Recruitment of mesenchymal stem cells and expression of TGF-beta 1 and VEGF in the early stage of shock wave-promoted bone regeneration of segmental defect in rats. J Orthop Res 2004; 22: 526–534
11 Chung B, Wiley JP. Effectiveness of extracorporeal shock wave therapy in the treatment of previously untreated lateral epicondylitis: a randomized controlled trial. Am J Sports Med 2004; 32: 1660–1667
12 Cleveland RO, Lifshitz DA, Connors BA, Evan AP, Willis LR, Crum LA. In vivo pressure measurements of lithotripsy shock waves in pigs. Ultrasound Med Biol 1998; 24: 293–306
13 Da Costa Gomez TM, Radtke CL, Kalscheur VL, Swain CA, Scollay MC, Edwards RB, Santschi EM, Markel MD, Muir P. Effect of focused and radial extracorporeal shock wave therapy on equine bone microdamage. Vet Surg 2004; 33: 49–55
14 Delius M, Draenert K, Al Diek Y, Draenert Y. Biological effects of shock waves: in vivo effect of high energy pulses on rabbit bone. Ultrasound Med Biol 1995; 21: 1219–1225
15 Demirbas M, Ergen A, Ozkardes H. Stone fragility in shock wave lithotripsy can be predicted in vitro. Int Urol Nephrol 1998; 30: 553–557
16 Forriol F, Solchaga L, Moreno JL, Canadell J. The effect of shockwaves on mature and healing cortical bone. Int Orthop 1994; 18: 325–329
17 Gerdesmeyer L, Maier M, Haake M, Schmitz C. Physical-technical principles of extracorporeal shockwave therapy (ESWT). Orthopaede 2002; 31: 610–617
18 Gerdesmeyer L, Wagenpfeil S, Haake M, Maier M, Loew M, Wortler K, Lampe R, Seil R, Handle G, Gassel S, Rompe JD. Extracorporeal shock wave therapy for the treatment of chronic calcifying tendonitis of the rotator cuff: a randomized controlled trial. JAMA 2003; 290: 2573–2580
19 Graff J. Die Wirkung hochenergetischer Stoßwellen auf Knochen und Weichteilgewebe. Ruhr-Universität Bochum, 1989
20 Haker E, Theodorsson E, Lundeberg T. An experimental model of tennis elbow in rats: a study of the contribution of the nervous system. Inflammation 1998; 22: 435–444
21 Harniman E, Carette S, Kennedy C, Beaton D. Extracorporeal shock wave therapy for calcific and noncalcific tendonitis of the rotator cuff: A systematic review. J Hand Ther 2004; 17: 132–151
22 Haupt G, Haupt A, Ekkernkamp A, Gerety B, Chvapil M. Influence of shock waves on fracture healing. Urology 1992; 39: 529–532.
23 Hausdorf J, Lutz A, Rohrig H, Maier M. Extracorporeal shock wave therapy and femur head necrosis – pressure measurements in the femur head. Z Orthop Ihre Grenzgeb 2004; 142: 122–126.
24 Hausdorf J, Schmitz C, Averbeck B, Maier M. Molecular basis for pain mediating properties of extracorporeal shock waves. Schmerz 2004; 18: 492–497
25 Hsu RW, Hsu WH, Tai CL, Lee KF. Effect of shockwave therapy on patellar tendinopathy in a rabbit model. J Orthop Res 2004; 22: 221–227
26 Ikeda K, Tomita K, Takayama K. Application of extracorporeal shock wave on bone: preliminary report. J Trauma 1999; 47: 946–950
27 Johannes EJ, Kaulesar Sukul DM, Matura E. High-energy shock waves for the treatment of nonunions: an experiment on dogs. J Surg Res 1994; 57: 246–252
28 Kaulesar Sukul DM, Johannes EJ, Pierik EG, van Eijck GJ, Kristelijn MJ. The effect of high energy shock waves focused on cortical bone: an in vitro study. J Surg Res 1993; 54: 46–51
29 Keller JC, Trancik TM, Young FA, St Mary E. Effects of indomethacin on bone ingrowth. J Orthop Res 1989; 7: 28–34
30 Kusnierczak D, Brocai DR, Vettel U, Loew M. Effect of extracorporeal shockwave administration on biological behavior of bone cells in vitro. Z Orthop Ihre Grenzgeb 2000; 138: 29–33
31 Ludwig J, Lauber S, Lauber HJ, Dreisilker U, Raedel R, Hotzinger H. High-energy shock wave treatment of femoral head necrosis in adults. Clin Orthop 2001; 119–126
32 Maier M, Averbeck B, Milz S, Refior HJ, Schmitz C. Substance P and prostaglandin E2 release after shock wave application to the rabbit femur. Clin Orthop 2003; 237–245
33 Maier M, Freed JA, Milz S, Pellengahr C, Schmitz C. Detection of bone fragments in pulmonary vessels following extracorporeal shock wave application to the distal femur in an in-vivo animal model. Z Orthop Ihre Grenzgeb 2003; 141: 223–226
34 Maier M, Hausdorf J, Tischer T, Milz S, Weiler C, Refior HJ, Schmitz C. New bone formation by extracorporeal shock waves. Dependence of induction on energy flux density. Orthopade 2004; 33: 1401–1410.
35 Maier M, Milz S, Tischer T, Munzing W, Manthey N, Stabler A, Holzknecht N, Weiler C, Nerlich A, Refior HJ, Schmitz C. Influence of extracorporeal shockwave application on normal bone in an animal model in vivo. Scintigraphy, MRI and histopathology. J Bone Joint Surg [Br] 2002; 84: 592–599

36 Maier M, Milz S, Wirtz DC, Rompe JD, Schmitz C. Basic research of applying extracorporeal shockwaves on the musculoskeletal system. An assessment of current status. Orthopaede 2002; 31: 667–677

37 Maier M, Saisu T, Beckmann J, Delius M, Grimm F, Hupertz V, Milz S, Nerlich A, Refior HJ, Schmitz C, Ueberle F, Weiler C, Messmer K. Impaired tensile strength after shock-wave application in an animal model of tendon calcification. Ultrasound Med Biol 2001; 27: 665–671

38 Maier M, Stabler A, Lienemann A, Kohler S, Feitenhansl A, Durr HR, Pfahler M, Refior HJ. Shockwave application in calcifying tendinitis of the shoulder — prediction of outcome by imaging. Arch Orthop Trauma Surg 2000; 120: 493–498

39 Maier M, Steinborn M, Schmitz C, Stabler A, Kohler S, Pfahler M, Durr HR, Refior HJ. Extracorporeal shock wave application for chronic plantar fasciitis associated with heel spurs: prediction of outcome by magnetic resonance imaging. J Rheumatol 2000; 27: 2455–2462

40 Maier M, Steinborn M, Schmitz C, Stabler A, Kohler S, Veihelmann A, Pfahler M, Refior HJ. Extracorporeal shock-wave therapy for chronic lateral tennis elbow — prediction of outcome by imaging. Arch Orthop Trauma Surg 2001; 121: 379–384

41 Maier M, Tischer T, Milz S, Weiler C, Nerlich A, Pellengahr C, Schmitz C, Refior HJ. Dose-related effects of extracorporeal shock waves on rabbit quadriceps tendon integrity. Arch Orthop Trauma Surg 2002; 122: 436–441

42 Maier M, Ueberle F, Rupprecht G. Physical parameters of extracorporeal shock waves. Biomed Tech (Berl) 1998; 43: 269–274

43 Martini L, Fini M, Giavaresi G, Torricelli P, de Pretto M, Rimondini L, Giardino R. Primary osteoblasts response to shock wave therapy using different parameters. Artif Cells Blood Substit Immobil Biotechnol 2003; 31: 449–466

44 Martini L, Giavaresi G, Fini M, Torricelli P, de Pretto M, Schaden W, Giardino R. Effect of extracorporeal shock wave therapy on osteoblast-like cells. Clin Orthop 2003; 269–280

45 McCormack D, Lane H, McElwain J. The osteogenic potential of extracorporeal shock wave therapy. An in-vivo study. Ir J Med Sci 1996; 165: 20–22

46 Melzack R, Wall PD. Pain mechanisms: a new theory. Science 1965; 150: 971–979

47 Mont MA, Jones LC, Einhorn TA, Hungerford DS, Reddi AH. Osteonecrosis of the femoral head. Potential treatment with growth and differentiation factors. Clin Orthop 1998; S314–335

48 Narasaki K, Shimizu H, Beppu M, Aoki H, Takagi M, Takashi M. Effect of extracorporeal shock waves on callus formation during bone lengthening. J Orthop Sci 2003; 8: 474–481

49 Ogden JA, Alvarez RG, Levitt RL, Johnson JE, Marlow ME. Electrohydraulic high-energy shock-wave treatment for chronic plantar fasciitis. J Bone Joint Surg [Am] 2004; 86: 2216–2228

50 Ogden JA, Toth-Kischkat A, Schultheiss R. Principles of shock wave therapy. Clin Orthop 2001; 8–17

51 Ohtori S, Inoue G, Mannoji C, Saisu T, Takahashi K, Mitsuhashi S, Wada Y, Yamagata M, Moriya H. Shock wave application to rat skin induces degeneration and reinnervation of sensory nerve fibres. Neurosci Lett 2001; 315: 57–60

52 Pauwels FE, McClure SR, Amin V, Van Sickle D, Evans RB. Effects of extracorporeal shock wave therapy and radial pressure wave therapy on elasticity and microstructure of equine cortical bone. Am J Vet Res 2004; 65: 207–212

53 Perlick L, Korth O, Wallny T, Wagner U, Hesse A, Schmitt O. The mechanical effects of shock waves in extracorporeal shock wave treatment of calcific tendonitis — an in vitro model. Z Orthop Ihre Grenzgeb 1999; 137: 10–16

54 Rompe JD, Bohl J, Riehle HM, Schwitalle M, Krischek O. Evaluating the risk of sciatic nerve damage in the rabbit by administration of low and intermediate energy extracorporeal shock waves. Z Orthop Ihre Grenzgeb 1998; 136: 407–411

55 Rompe JD, Buch M, Gerdesmeyer L, Haake M, Loew M, Maier M, Heine J. Musculoskeletal shock wave therapy–current database of clinical research. Z Orthop Ihre Grenzgeb 2002; 140: 267–274

56 Rompe JD, Decking J, Schoellner C, Theis C. Repetitive low-energy shock wave treatment for chronic lateral epicondylitis in tennis players. Am J Sports Med 2004; 32: 734–743

57 Rompe JD, Kirkpatrick CJ, Kullmer K, Schwitalle M, Krischek O. Dose-related effects of shock waves on rabbit tendo Achillis. A sonographic and histological study. J Bone Joint Surg [Br] 1998; 80: 546–552

58 Rompe JD, Rosendahl T, Schollner C, Theis C. High-energy extracorporeal shock wave treatment of nonunions. Clin Orthop 2001; 102–111

59 Sakamoto W, Kishimoto T, Takegaki Y, Sugimoto T, Wada S, Yamamoto K, Maekawa M, Ochi H. Stone fragility — measurement of stone mineral content by dual photon absorptiometry. Eur Urol 1991; 20: 150–153

60 Schelling G, Delius M, Gschwender M, Grafe P, Gambihler S. Extracorporeal shock waves stimulate frog sciatic nerves indirectly via a cavitation-mediated mechanism. Biophys J 1994; 66: 133–140

61 Silcox DH 3rd, Daftari T, Boden SD, Schimandle JH, Hutton WC, Whitesides TE Jr. The effect of nicotine on spinal fusion. Spine 1995; 20: 1549–1553

62 Soslowsky LJ, Thomopoulos S, Tun S, Flanagan CL, Keefer CC, Mastaw J, Carpenter JE. Neer Award 1999. Overuse activity injures the supraspinatus tendon in an animal model: a histologic and biome-

chanical study. J Shoulder Elbow Surg 2000; 9: 79–84

[63] Takahashi N, Wada Y, Ohtori S, Saisu T, Moriya H. Application of shock waves to rat skin decreases calcitonin gene-related peptide immunoreactivity in dorsal root ganglion neurons. Auton Neurosci 2003; 107: 81–84

[64] Tischer T, Milz S, Anetzberger H, Muller PE, Wirtz DC, Schmitz C, Ueberle F, Maier M. Extracorporeal shock waves induce ventral-periosteal new bone formation out of the focus zone — results of an invivo animal trial. Z Orthop Ihre Grenzgeb 2002; 140: 281–285

[65] Ueberle F. Acoustic parameters of pressure pulse sources used in lithotripsy and pain therapy. In: High energy shock waves used in medicine, Chaussy C et al. (ed), Thieme, Stuttgart, New York 1997, pp 76–85

[66] Uslu MM, Bozdogan O, Guney S, Bilgili H, Kaya U, Olcay B, Korkusuz F. The effect of extracorporeal shock wave treatment (ESWT) on bone defects. An experimental study. Bull Hosp Jt Dis 1999; 58: 114–118

[67] Valchanou VD, Michailov P. High energy shock waves in the treatment of delayed and nonunion of fractures. Int Orthop 1991; 15: 181–184

[68] Van Arsdalen KN, Kurzweil S, Smith J, Levin RM. Effect of lithotripsy on immature rabbit bone and kidney development. J Urol 1991; 146: 213–216

[69] Vaterlein N, Lussenhop S, Hahn M, Delling G, Meiss AL. The effect of extracorporeal shock waves on joint cartilage — an in vivo study in rabbits. Arch Orthop Trauma Surg 2000; 120: 403–406

[70] Wang CJ, Chen HS, Chen CE, Yang KD. Treatment of nonunions of long bone fractures with shock waves. Clin Orthop 2001; 95–101

[71] Wang CJ, Huang HY, Chen HH, Pai CH, Yang KD. Effect of shock wave therapy on acute fractures of the tibia: a study in a dog model. Clin Orthop 2001; 112–118

[72] Wang CJ, Huang HY, Pai CH. Shock wave-enhanced neovascularization at the tendon-bone junction: an experiment in dogs. J Foot Ankle Surg 2002; 41: 16–22

[73] Wang CJ, Wang FS, Yang KD, Weng LH, Hsu CC, Huang CS, Yang LC. Shock wave therapy induces neovascularization at the tendon-bone junction. A study in rabbits. J Orthop Res 2003; 21: 984–989

[74] Wang CJ, Wang FS, Yang KD, Weng LH, Sun YC, Yang YJ. The effect of shock wave treatment at the tendon-bone interface — a histomorphological and biomechanical study in rabbits. J Orthop Res 2005; 23: 274–280

[75] Wang CJ, Yang KD, Wang FS, Hsu CC, Chen HH. Shock wave treatment shows dose-dependent enhancement of bone mass and bone strength after fracture of the femur. Bone 2004; 34: 225–230

[76] Wang FS, Wang CJ, Chen YJ, Chang PR, Huang YT, Sun YC, Huang HC, Yang YJ, Yang KD. Ras induction of superoxide activates ERK-dependent angiogenic transcription factor HIF-1alpha and VEGF-A expression in shock wave-stimulated osteoblasts. J Biol Chem 2004; 279: 10331–10337

[77] Wang FS, Wang CJ, Huang HJ, Chung H, Chen RF, Yang KD. Physical shock wave mediates membrane hyperpolarization and Ras activation for osteogenesis in human bone marrow stromal cells. Biochem Biophys Res Commun 2001; 287: 648–655

[78] Wang FS, Wang CJ, Sheen-Chen SM, Kuo YR, Chen RF, Yang KD. Superoxide mediates shock wave induction of ERK-dependent osteogenic transcription factor (CBFA1) and mesenchymal cell differentiation toward osteoprogenitors. J Biol Chem 2002; 277:10931–10937

[79] Wang FS, Yang KD, Chen RF, Wang CJ, Sheen-Chen SM. Extracorporeal shock wave promotes growth and differentiation of bone-marrow stromal cells towards osteoprogenitors associated with induction of TGF-beta1. J Bone Joint Surg [Br] 2002; 84: 457–461

[80] Wang FS, Yang KD, Kuo YR, Wang CJ, Sheen-Chen SM, Huang HC, Chen YJ. Temporal and spatial expression of bone morphogenetic proteins in extracorporeal shock wave-promoted healing of segmental defect. Bone 2003; 32: 387–396

[81] Yeaman LD, Jerome CP, McCullough DL. Effects of shock waves on the structure and growth of the immature rat epiphysis. J Urol 1989; 141: 670–674

[82] Haupt G. Animal studies and radial shock wave therapy. In: Extracorporeal shock wave therapy, Gerdesmeyer L (ed), Verlag Books on Demand, Norderstedt, Germany, 2004 (ISBN 3-8334-1088-4)

Manufacturers' Update on Lithotripter Concepts

Dornier MedTech: Products and New Developments — An Overview

H. Hermeking

Introduction

The timing of the present consensus meeting almost exactly coincides with the 25th anniversary of the first ESWL of a kidney stone patient by Christian Chaussy on a Dornier lithotripter on February 20, 1980. This was the beginning of a revolution in the treatment of kidney stone disease. The objective of Dornier MedTech as the inventor/manufacturer has been to serve the user's needs with regard to this new technology ever since. Today Dornier MedTech produces lithotripters, urotables, orthopedic shock wave devices, and medical lasers. The Dornier Epos Ultra orthopedic shock wave device was approved by the FDA in 2002 for the treatment of plantar fasciitis. With an installed base of over 1000 lithotripters, Dornier MedTech is offering worldwide a diverse range of high-quality lithotripters, as well as an advanced, digital urology imaging system. Dornier's comprehensive lithotripter product-line ranges from more compact units suitable for mobile service providers or smaller health-care settings:
– Dornier Compact Delta and Dornier Compact Sigma

to high-end devices appropriate for larger medical institutions or university settings:
– Dornier Lithotripter S II.

Regardless of model, all Dornier lithotripters are renowned for their efficiency, low retreatment rates, user-friendliness, and high value.

In this chapter we will focus on the presentation of new features of the most recently launched lithotripters, Dornier Compact Sigma and Dornier Lithotripter S II. In addition we want to address the most significant new features of the Compact Delta II, which will be introduced at the EAU on March 16–19, 2005 in Istanbul, Turkey.

Modular Lithotripter Dornier Compact Sigma

The Dornier Compact Sigma is a modular lithotripter (Fig. 1). Together with the Dornier *Relax+* patient table it may be combined with X-ray, ultrasound, and endoscopic equipment to form a truly comprehensive urological workstation. The fully motorized, four-axis Dornier *Relax+* patient table is ideal for both extracorporeal shock wave lithotripsy (ESWL) and endourology. It features a radiolucent table top offering a wide range of movement as well as Trendelenburg tilting capability. Extensive urological accessory options are also available.

C-arms can be mechanically linked to the Dornier Compact Sigma either with or without mechanical coupling to create a single stable unit. This provides high quality imaging for lithotripsy as well as for other applications. An innovatively designed laser pointer system offers reliable alignment control for ESWL. The Merlin ultrasound scanner from B-K Medical is well suited for general urological diagnosis and shock wave applications. A range of ultrasound transducers can be configured for general urological diagnosis. Attachments for brachytherapy are offered in addition.

The Dornier Compact Sigma's isocentric design allows both the shock wave and the imaging systems to revolve around a single focal point resulting in the easy and precise alignment of the targeting system with the shock wave focus. The projection angles of the X-ray localization and the ultrasound windows can be varied over a wide range for optimal imaging, without losing the relationship to the therapy focus. Thanks to this isocentric design, elaborate and costly navigation systems for stone localization are unnecessary with the Dornier Compact Sigma.

The Dornier Compact Sigma features optimized indication settings for shock wave and localization. Proximal ureteral stones can be localized by both vertical and oblique X-ray projections providing posterior lateral coupling for shock wave treatment. This leaves the X-ray

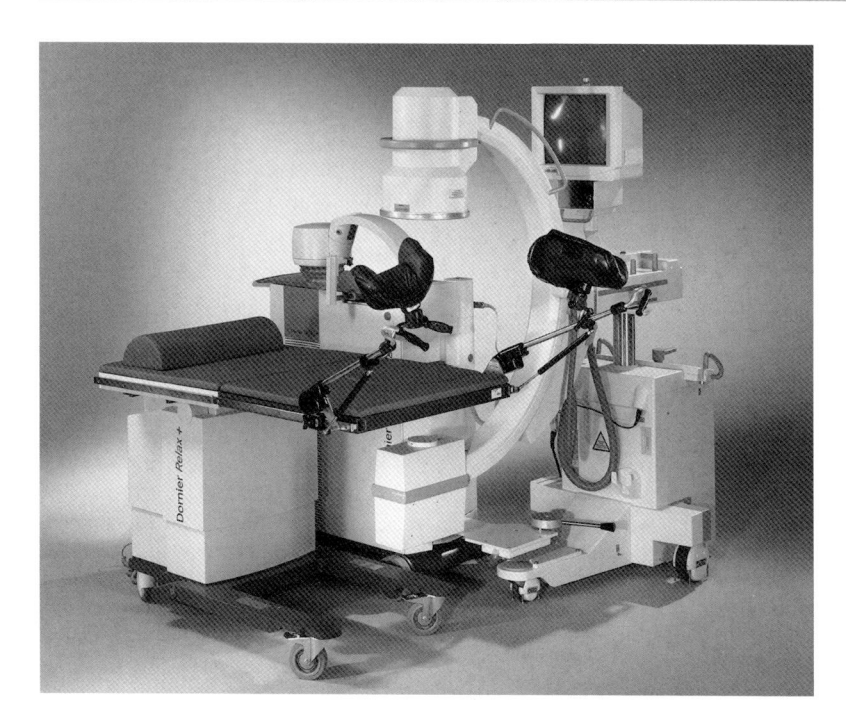

Fig. 1 Modular lithotripter Dornier Compact Sigma.

image clear and unobstructed. Avoidance of bone or intestinal gas is simple thanks to the flexible imaging design. Lithotripsy in the medial and distal ureter is typically performed ventrally due to the osseous pelvis. The over-table position of the therapy unit provides excellent access while patients remain comfortably in supine position.

Urological Workstation Dornier Lithotripter S II

The Dornier Lithotripter S II is a fully integrated urological workstation. It provides a high level of efficiency over a wide range of applications as well as simple operation – everything that is required for a quick and successful performance of ESWL and endourology. The Dornier Lithotripter S II combines a proven concept with the latest digital X-ray and information technology. The fully digital X-ray chain developed by Dornier MedTech represents the latest in imaging technology. The high-quality components function as an integrated system resulting in superior image quality and low radiation dose. The 50 to 80 kilowatt high-frequency generator works in dose-saving pulsed operation, even during continuous fluoroscopy. The high resolution CCD camera provides superior high-contrast images. In addition, high-level fluoroscopy and digital spot images are also available. Optional color LCD monitors round up the system providing display flexibility. Easy-to-read menus for X-ray operation, image processing, image storage, and documentation allow quick familiarity with the system.

Fully Integrated, Transportable Dornier Compact Delta II

The Compact Delta II (Fig. 2) is a fully integrated, transportable lithotripter like its predecessor, the Compact Delta. The versatile, modular design makes the Delta II the optimal solution for all areas of urological diagnosis and therapy, including lithotripsy, endourology, percutaneous procedures, and diagnostic X-ray. The Dornier Compact Delta II's isocentric design allows both shock wave and imaging systems to revolve around a single point making it easier to target under difficult conditions.

Different from its predecessor, the Compact Delta II features the newly developed Urology Information Management System (UIMS) offering superior image management and connectivity. In addition, like no other lithotripter, it offers

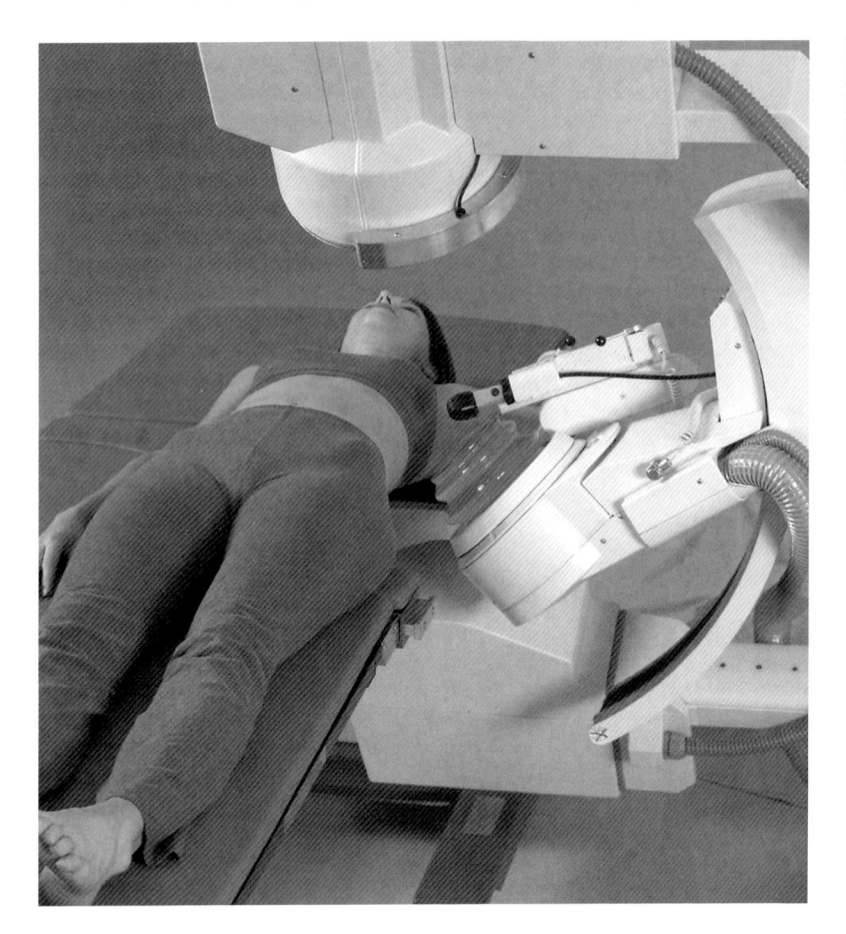

Fig. 2 Dornier Compact Delta II's unique isocentric shock wave therapy, X-ray and ultrasound imaging systems.

tri-mode imaging with the newly developed ultrasound imaging system FarSight, X-ray imaging, and isocentric ultrasound resulting in unsurpassed flexibility in imaging and therapy.

The FarSight ultrasound imaging system is a specially developed locating system. Its transducer is integrated in the lens of the therapy head of the Compact Delta II. This way it is protected against shock wave exposure. To guarantee optimum image quality the transducer was developed especially for these specific requirements. The viewing axis of FarSight coincides with the shock wave propagation axis. Unlike with traditional in-line ultrasound systems in lithotripters, the transducer of FarSight does not have to be retracted during shock wave application allowing real-time imaging during shock wave application in the direction of shock wave propagation.

Unique tri-mode imaging capabilities increase the shock wave treatment efficiency of the Delta II. Its digital image acquisition, processing and connectivity to hospital data management systems lead to enhanced system flexibility with improved workflow.

Siemens Medical Solutions: LITHOSKOP: A New Era in Stone Therapy and Overall Urology

M. Lanski

Introduction

With the introduction of the multifunctional urology system LITHOSKOP® in March 2005, Siemens Medical Solutions has set new standards in urology. LITHOSKOP focuses on highly efficient extracorporeal shock wave lithotripsy (ESWL) with its new shock wave system Pulso™ and enhanced workflow throughout virtually all urologic applications and interventions.

In times of globally changing healthcare systems, financial aspects are also an important consideration. LITHOSKOP represents the ideal solution to address these changes, and to ensure efficient therapy at the highest level.

LITHOSKOP — A "Revolutionary" Concept

Major progress in workflow and patient handling was made by focusing the entire system's philosophy on the daily clinical routine.

LITHOSKOP fully adapts to the patient. For lithotripsy, both the X-ray C-arm and the shock wave head revolve around the patient, therefore any stone location can be reached without repositioning the patient. With the patient always in the supine position, the shock wave head reaches both kidneys from two under-table positions (see Figs. **1** and **2**). Ureteral stones are typically treated with the shock wave head in an over-table position (see Fig. **3**).

LITHOSKOP provides far more degrees of freedom. Given that it can bypass obstructions to the shock wave, such as ribs or bowel gas. This also facilitates any other shock wave application, e. g., extracorporeal shock wave therapy (ESWT), treatment of Peyronie's disease, biliary ESWL, etc.

LITHOSKOP's one-time patient positioning ensures a constant patient position throughout most applications. For endourologic procedures, such as cystoscopy, TURP, etc., as well as ESWL

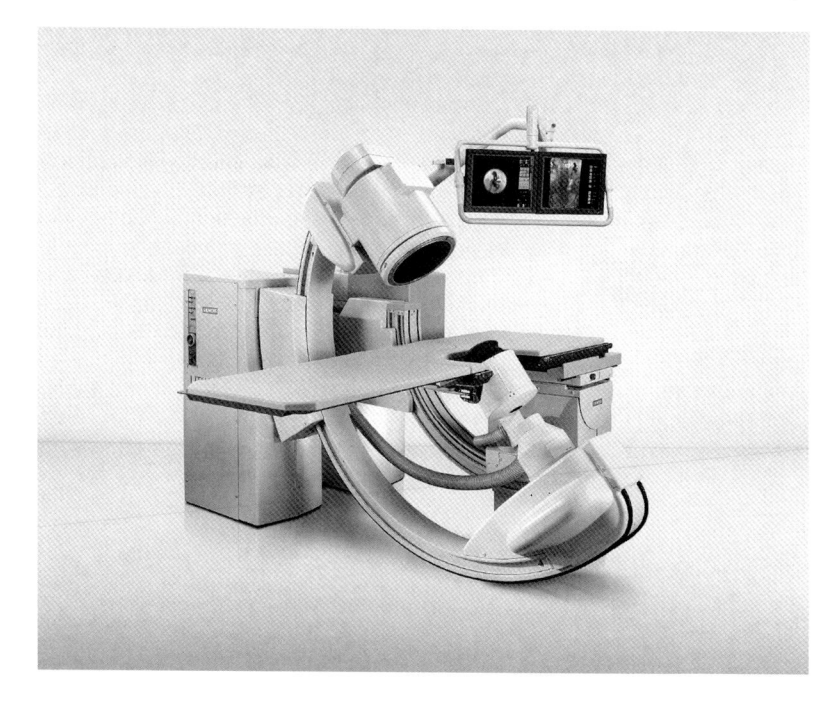

Fig. 1 Shock wave head in under-table position for treatment of, e. g., a left kidney stone.

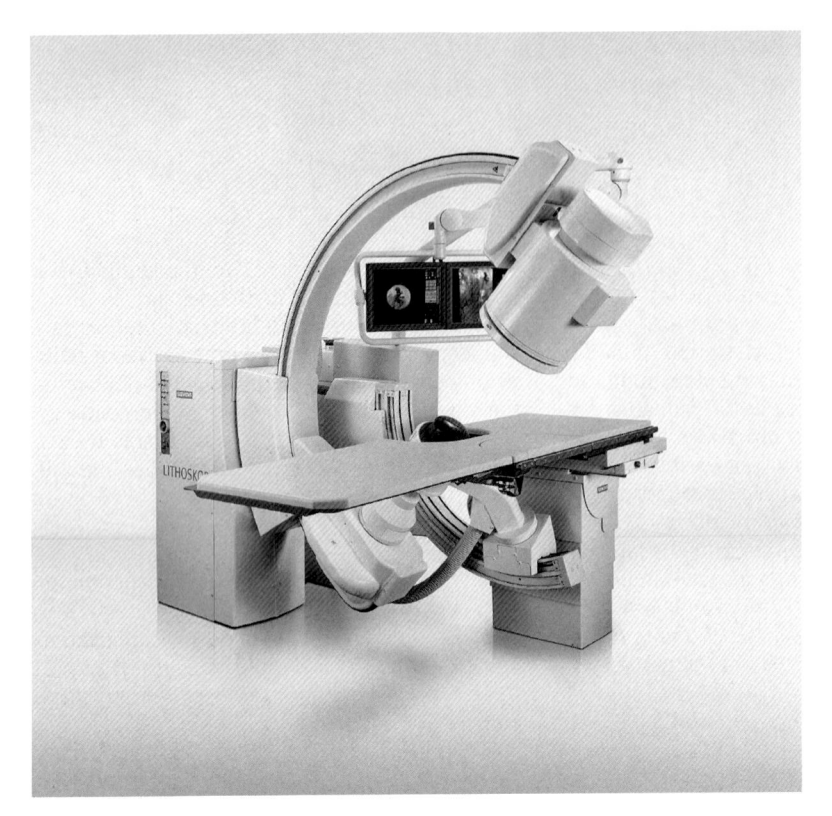

Fig. 2 Shock wave head in under-table position for treatment of, e. g., a right kidney stone.

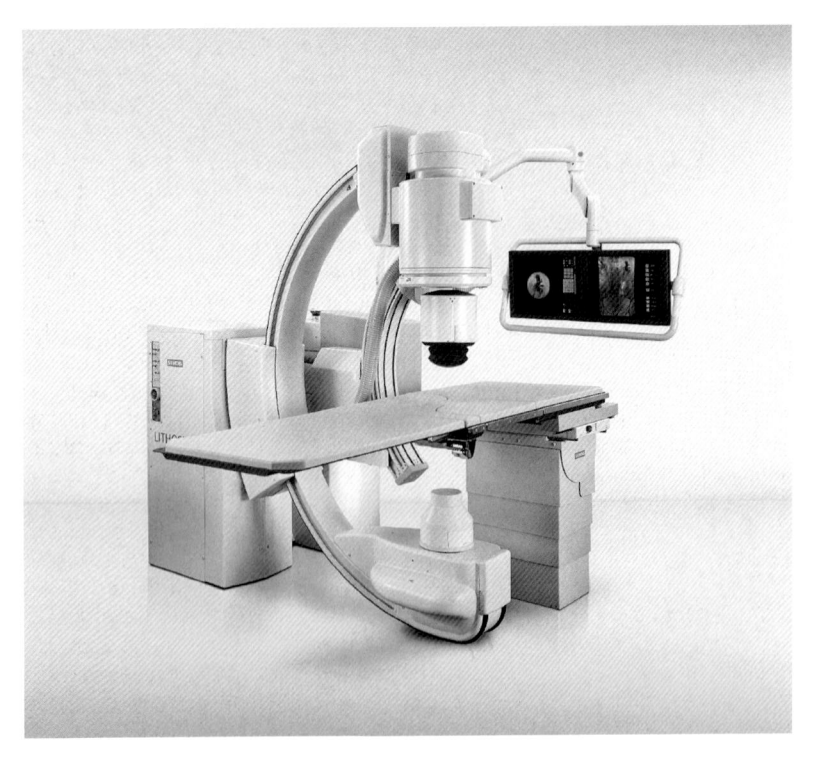

Fig. 3 Shock wave head in over-table position for treatment of, e. g., a ureteral stone.

including all auxiliary procedures, the patient is always in a supine position.

Due to the table's single column design, all anesthesia equipment may remain on one side of the system.

By placing the patient's perineum over the table's perineal end, both kidneys are instantly centered within the bilateral ESWL cutouts of the table. At the same time, the patient's head is located on the table's head end allowing optimal access by the anesthetist.

A counterbalanced, highly flexible monitor arm permits positioning of the dual monitors wherever needed. For endourologic and percutaneous procedures, both monitors may be individually placed for optimal visibility. The monitors display X-ray, ultrasound, and endoscopic images and sequences.

These important features lead to simplified patient handling. Cumbersome and time-consuming patient repositioning is now an issue of the past. Above all, these functional product characteristics contribute to better patient care.

For ESWL, the entire system can be operated from a remote desk. Comprehensive software guides the user through the patient's workflow – patient registration, diagnosis, image processing, therapy, and documentation of therapy data.

This software also incorporates LithoReport™, a software tool designed to precisely track the overall ESWL procedure. It serves for documentation of stone locations, stone size, all ESWL parameters, etc. LithoReport also allows for statistical analysis of previously performed shock wave treatments and full DICOM connectivity assists in patient data handling.

Pulso – Siemens Shock Wave Technology for Efficient Stone Therapy

The electromagnetic Siemens shock wave system Pulso was designed to maximize therapeutic efficiency in terms of increased stone fragmentation and decreased side effects. The main design objectives were to reduce retreatment rates, need for anesthesia and auxiliary measures while increasing the stone-free rate and patient comfort and safety.

The shock wave system's effective energy ranges from very low energy levels for ESWT and pediatric ESWL to highest levels for reliable and rapid stone fragmentation of even hardest calculi.

By widening the lateral focal extent, the energy density was lowered in order to ensure tissue-sparing stone therapy. A larger size therapy focus also contributes to an increased hit ratio, thus compensating for respiratory stone excursion.

In addition, LITHOSKOP provides a soft operation mode for shock wave treatments with minimal pain and maximal patient comfort.

A focal depth of 16 cm accommodates effective treatments on even obese patients.

Exchangeable coupling bellows allow for tailoring the shock wave system towards specific applications. A dedicated bellows for ESWL provides a large coupling area for optimal energy transfer to the stone. For superfacial treatments, a tapered bellows provides best possible visibility of the area to be treated.

Reliable and Precise Imaging with Siemens X-Ray and Ultrasound

Since best image quality is crucial for the therapeutic success, LITHOSKOP's isocentric X-ray C-arm is equipped with high quality X-ray components.

For stone localization, LITHOSKOP provides an orbital movement of the X-ray C-arm. For localization, one projection always runs directly through the shock wave head and is in-line with the shock wave path. The second projection is tangential to the shock wave head. An angle of approximately 40° between both projections ensures precise stone localization.

Synchronized and isocentric movements of the X-ray C-arm and the shock wave head provide accurate stone localization at all times, regardless of the stone location.

To ease the stone positioning process, LITHOSKOP features AutoPos™, a computerized 3D localization. By simply identifying the stone on the X-ray monitor in both projections, the calculi is automatically positioned in the therapy focus.

Within seconds one can switch between X-ray and ultrasound localization. The Siemens ultrasound unit SONOLINE G50 is equipped with a phased array transducer ensuring excellent image quality even in large penetration depths. For in-line ultrasound localization, the transducer is mounted within the shock wave head. All its movements can also be controlled from the remote desk. Respective ultrasound images are transferred and displayed on the desk's monitors and may be archived together with X-ray images in one patient folder.

Physicians and patients are not exposed to X-ray radiation with the use of ultrasound. This opens up the possibility for continuous monitoring of the stone's disintegration process.

The SONOLINE G50 can be detached from the LITHOSKOP at any time and may be used as a stand-alone system. A large variety of additional transducers is available for different applications. A biplane endorectal probe facilitates ergonomic prostate diagnosis and can also be used for, e. g., brachytherapy.

Superior in-line localization

LITHOSKOP features the renowned in-line localization principle for X-ray and ultrasound imaging modalities. It enables stone visualization coaxially with the propagation of the shock wave for accurate stone localization. Obstructing objects within the shock wave path can be recognized and avoided.

Multifunctional

LITHOSKOP is the perfect symbiosis of a lithotripter and a urologic diagnostic system. It smoothly blends in the daily clinical work-flow by supporting each step, from patient registration through patient treatments to accounting.

LITHOSKOP is ideally tailored towards the following applications and interventions:
- extracorporeal shock wave applications,
- endourologic applications,
- percutaneous interventions,
- urological diagnosis.

Extracorporeal shock wave applications

LITHOSKOP's shock wave system Pulso covers virtually all shock wave applications. Its wide range of energy, combined with its unique mechanism for flexible shock wave head positioning, also facilitates interdisciplinary shock wave therapy. Therefore, the system can be applied for urologic, orthopedic (pain therapy), and gastroenterologic shock wave applications.

Physicians benefit from easy and virtually safe patient handling, in addition to reduced treatment times.

Endourologic applications

LITHOSKOP is designed for conveniently performing all endourologic interventions without any restrictions.

A head-supported table top provides optimal clearance for the urologist's legs. This allows convenient control of all table movements including operation of various imaging functions via the footswitch. The carbon fiber table top is highly radiolucent and provides unobstructed imaging of the entire urinary tract without bladder cutoff. It accommodates safe positioning of patient's weighing up to 203 kilograms. Moreover, the table provides a ± 15° Trendelenburg tilt to ease endourologic procedures.

A wide range of dedicated accessories ensures application-oriented patient positioning and supports the clinical work-flow.

Percutaneous interventions

To facilitate percutaneous interventions, LITHOSKOP provides ideal access to the patient from all sides of the system.

A dedicated interface transfers endoscopic images from the physician's endo-equipment to the system's monitors for optimal viewing.

LITHOSKOP's orbital C-arm movement, which may also be controlled by a footswitch, supports X-ray based percutaneous procedures.

Urological diagnosis

For diagnostic purposes, LITHOSKOP is equipped with a high resolution X-ray imaging chain in combination with sophisticated imaging software. A large image intensifier and a powerful X-ray generator further contribute to brilliant images.

LITHOSKOP does not compromise in any respect.

Economic aspects

LITHOSKOP is in sync with the global trend towards economic solutions. Its cost-effectiveness is a result of, amongst others, low operational costs. This is based on, e. g., the shock wave head and the integrated semiconductor switch for energy generation both providing maximum longevity.

Furthermore, the shock wave system's outstanding performance leads to reduced retreatment rates and less auxiliary measures, making ESWL even more financially lucrative.

The economic benefits are a result of optimized work-flow. Time-consuming patient positioning and the need for additional personnel is now reduced to a minimum due to LITHOSKOP's one-time positioning philosophy.

Above all, LITHOSKOP ensures maximum utilization since it allows for multifunctional and interdisciplinary application.

Summary

LITHOSKOP is a highly multifunctional urologic system offering maximal patient safety and ease of applications.

Its elaborate concept facilitates every detail within the daily clinical routine. The design has been fine-tuned to meet all the urologists' and the patients' needs and expectations.

By focusing on economic aspects, LITHOSKOP becomes the solution for today's urology as well as urology for the future.

Storz Medical: Shock Waves for Stone Treatment and Tissue Engineering

O. Wess

Introduction

Extracorporeally generated shock waves are well established in stone treatment, mainly for stones in the urinary tract. Also common bile duct stones, pancreatic stones, and salivary duct stones may be fragmentized without open surgery. Without doubt, shock waves are a noninvasive and most gentle treatment option. Although usually negligible, shock waves may, however, cause a certain amount of tissue damage. Careful focusing of the shock wave energy exactly to the treatment area is important. Modern lithotripsy devices, therefore, make use of large apertures providing optimal field parameters with precise focal zones and utmost protection of surrounding tissue. The acoustic energy is optimally concentrated on the treatment area to develop sufficient power for fragmentation even of very hard or impacted stones. However, due to imperfections in localization, small movements of the patient, or for other reasons, sometimes a larger focus distribution may be appropriate. Storz Medical is the only company who has developed a dual focus feature, capable of switching the focal size from precise to extended dimensions according to medical requirements. Individually matched treatment options may be applied to specific indications and/or anatomical conditions.

Since the early 1990s, shock waves were found not only to break body concrements but are also well suited to stimulate healing processes of soft tissue. Different indications such as heel spur, pseudarthrosis, or prostatitis require different shock wave devices with or without localization modalities.

Storz Medical offers highly specialized shock wave devices for almost any medical application. The most advanced developments for urinary stone treatment and for tissue engineering are presented below:

MODULITH SLX-F2, Dual Focus Technology to Match Medical Needs

Lithotripters changed from bulky bath tubs of the 1980s to multifunctional dry coupling devices of the present day. Side effects were reduced, anesthesia requirements were lowered, and the localization modalities ultrasound and/or X-ray were further utilized for diagnostic purposes. Only few systems, however, reach or surpass the fragmentation efficacy of the early bath-tub system HM3. Beside the extended care required for dry coupling compared to wet coupling of an open water-bath, the smaller focus is often blamed for a reduction of efficiency. Although no rational reason could be appointed to that, applicational features and treatment strategies may have an important influence on performance data of lithotripters. A precise focus is still the first choice if high fragmentation efficiency has to go hand in hand with gentle shock wave application. Larger focal zones with lower peak pressure may be appropriate if kidneys move significantly with respiration and if continuous on-line control of stone positions is not possible due to a lack of real-time ultrasound. Whatever reason may be valid, Storz Medical is the only company to offer both options at a tip of a finger. The operator has the choice of high pressure values and precisely confined treatment zones for hard and impacted ureteral stones, e. g., or moderate pressure values with a more extended focal zone when requested.

Storz Medical shock wave technology, the proven platform for innovations

The Modulith SLX-F2 is based on the proven electromagnetic cylinder source as implemented in all Storz Medical shock wave devices. When Storz Medical entered the market in 1989 with the MODULITH SL10/20, the electromagnetic cylinder source was, and is still today, a milestone in lithotripsy technology. The proprietary Storz Medical source with a cylindrical coil and a parabolic reflector configuration has proven again unsurpassed fragmentation efficiency [1]. The unique design features a coaxial opening for easy integration of in-line ultrasound and in-line X-ray localization devices without affecting free energy transmission. Accordingly, the new MODULITH SLX-F2 does not only provide the dual focus capability but in-line X-ray and ultrasound localization. In-line configurations for localization offer the highest possible precision and coaxial view of the treatment area. Therefore only in-line localization guarantees a perfect control of the shock wave pathway.

The MODULITH SLX-F2 Concept

The MODULITH SLX-F2 is based on the successful predecessor MODULITH SLX built as a superb lithotripter and multifunctional urological workstation. Cysto table functions for most of the endourological procedures as requested by modern urology departments are integrated. Besides offering all lithotripsy functions on the highest level, Trendelenburg inclination and further uro-options, such as leg holders and uro-sink, make the device a universal workstation for almost any urological application. Easy and ergonomical patient positioning and high quality X-ray components provide diagnostic tools for fluoroscopic images of the highest contrast and resolution.

Modular design for tailor-made solutions

The design of the MODULITH SLX-F2 is based on building blocks for the lithotripsy table, including optional endoscopy equipment, various X-ray localization, and diagnostic options as well as a limited number of in-line ultrasound devices. Depending on the individual needs, the system architecture is open for networking, DICOM interfacing, etc. Mobile and fixed installations with remote control options are available.

DUOLITH SD_1, Dual Technology Device for ESWT

Shock waves for tissue engineering require a different approach compared to shock waves for lithotripsy. Shock waves in orthopedics were initially used with the intention to disintegrate calcium deposits at the insertion points of tendons and to refresh fracture gaps of nonunions. ESWT turned out to be successful in various different applications such as tendinosis calcarea, nonunions, heel spur, etc. Also IPP and possibly prostatitis seem to be potential indications for ESWT. The concept of the underlying working mechanism, however, was significantly modified. Instead of primary disintegration effects of shock waves, the biological response to shock waves followed by NOS and VEGF production is shifted into the center of interest [2]. Accordingly, shock

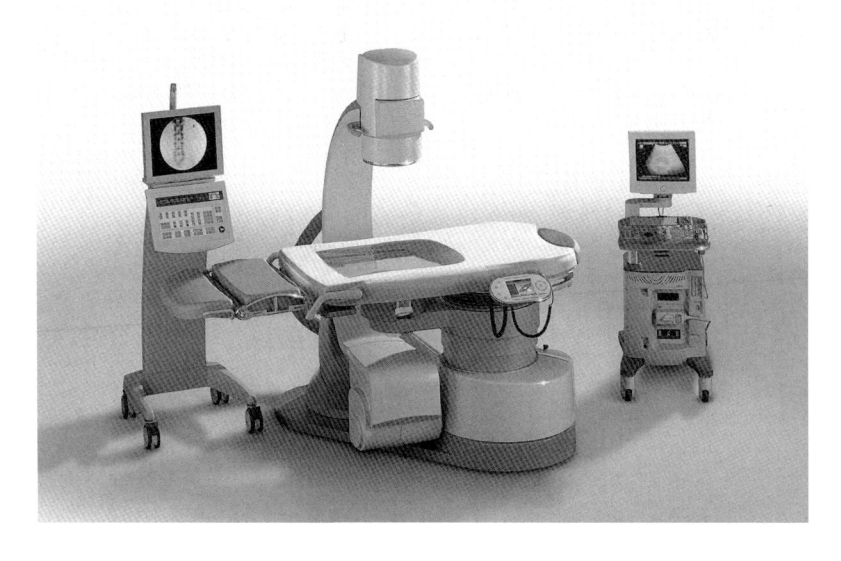

Fig. 1 MODULITH SLX-F2.

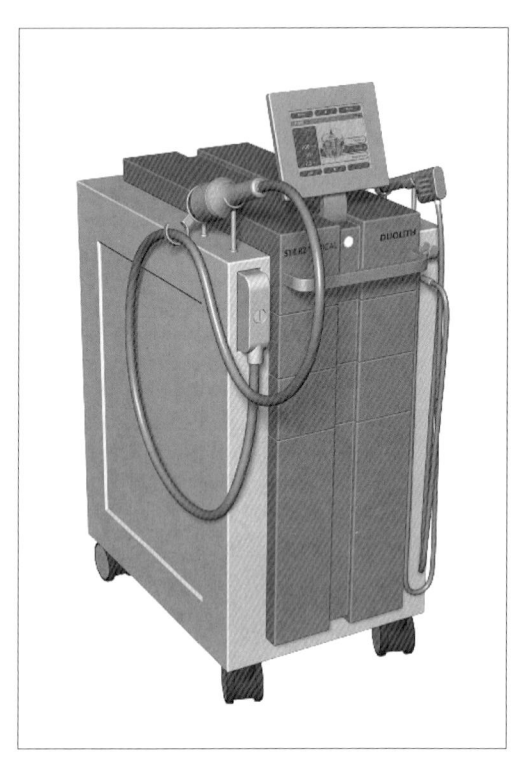

Fig. 2 DUOLITH SD$_1$.

wave field parameters are not necessarily as high as for fragmentation purposes and the method of localization and targeting may be different.

Focused shock waves are generally used for targeting treatment areas laying a few cm below the skin surface. Superficial tissue areas, however, are well treated by locally applied pressure waves generated by contact with a ballistic pressure device. The working area is clearly defined by the point of direct contact.

Storz Medical have developed a new concept combining both technologies within one device. The Duolith SD$_1$ (Figure 2) is an office- and clinic-based system with two independent applicators, one for focused shock waves and the second one for unfocused, radial pressure waves. Both therapy heads are flexible hand-held units easily applied to the various body regions. They are small enough to reach even hidden body areas not accessible to larger shock wave heads. Therapeutic penetration is up to 50 mm for the focused shock wave head thus reaching most of targets in this field.

The pressure pulse unit is offered with different applicator dimensions and repetition frequency up to 15 pulses per second.

Both treatment techniques do not require any localization devices. The area of interest is diagnosed by different means and marked at the skin surface. Application is controlled by direct view of the point of application and/or by feedback of the patient.

References

[1] Teichmann JMH et al. In vitro comparison of shock wave lithotripsy machines. J Urol 2000; 164: 1259–1264
[2] Wang CJ. An overview of shock wave therapy in musculoskeletal disorders. Chang Gung Med J 2003; 26: 220–231

Wolf: Innovative Piezoelectric Shock Wave Systems — PIEZOLITH 3000 and PIEZOSON 100 *plus*

S. Ginter, W. Krauß

Introduction

Since 1986, the piezoelectric shock wave systems for ESWL manufactured at Richard Wolf have been successful in clinical use worldwide. In the following years it was shown that shock waves (SW) are effective not only for lithotripsy of stones in the body but for many other medical indications such as, for example, orthopedic ESWT for pain and bone regeneration. In the future one hopes to be able to use shock waves successfully in other areas as well, e. g., for vascularization or drug delivery. For previous piezoelectric shock wave sources, large units with an aperture of 50 cm were necessary, such as used in our older lithotripters. The objective for the future of our piezoelectric systems for more convenient shock wave systems with reduced weight and smaller design was the development of a basic technology with the following requirements:
– *Compact and high-performance SW sources* are required to facilitate, for instance, smooth working with sufficient power reserves for orthopedic indications.
– *Controlled and reliable working* by fine energy graduation, exact focusing, and long-term stability of the SW source are indispensable for accurate dosage.
– *Flexible and simple adaptability* to widely differing sound field requirements opens the door to new indications.
– *Technology at favorable costs.*

Our new double-layer technology, which represents the main item in all our current SW systems, makes the most important contribution to fulfilling these requirements.

Double-Layer Technology — Performance and Flexibility

Figure **1** shows schematically the basic construction of a self-focusing SW source in double-layer technology. Two active piezoceramic layers, a front layer and a back layer, are mounted on a metallic bowl. Both the front layer and the back layer are actuated with high-voltage pulses through their own separate networks. They are actuated in such a way that the single pulses

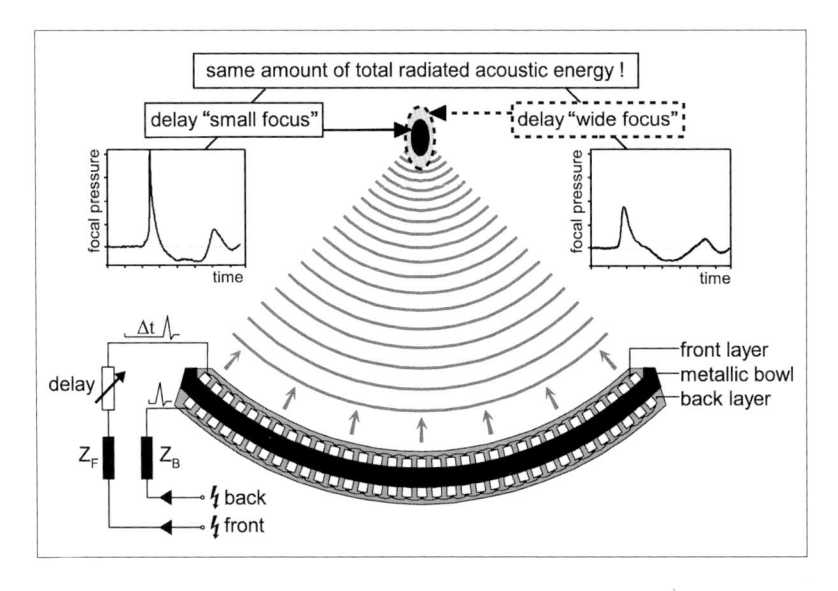

Fig. **1** Principle of the double-layer technology. Superposing the front and back pulse of the SW source the same amount of radiated energy can be focused with high ("small focus") or with less energy density ("wide focus").

generated in the layers are superposed additively at the surface of the SW source. Thus, the acoustic energy and power radiated per area are practically doubled. With unchanged acoustic power values, the size of the therapy source, and thus also its weight, can be reduced compared to the conventional SW sources in single-layer technology. The patented double-layer technology is the key to our compact and high-performance SW systems, the mobile PIEZOLITH 3000 and the portable PIEZOSON 100 *plus*. A controllable and reliable pulse superposition is decisive for the quality of the double-layer technology. The high-voltage pulses can be matched exactly to one another in time by highly accurate power thyristor switches. A further strength of the double-layer technology lies in its extraordinary flexibility. With the double-layer technology, the sound field acting in the focal region can be changed selectively on several areas with regard to the different requirements (lithotripsy, orthopedics, future applications).

At first the pulse form of each piezoelectric layer can be influenced specifically through the network. Thus the same or two completely different acoustic signals can be superposed. The freely selectable and exactly adjustable time delay between the front and back actuation can be used not only to superpose the pulses optimally constructively, which leads to an optimum energy concentration, to high pressure amplitudes, and high energy densities in the focal area ("small focus" delay setting). It can also be used for a wanted time shift between the two pulses ("wide focus" delay setting). This setting leads to a widening of the focal zone, a reduction of the maximum occurring pressure amplitudes and energy densities, however, at unchanged total radiated energy! The delay can be chosen variably according to therapy requirements and treatment wishes. With an even greater time delay between the two pulses, they are no longer superposed additively, but result in tandem pulses. Cavitation effects can be controlled in wide areas in this manner.

PIEZOLITH 3000 — Modular and Optimal

Figure **2** shows the PIEZOLITH 3000 with shock wave source, treatment table, X-ray unit, WOLF-LITHOARM, and ultrasound unit. The modular approach, which permits different components to be combined to form an optimal total system, is characteristic for the system.

Shock wave source

The new double-layer technology enables a variable focus size from small to wide, with a conspicuously small and ergonomic design of the piezoelectric shock wave source. The most important quality features are its penetration depth of up to 165 mm, its excellent power data, and the extremely long lifetime of more than 5 million shock wave pulses. Dosing is in 20 intensity levels up to a maximum of

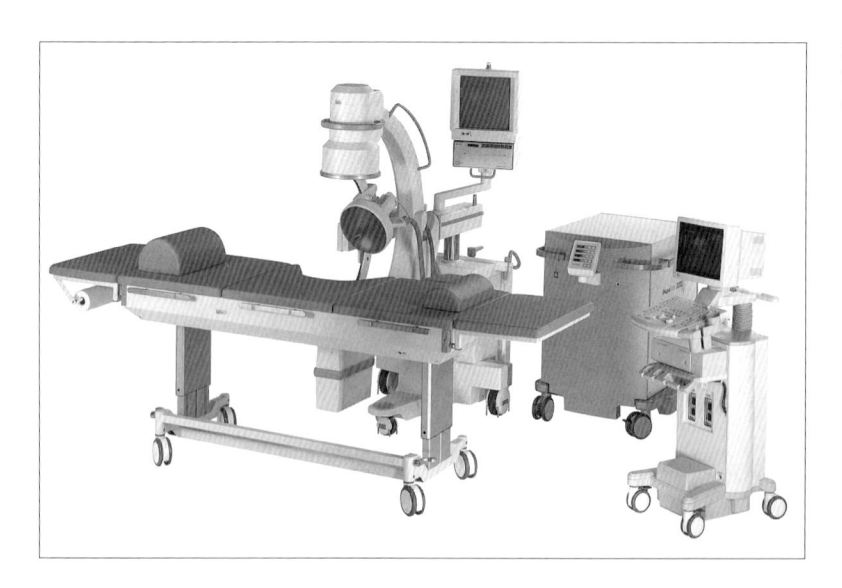

Fig. **2** PIEZOLITH 3000 — System overview.

115 mJ ($E_{5\,MPa}$) and 120 MPa peak pressure amplitude.

Localization systems

For real-time ultrasound localization during therapy an ultrasound probe is arranged in the center of the shock wave source. It can be rotated and moved axially inside the shock wave source by an electric motor drive. The in-line ultrasound localization is close to optimum, since the direction of view and therapy direction coincide. The electronic ultrasound probe can also be operated optionally with high-quality color Doppler ultrasound devices. The shock wave source can be easily moved by a swiveling device weight counter-balanced confocally from the under-table arrangement into the over-table position. The WOLF-LITHOARM adaptation of the shock wave source to the X-ray unit ensures stable and precise assignment of the therapy focus to the X-ray isocenter. This guarantees optimum accuracy even in the case of small ureteral calculi. X-ray localization itself is done by two projections in AP and CC by lateral swiveling of the C-arm.

PIEZOSON 100 plus — Gel-Pad Technology for the Smallest ESWT Desktop Unit in the World

Figure 3 shows the smallest ESWT unit worldwide. The PIEZOSON 100 *plus*. It combines all advantages that are necessary for effective ESWT: convenience, flexibility, and high performance. Three different therapy sources FB7, FB10, and FB12, equipped with the advantages of the double-layer technology, can be connected through a multi-connector corresponding to the required indication. The key data of the SW sources are listed in Table 1. The wanted dosage from low through medium up to high energy at pulse frequencies of 1 to 8 Hz can be applied in 25 intensity levels. Due to our patented gel-pad technology, the shock waves can be coupled into the body without a water path normally needed therefore. A soft plastic gel with specially selected acoustic properties serves as coupling medium. Expensive water conditioning and the problem of microbic water contamination thus no longer apply. The gel-pad technology is the key to a compact, maintenance-free and above all very inexpensive ESWT unit. Different penetration depths can be varied by simply changing gel pads of different height. Special anatomical gel pads (Figure 3) can be used for new indications for optimum therapy.

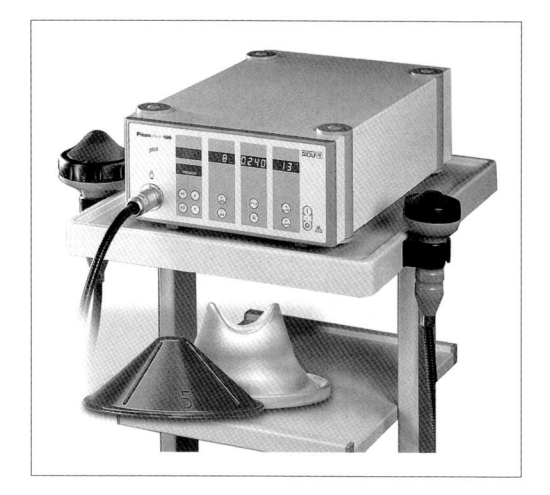

Fig. 3 PIEZOSON 100 *plus* with two different SW sources and changeable gel pads.

Table 1 Characteristics of the different orthopedic SW sources

Parameter	FB7	FB10	FB12
Aperture (mm)	70	100	120
Penetration depth (mm)	0–22	0–40	0–55
Max. pressure (MPa)	58	126	122
Energy 5 MPa zone (mJ)	20.2	48.7	66.2

Participants of the 4th Consensus Meeting of the German Society of Shockwave Lithotripsy, Speyer, 17th–19th February 2005

Bodo Beck
Division of Pediatric Nephrology
University of Cologne
Kerpener Str. 62
50937 Köln
Germany

Richard Berges
PAN-Klinik Cologne
Zeppelinstraße 1
50667 Köln
Germany

Thorsten Bergsdorf
Department of Urology
Städtisches Krankenhaus München-Harlaching
Sanatoriumsplatz 2
81545 München
Germany

Andreas Blana
Department of Urology
University of Regensburg
St. Josef Hospital
Landshuter Straße 65
93053 Regensburg
Germany

Moritz Braun
Department of Urology and Pediatric Urology
Klinikum Fulda
Pacelliallee 4
36043 Fulda
Germany

Bernhard Brehmer
Department of Urology
University of Aachen
Pauwelsstraße 30
52074 Aachen
Germany

Christian Chaussy
Department of Urology
Städtisches Krankenhaus München-Harlaching
Sanatoriumsplatz 2
81545 München
Germany

Siegfried Ginter
Department of Research
Richard Wolf GmbH
Pforzheimer Straße 32
75438 Knittlingen
Germany

Bernd Granz
R&D Urology
Siemens AG
Med SP PLM U1
Postfach 3260
91052 Erlangen
Germany

Axel Häcker
Department of Urology
University Hospital Mannheim
Faculty of Clinical Medicine Mannheim
Ruprecht-Karls-University Heidelberg
Theodor-Kutzer-Ufer 1–3
68135 Mannheim
Germany

Georgios Hatzichristodoulou
Department of Urology
Hospital St. Trudpert
Wolfsbergallee 50
75177 Pforzheim
Germany

Ekkehard W. Hauck
Department of Urology and Pediatric Urology
Justus Liebig University Gießen
Rudolf-Buchheim-Str. 7
35385 Gießen
Germany

Gerald Haupt
Department of Urology
St.-Vincentius-Hospital
Holzstraße 4a
67346 Speyer
Germany

Albrecht Hesse
Division of Experimental Urology
Department of Urology
University of Bonn
Sigmund-Freud-Straße 25
53105 Bonn
Germany

Rainer Hofmann
Department of Urology
Philipps-Universität Marburg
Baldingerstraße
35043 Marburg
Germany

Dieter Jocham
Department of Urology
UKSH Campus Lübeck
Ratzeburger Allee 160
23538 Lübeck

Thomas Knoll
Department of Urology
University Hospital Mannheim
Faculty of Clinical Medicine Mannheim
Ruprecht-Karls-University Heidelberg
Theodor-Kutzer-Ufer 1–3
68135 Mannheim
Germany

Kai Uwe Köhrmann
Department of Urology
Theresien-Krankenhaus
Bassermannstraße 1
68135 Mannheim
Germany

Sven Lahme
Department of Urology
Hospital St. Trudpert
Wolfsbergallee 50
75177 Pforzheim
Germany

Andreas Lutz
Department of Research
Dornier MedTech Systems
82234 Weßling
Germany

Markus Maier
Department of Orthopaedic Surgery
and Institute for Surgical Research
Ludwig-Maximilians-University Munich
Hermann-Hummel-Str. 33
82166 Gräfelfing bei München
Germany

Dietmar Neisius
Department of Urology
Krankenhaus der Barmherzigen Brüder
Nordallee 1
54292 Trier
Germany

Stephan Neubauer
West German Prostate Center and
Department of Urology
Klinik am Ring
Hohenstaufenring 28
50674 Köln
Germany

Jens J. Rassweiler
Department of Urology
Klinikum Heilbronn
SLK Kliniken Heilbronn
Am Gesundbrunnen 20
74074 Heilbronn
Germany

Michael Straub
University of Ulm
Department of Urology and Pediatric Urology
Urolithiasis Research Group
Prittwitzstraße 43
89075 Ulm
Germany

Walter Ludwig Strohmaier
Department of Urology and Paediatric Urology
Klinikum Coburg gGmbH
Ketschendorfer Str. 33
96450 Coburg
Germany

Stefan Thüroff
Department of Urology
Städtisches Krankenhaus München-Harlaching
Sanatoriumsplatz 2
81545 München
Germany

Christian Türk
Department of Urology
Krankenanstalt Rudolfstiftung
Juchgasse 25
1030 Vienna
Austria

Othmar Wess
Department of Research
STORZ Medical AG
Unterseestrasse 47
8280 Kreuzlingen
Switzerland

Dirk Wilbert
Department of Urology
Kantonales Spital
Gasterstrasse 25
8730 Uznach
Switzerland

Ulrich K. F. Witzsch
Department of Urology and Pediatric Urology
Krankenhaus Nordwest
Stiftung Hospital zum Heiligen Geist
Steinbacher Hohl 2–26
60488 Frankfurt/Main
Germany

Index

A

ABLASONIC® 98
Ablatherm® 98ff
– side effects 101
acetaminophen 49
acetohydroxamic acid 82
acoustic impedance 149f
adenine-phosphoribosyl-transferase deficiency 90
alkaline citrates 78
allopurinol 82
alternative energies 92ff
– report of working group 92ff
ammonium urate stones
metaphylaxis 82
anesthesia requirements 32
antegrade ureteropyelography 69
aseptic pseudarthrosis 156
– extracorporeal shock waves 156
Autopos™ 169

B

bacteria
– urea-degrading 76
– urease-forming 76
ballistic lithotripsy 46
– proximal ureteral stones 46
Bartter's syndrome 86, 90
benign prostatic hyperplasia 103
– TUMT 117ff
bioheat equation 117
biological tissues 150f
– effect of shock waves 150f
blind basket extraction 52
– distal ureteral stones 52
bone 158
– application of extracorporeal shock waves 158
brachytherapy
– 3D-isodose calculation 106
– definition 106
– high-dose rate 106
– intraoperative planning 106
– low-dose rate 106
– permanent seed implants 106
– post-implant X-ray 107
– prostate 106ff
– – advantages 106
– – clinical results 108
– – complications 112
– – management 112
– – modern techniques 106f
– – patient selection 107
– – rectal morbidity 112
– – sexual function 113
– – technical considerations 108
– – temporary seed implants 107
– – urinary morbidity 112
– transrectal ultrasound 106
brushite 80
β-blockers 132
– Peyronie's disease 132

C

Ca antagonists 49
calcific tendinitis of the shoulder 144
– ESWT 144
calcium oxalate stones 75
– metaphylaxis 78
calcium phosphate stones 75
– metaphylaxis 79
carbonate apatite 80
cartilage 159
– application of extracorporeal shock waves 159
cavitation 1, 150
– bubbles 145
children 86ff
– nephrocalcinosis 86ff
– – presentation 86
– nephrolithiasis 86ff
– normal values for spot urine analysis 89
coil configuration 9
– optimization 9
collagen metabolism 133
– Peyronie's disease 133
consensus statements
– alternative energies 94
– ESWL in urology 131
– metabolic evaluation of stone disease 72ff
– metaphylaxis of stone disease 72ff
– outpatient vs. inpatient ESWL 64
– treatment of urinary stones 36ff
conservative therapy 49
– distal ureteral stones 49
cortical nephrocalcinosis 86
coupling 10
– optimal 10
Crohn's disease 86
cryoablation 103
cryotherapy
– approaches to the kidney 127

– history 103
– mechanism of action 103
– principles 126
– prostate 103ff
– renal cell carcinoma 126ff
– – results 126f
– salvage 103
– third generation devices 127
current technologies
– future perspectives 93
cylinder source 30
– with parabolic reflector 30
– – affected tissue 31
cystine stones 77
– metaphylaxis 82
cystinuria 90

D

6 dB focal area 28
6 dB shock wave focus 145
delayed bone healing 154
Dent's disease 86, 90
diagnosis 78
– urolithiasis 65ff
diet 78
– stone-neutral 78
diffuse nephrocalcinosis 86
2,8-dihydroxyadenine stones 77
distal ureteral stones 37, 49ff
– alternative therapy 52
– blind basket extraction 52
– conservative therapy 49
– definitions 49
– ESWL 49
– – analgesia 50
– – results 50
– – stone-free rates 50
– laparoscopy 52
– loop extraction 52
– open surgery 52
– retroperitoneoscopy 52
– splints 53
– ureteroscopy 51
– – analgesia 51
– – results 51
Dornier MedTech, products 164ff
– Dornier Compact Delta II® 165
– Dornier Compact Sigma® 164
– Dornier Lithotripter S II® 165
double-layer technology 175
DUOLITH SD$_1$ 173
Dupuytren's contracture 132f
dynamic fatigue 5

E

electrohydraulic generator 27
– affected tissue and organs 27
– focused shock wave field 27

electrohydraulic lithotripsy 46
– proximal ureteral stones 46
endoscopic therapy 45
– proximal ureteral stones 45
endourological techniques 55ff
epicondylitis humeri radialis 154
– ESWT 144
ESWL (extracorporeal shock wave lithotripsy)
– complications 56
– – caused by passing fragments 56
– – caused by shock waves 56
– contraindications 55
– indications 55
– outpatient treatment 64
– proximal ureteral stones 45
– risk factors for renal hematoma 56
– side effects 56
– tables 1
– technique 55
– treatment 55
– – distal ureteral stones 49
– – – analgesia 50
– – – results 50
– – – stone-free rates 50
– urology
– – consensus statement 131
ESWT (extracorporeal shock wave treatment)
– applications 144
– calcific tendinitis of the shoulder 144
– epicondylitis humeri radialis 144
– gallstones 144
– non-union of long bones 144
– pancreatic stones 144
– Peyronie's disease 135, 137ff
– – clinical studies 137f
– – explorative meta-analysis 139f
– – mode of action 137
– – patient characteristics 138
– – results 138ff
– – – placebo-controlled, prospective, randomized, single-blind study 140
– – safety 138
– – technical parameters 139
– physical-technical principles 144ff
– plantar fasciitis 144
– salivary stones 144
evidence-based medicine 44
– data sources 44
– system 44
evidence-based guidelines 44
– proximal ureteral stones 44ff
ex vivo models 16ff
– evaluation of SW-induced renal injury 16ff
– – histologic evaluation 16
– – kidney preparation 16
– – radiological evaluation 18
external beam radiotherapy (EBRT) 108
– prostate 108
extracorporeal HIFU (high intensity focused ultrasound) 128ff

– clinical applications 129f
– renal tumor ablation 128ff
– results 129
– side effects 129
– technical principle 128f

F

familial hypomagnesemia 90
fatigue
– dynamic 5
fiberoptic hydrophone 149
flexible URS 36, 59
fluoroscopy 12
– AP projection 12
– 3D navigation 12
– cranial caudal projection 12
– digital imaging 12
– isocentric C-arm 12
– lateral projection 12
– passing by shock wave source 12
– passing through shock wave source 11
– use of air-bags 12
focal nephrocalcinosis 86
focal size 26
– shock wave lithotripsy 26ff
focal zone 27
– definition 11
– different devices 32
– enlargement 8
– – principles 8
– fragmentation 29
– optimized 29
fracture healing 154, 156
– extracorporeal shock waves 156
FREDDY 59

G

gallstones 144
– ESWT 144
gel-pad technology 177
German Society of Shock Wave Lithotripsy 36, 64
– consensus statement
– – outpatient vs. inpatient ESWL 64
– – treatment of urinary stones 36ff

H

hematuria 56
hemospermia 56
HIFU (high intensity focused ultrasound)
– antibiotic prophylaxis 99
– contraindications 99
– current status in urology 98ff
– current technique 96
– definition 95
– extracorporeal application 128ff
– – renal tumors 128ff

– follow-up 99
– generation 95
– indications 99
– – neoadjuvant local debulking 99
– – partial therapy in low-volume, low-Gleason cases 101
– – primary therapy 99
– – salvage in recurrent Pca 101
– mechanical effects 95
– München-Harlaching prospective database 100
– preparation 98
– prostate cancer 96, 101
– system components 128
– technical equipment 98
– technical principles 95ff
– therapy 99
– thermal effects 95
– transrectal probe 96
– treatment planning 98
Ho:YAG laser 45, 49
hydrophones
– current situation 20
– fiberoptic 6, 20, 149
– laser fiber 149
– light-spot 6, 20ff
– – bandwidth estimation 22
– – basic considerations 20
– – calculation of sensitivity 21
– – calibration 23
– – construction 22
– – – calibration control 23
– – – glass block 22
– – – optical head 22
– – – optoelectronics 23
– – design considerations 21
– – measurement set-up 23
– – measurements 24
– – sensitivity 23
– piezoelectric crystal 148
– PVDF (polyvinylidine fluoride) 20
hypercalcemic hypercalciuria 90
hypercalciuria syndrome 90
hyperparathyroidism 79
hyperuricosia 90

I

idiopathic hypercalciuria 90
imaging techniques 67f
– assessment of function 67
– availability 67
– cost effectiveness 68
– costs 68
– follow-up examinations 67
– radiological protection 67
– sensitivity 67
– specificity 67
– therapeutic relevance 68
– untoward effects 67
incontinence 112

infection stones 76
– metaphylaxis 81f
intracorporeal lithotripsy 59
– electrohydraulic probe 59
– laser-based systems 59
– pneumatic probe 59
– ultrasound probe 59

J

jitter effect 10

K

kidney
– approaches for cryotherapy 127
– radiofrequency therapy 122ff
– – clinical studies 122f
– – indications 122ff
– – outcome 122ff
– – technique 122ff
kidney cancer 92
– application of alternative energies 92
– – indications 92
– – technique 93

L

laparoscopy
– distal ureteral stones 52
laser fiber hydrophone 149
laser lithotripsy 45
– proximal ureteral stones 45
Lithoreport® 169
LITHOSKOP® 167ff
– endourologic applications 170
– in-line localization 170
– multifunctional 170
– percutaneous interventions 170
– urological diagnosis 170
lithotripsy
– ballistic 46
– electrohydraulic 46
– laser 45
– pneumatic 46
– ultrasonic 46
lithotripter
– actual concepts 1
– characteristics of current systems 2
– comparison 32
– – 6 dB zone 33
– – equal pressure limits 33
– – equal pressure values 34
– – focal zone 32
– – treatment zone 32
– ESWL-tables 1
– history 26
– localization principles 3
– modular 164
– spark gap 26

– technology 1ff
– transportable 165
– uro-lithotripters 1
localization
– optimal 10
– systems 11
– – fluoroscopy 12
– – ultrasound 13
loop extraction
– distal ureteral stones 52f
lower calyx stones 37
lower pole stones 39ff
– alternative management 41
– ESWL treatment 39
– – stone-free rate 39
– flexible URS 41
– incidence 39
– problems 39ff
– recommendations 42

M

magnetic resonance urogram 68
– urolithiasis 68
medullary nephrocalcinosis 86
metabolic evaluation 72, 88
– initial 88
– – pediatric nephrocalcinosis 88
– – pediatric nephrolithiasis 88
– stone disease 72ff
metaphylaxis
– ammonium urate stones 82
– calcium oxalate stones 78
– calcium phosphate stones 79
– consented clinical pathway 74
– cystine stones 82
– infection stones 81f
– stone disease 72ff
– – current concepts 78
– – general measures 78
– stone-specific 78
– uric acid stones 82
L-methionine 79
microtrauma
– Peyronie's disease 132
microwaves 117ff
mini-PNL 58
MODULITH SL10/20 172
MODULITH SLX 173
MODULITH SLX-F2 172
– modular design 173
München-Harlaching prospective HIFU database 100
musculoskeletal system 154f
– application of extracorporeal shock waves 154f
– – animal models 155f
– – cell cultures 155f

N

Nd:YAG laser   59
negative maximum pressure   144
– shock wave   144
negative pressure bubbles   145
nephrocalcinosis   76, 86ff
– pediatric aspects   86ff
– specific evaluation program   76
nephrolithiasis   65, 68ff
– pediatric aspects   86ff
nephron-sparing surgery   126
– renal cell carcinoma   126
new technologies
– problems of introduction   93
nitinol basket   36, 59
non-union of long bones   154
– ESWT   144
normocalcemic hypercalciuria   90

O

open surgery
– distal ureteral stones   52
– proximal ureteral stones   47
orthopedics
– application of extracorporeal shock waves   154ff
osteoblastic stimulation   154

P

pancreatic stones   144
– ESWT   144
parabolic reflector   30
paracetamol   49
PCNL (percutaneous nephrolithotomy)   36
pediatric nephrocalcinosis   86ff
– copresenting disorders   90
– imaging   88
– initial metabolic evaluation   88
– therapy   89
pediatric nephrolithiasis   86ff
– copresenting disorders   90
– imaging   88
– initial metabolic evaluation   88
– presentation   86
– therapy   89
penile deviation   132
penis
– erectile dysfunction   132
– pain on erection   132
– plaque formation   132
percutaneous antegrade lithotripsy   36
percutaneous nephrolithotomy (PNL)   57
– complications   58
– indications   57
– technique   57
– treatment   57
permanent seed implants
– brachytherapy of prostate   106

Peyronie's disease   132ff
– clinical implications   132ff
– collagen metabolism   133
– definition   132
– diagnostics   134
– epidemiology   132
– etiology   132ff
– EWST   135, 137ff
– – clinical studies   137f
– – explorative meta-analysis   139f
– – mode of action   137
– – patient characteristics   138
– – results   138ff
– – – placebo-controlled, prospective, randomized, single-blind study   140
– – safety   138
– – technical parameters   139
– microtrauma   132
– pathophysiology   132f
– Potaba®   134
– potassium *para*-aminobenzoate   134
– surgical treatment   135
– symptomatology   133
– therapy   134f
– vitamin E   134
piezoelectric crystal hydrophone   148
piezo-electric elements
– double-layer   9
piezoelectric polymembranes from polyvinylidine fluoride   149
PIEZOLITH 3000   176
PIEZOSON 100 plus   176
plantar fasciitis   154
– ESWT   144
pneumatic lithotripsy   46
– proximal ureteral stones   46
Polyvinylidine fluoride (PVDF)   149
positive maximum pressure
– shock wave   144
Potaba®   134
potassium *para*-aminobenzoate   134
premature neonate   90
primary hyperoxaluria   78, 90
– type I   90
– type II   90
proctitis   112
Prostalund®   118
Prostalund-feedback treatment PLFT®   118f
prostate
– brachytherapy   106ff
– – advantages   106
– – complications   112
– – management   112
– – rectal morbidity   112
– – sexual function   113
– – urinary morbidity   112
– combined HDR-afterloading and EBRT   110
– combined permanent seed implant and EBRT   109
– cryotherapy   103ff

- external beam radiotherapy   108
- HDR-afterloading monotherapy   110
- LDR brachytherapy   111
- temporary implants   110
prostate adenoma
- application of alternative energies   93
- - indications   93
- - technique   93
prostate cancer
- application of alternative energies   92
- - indications   92
- - technique   92
- HIFU   96, 101
- risk groups   107
Prostatron®   118
proximal ureteral stones   37, 44ff
- ballistic lithotripsy   46
- definitions   44
- electrohydraulic lithotripsy   46
- endoscopic therapy   45
- epidemiology   44
- evidence-based guideline   44ff
- extracorporeal shock wave lithotripsy   45
- laser lithotripsy   45
- open surgery   47
- pneumatic lithotripsy   46
- recommendations   47
- therapy   44ff
- ultrasonic lithotripsy   46
- ureterorenoscopic therapy   45
pulse amplitude
- shock wave   144
Pulso
- Siemens shock wave technology   169
PVDF 48
- hydrophone   20
PVDF
- pressure transducer   149
pyridoxine   78
Pyrotech®   98

Q

quasistatic squeezing   3f

R

radiofrequency ablation   122
radiofrequency therapy   122ff
- basic technical aspects   122
- kidney   122ff
- - clinical studies   122f
- - contraindications   122
- - indications   122ff
- - outcome   122ff
- - technique   122ff
rectal morbidity   112
- prostate brachytherapy   112
renal cell carcinoma   122
- contraindications for radiofrequency therapy   122
- cryotherapy   126ff
- - results   126f
- indications for radiofrequency therapy   122
- nephron-sparing surgery   126
- surgical resection   122
renal function scintigraphy
- urolithiasis   69
renal lesions
- correlation with energy density   11
renal pelvis stones   37
renal trauma   16ff
- shock wave-induced   16ff
- *ex vivo* models   16ff
- - minimization   11
renal tubular acidosis   78, 90
renal tumors   126, 128
- ablation   128
- - extracorporeal HIFU   128ff
- treatment   126
retrograde ureteropyelography   69
retroperitoneoscopy   34
- distal ureteral stones   52
rise time 144
- shock wave   144

S

salivary stones   43
- ESWT   144
salvage cryosurgery   103
salvage cryotherapy   103f
- indications   104
- results   104
secondary hyperoxaluria   90
sexual function
- prostate brachytherapy   113
shock wave lithotripsy
- focal size   26ff
- perspectives   14
- renal stones   16
- ureteral stones   16
shock waves
- combination of sources   10
- cylinder source with parabolic reflector   30
- 6 dB focus   145
- 3D shock wave field   145
- different pulse durations   9
- efficacy   26
- electrohydraulic sources   101
- extracorporeal
- - application in cell culture models   158
- - application in orthopedics   154ff
- - application to bone   158
- - application to cartilage   159
- - application to intact tissue   158
- - application to musculoskeletal system   154f
- - - animal models   155f
- - - cell cultures   155f
- - application to pathologically altered tissue   156
- - application to tendon   14

– – definition 144
– – effect on biological tissues 150f
– – fracture healing 156
– – physical characteristics 144
– – principles of generation 147f
– – propagation 149
– – pseudarthrosis 156
– – technique of pressure measurement 148f
– – tendinitis 158
– – tendinosis calcarea 158
– focus 145
– – energy 146
– focused field 27
– focusing 26
– generation 26
– – ballistic principle 148
– – electrohydraulic principle 147
– – electromagnetic principle 148
– – piezoelectric principle 148
– importance of energy 7
– minimization of renal trauma 11
– negative maximum pressure 144
– parameters 5
– positive maximum pressure 144
– precise ultrasonic measurements 20ff
– pressure measurement 5
– pulse amplitude 144
– rise time 144
– side effects 26
– unfocused field 27
Siemens Medical Solutions 167ff
– Pulso shock wave technology 169
– products 167ff
Sonablate® 98ff
SONOLINE G50 169
spark gap 10
speed of sound 150
splints 53
– distal ureteral stones 53
squeezing 3
– quasistatic 3f
staghorn stones 37
– treatment options 37
steroids 49
stone disease
– algorithm for current management 73
general metaphylactic measures 74
– high risk patients 73
– metabolic evaluation 72ff
– metaphylaxis 72ff
– – current concepts 78
– – general measures 78
– patient selection 72
stone formers
– basic evaluation program 73
– calcium oxalate stones 75
– calcium phosphate stones 75
– cystine stones 77
– 2,8-dihydroxyadenine stones 77
– infection stones 76

– metabolic evaluation 74f
– – basic 74
– – elaborate 75
– stone analysis 74
– stones of unknown composition 77
– urate stones 76
– uric acid stones 76
– xanthine stones 77
stone-neutral diet 78
stones
– ammonium urate 82
– – metaphylaxis 82
– analysis 74
– calcium oxalate 75
– – metaphylaxis 78
– calcium phosphate 75
– – metaphylaxis 79
– cystine 77
– – metaphylaxis 82
– destruction 1, 5
– – mechanisms 1
– – physical parameters 5
– – theories 1
– 2,8-dihydroxyadenine 77
– fragmentation 1
– infection 76
– – metaphylaxis 81f
– mechanism of destruction 1
– shear stress 1
– tensile stress 1
– unknown composition 77
– urate 76
– uric acid 76
– – metaphylaxis 82
– xanthine 77
Storz Medical
– products 172ff
struvite 81

T

Tamm-Horsefall kidney 87
tamsulosin 49
Targis® 118
tendinitis 158
– extracorporeal shock waves 158
tendinosis calcarea 154
– extracorporeal shock waves 158
tendon 159
– application of extracorporeal shock waves 159
thermal ablation 128
– renal tumors 128
– – extracorporeal HIFU 128ff
thiazides 79
transrectal ultrasound
– brachytherapy 106
transurethral microwave therapy, see TUMT
treatment zone 27
– different devices 32
TUMT

– adverse events 119f
benign prostatic hyperplasia 117ff
– high energy 118
– – outcome 119
– low energy 118
– – outcome 118
– outcome 118
– techniques 117

U

ultrasonic lithotripsy 46
– proximal ureteral stones 46
ultrasound localization
– advantages 13
– disadvantages 13
– technical aspects 13
urate stones 76
ureterorenoscopic therapy
– proximal ureteral stones 45
ureterorenoscopy (URS) 58
– complications 60f
– endoscopes 58
– – flexible 59
– – semi-rigid 58
– indications 58
– – renal stones 58
– – ureteral stones 58
– intracorporeal lithotripsy 59
– stone extraction 59
– – basket 59
– – forceps 59
– technique 58
– treatment 59f
ureterorenoscopy 36
ureteroscopy 52
– distal ureteral stones 51
uric acid stones 76
– metaphylaxis 82
urinary morbidity 11
– prostate brachytherapy 112
urinary stones 36
– principle of treatment decision 36
– treatment 36
– – consensus statement 36ff
urine analysis 65, 88
– normal values for children 89
urolithiasis 44
– antegrade ureteropyelography 69
– diagnosis 65ff
– imaging techniques 66
– – assessment of function 67
– – availability 67
– – computed tomography 67
– – conventional radiology 66
– – – excretory urography 66
– – – plain renal film 66
– – cost effectiveness 68
– – costs 68
– – follow-up examinations 67
– – radiological protection 67
– – sensitivity 67
– – sonography 66
– – specificity 67
– – therapeutic relevance 68
– – untoward effects 67
– laboratory examinations 65
– – blood analysis 66
– – urine analysis 65
– magnetic resonance urogram 68
– other diagnostic techniques 68f
– patient's family history 65
– patient's history 65
– patient's previous history 65
– physical examination 65
– renal function scintigraphy 69
– retrograde ureteropyelography 69
– symptoms 65
uro-lithotripters 1
urological workstation 165
Urologix® 118
Urology
– consensus statement on ESWL 131
– current status of HIFU 98ff

V

vitamin E 134

W

weddellite 79
whewellite 79
whitlockiter 80
Williams-Beuren syndrome 90
Wolf
– products 175ff
WOLF-LITHOARM 177
working group "alternative energies" 92ff

X

xanthine stones 77
xanthinuria 90
X-rays
– brachytherapy 107
– – post-implant 107

Z

Zeiss' loop 52